Otto Rank and the Creation of Modern Psychotherapy

Otto Rank and the Creation of Modern Psychotherapy

ROBERT KRAMER

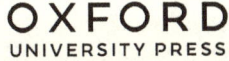
OXFORD
UNIVERSITY PRESS

OXFORD
UNIVERSITY PRESS

Oxford University Press is a department of the University of Oxford.
It furthers the University's objective of excellence in research, scholarship,
and education by publishing worldwide. Oxford is a registered trade mark of
Oxford University Press in the UK and in certain other countries.

Published in the United States of America by Oxford University Press
198 Madison Avenue, New York, NY 10016, United States of America.

Library of Congress Cataloging-in-Publication Data
Names: Kramer, Robert, 1953- author.
Title: Otto Rank and the creation of modern psychotherapy / Robert Kramer.
Description: New York : Oxford University Press, [2025] |
Includes bibliographical references and index.
Identifiers: LCCN 2024044433 (print) | LCCN 2024044434 (ebook) | ISBN 9780197698273 (hardback) |
ISBN 9780197698297 (epub) | ISBN 9780197698280 | ISBN 9780197698303
Subjects: MESH: Rank, Otto, 1884-1939. | Psychoanalysis–history |
Psychotherapy–history | Psychoanalytic Theory
Classification: LCC RC480.5 (print) | LCC RC480.5 (ebook) | NLM WM 11.1 |
DDC 616.89/14–dc23/eng/20241209
LC record available at https://lccn.loc.gov/2024044433
LC ebook record available at https://lccn.loc.gov/2024044434

DOI: 10.1093/9780197698303.001.0001

Printed by Marquis Book Printing, Canada

In memory of my parents, Margaret and Francis Kramer

I was born beyond psychology and want to die beyond it, but first and foremost, I want to live beyond it—and formerly it has been in my way.[1]

Otto Rank

[The] creative will was Rank's great contribution to the psychology of woman.[2]

Anaïs Nin

Therapy is a process in which a person who has been unable to go on with living without more fear or guilt than he is willing or able to bear, somehow gains courage to live again, to face life positively instead of negatively.[3]

Jessie Taft

I remember today the sense of illumination when [Rank] said "perhaps what the self really seeks is identity; does it ever accept difference?"[4]

Virginia Robinson

Rank's own writings [are] still an unknown language. Never mind. *He* changed me, if his writings don't. And his change in me was from black to red. From ink to blood. From trying to work things out intellectually to giving myself more to feeling. So—*he* won't mind if I can't read him.[5]

Phoebe Crosby

Contents

List of figures	x
Foreword by Matthew Fox	xii
Preface	xvii
1. Creating modern psychotherapy	1
2. Self-leadership	13
3. The denial of death	27
4. Immortality	40
5. Difference versus likeness	52
6. "David and Goliath"	64
7. The will of the father	78
8. The will of the mother	90
9. Transference versus relationship	102
10. Feelings	115
11. How did Rank practice therapy?	130
12. Carl Rogers meets Otto Rank	147
13. Willing = feeling alive = guilt-feeling	160
14. I–Thou . . . Thou–I	174
15. Client-centered therapy	185
16. The daimonic, counter-willing, and an "other world"	197
17. Empathy and *agape*	210
Epilogue: "I was born beyond psychology"	222
Appendix A Chronology of Rank's life and work	235
Appendix B Annotated Bibliography of Selected Writings on Rank	240
Notes	276
References	282
Author's Note	305
Index	306

List of figures

Figure 1.1. Rank with his dog Spooky   3

Figure 2.1. Goddess of Reason   21

Figure 3.1. Ernest Becker   29

Figure 3.2. The soul exploring the recesses of the grave   34

Figure 3.3. Sigmund Freud, c. 1921   37

Figure 4.1. The planet Earth   47

Figure 5.1. Otto Rank, c. 1930   54

Figure 5.2. Nella Larsen, 37, in 1928   60

Figure 6.1. Otto Rank, in the early 1920s   64

Figure 6.2. The Secret Committee, 1922   67

Figure 6.3. David holding the head of Goliath   69

Figure 7.1. Oedipus and the Sphinx (after Ingres)   79

Figure 8.1. Freud and his mother, 1925   92

Figure 8.2. Martha Freud, 1882   100

Figure 9.1. Sándor Ferenczi, 1909   102

Figure 9.2. Tola Rank holding her newborn, Helene—named after Helen
            of Troy—with photo of Freud behind her, 1919   108

Figure 10.1. The Zuider Zee dam   119

Figure 10.2. Freud and Anna, 1913   125

Figure 10.3. Betty Friedan   128

Figure 11.1. Rank's invoice, 1927. In Paris, Rank charged five dollars less
            than Freud, but triple what New York analysts were then
            charging. He offered a reduced fee to social workers.   132

Figure 11.2. Jessie Taft and Virginia Robinson with adopted children,
            Martha and Everett, 1923. From left to right: Jessie, Martha,
            Everett, Virginia.   137

Figure 11.3. Henry Miller and Anaïs Nin   143

Figure 12.1. Carl Rogers, c. 1930   148

Figure 12.2. Martha Graham, 1922   158

Figure 13.1. Anxiety   163

Figure 13.2. NASA describes the Webb Telescope's "First Deep Field," galaxy cluster SMACS 0723, as "approximately the size of a grain of sand held at arm's length, a tiny sliver of the vast universe."   170

Figure 14.1. Friedrich Nietzsche   177

Figure 15.1. Rank in his Paris library, with a portrait of Freud behind him   186

Figure 16.1. *Agathos daimon*, a deity of ancient Egyptian-Greek religion   198

Figure 17.1. A man crawls out from under the world to wonder at "the Beyond," a *terra incognita*   213

Figure 17.2. Søren Kierkegaard   219

Figure E.1. The trauma of birth   228

Figure E.2. Human blastocyst within the zona pellucida   233

Foreword

I am honored to write a Foreword to this important book by Robert Kramer, who has devoted much of his impressive career to rediscovering and resuscitating the genius of Otto Rank.

This latest of his many writings on Rank is a tour de force placing Rank in his cultural and historical setting and demonstrating how profoundly he influenced psychology—both humanistic and existential—and also social work, art, religion, and culture.

It is not easy to write a book that illuminates a mind and spirit as lively and dispersed and deep as Rank's.

As reflected in the teachings of pioneer feminists and social workers Jessie Taft and Virginia Robinson, Rank's critique of "masculine ideology" acknowledged women's powerful will to create and lead social change, making him an important precursor of both female and male liberation.

One cannot pigeonhole Rank's profound achievements for he was uniquely broad in his interests and he impacts the reader as a student of culture and the history of humanity. He does not restrict himself to focus on one specialty alone. Indeed, Freud himself, to his credit, recognized this dimension of breadth as well as depth in Rank as a young thinker by inviting him to edit his two journals, one on psychoanalytic theory and practice and the other on culture and the arts.

By way of transparency, I confess that I am neither a medical doctor nor a psychologist by trade but rather a spiritual theologian whose gift it has been to resuscitate and offer ways to interpret our Western mystical and prophetic heritage.

It was in the process of doing this that I ran across Ernest Becker's classic work, *The Denial of Death*, wherein he says Rank's book on *Art and Artist* was the most important book he had read in his life. That was my introduction to Rank. My response was to write a major review of *Art and Artist* in the journal *Spirituality Today* entitled "Otto Rank on the Artistic Journey as a Spiritual Journey, the Spiritual Journey as an Artistic Journey" in 1979. That is how long I have been living with and learning from Rank—some 46 years now.

I have written several additional articles about him since and devoted a chapter in my book *Meister Eckhart: A Mystic-Warrior for Our Times* to Rank and Meister Eckhart. I believe Rank has much to say about moving *beyond* religion to spirituality and have taught many classes on him, including one memorable one alongside Robert Kramer at the University of Creation Spirituality.

For me, Rank never grows old, is never overly familiar, always breaks through with insights that demand one's attention. He plays a key role in my book *Creativity: Where the Divine and the Human Meet.*

I consider Rank to be not just a genius in the field of psychology and what he called "the philosophy of healing," but also in the field of spirituality. Such themes as "the Beyond," "*unio mystica,*" the birth trauma as "the original wound" (instead of "original sin"); "rebirth" as a democratizing of the immortality quest; and his focus on the "Now" gift us with a vocabulary that is real, grounded, earthy. His spiritual themes are exceptionally valuable for probing more deeply our life's work, both inner and outer, in a traumatized world.

His passion for justice—exemplified by his opening chapter in *Beyond Psychology* on why Karl Marx was so influential in the twentieth century (hint: because he offered hope, which is something irrational, beyond reason, to the struggling masses)—and his later chapter on feminism give ample evidence of why schools of social work understood his contributions to societal healing long before psychology schools grasped what he was telling us about the meaning of the soul.

As Anaïs Nin said, "Rank was preoccupied with social problems and felt individual therapy was not enough to solve our problems." Educating female social workers for leading change to promote social justice was a special passion of his, as was encouraging self-leadership for their poor, minority, and disadvantaged clients.

Rank was far ahead of his time in critiquing what we now call patriarchy and its deleterious impact on women and children and, as we now are waking up to, Mother Earth herself. His advice to women that they create their own psychology and avoid Freud's, because it was "man's last attempt to control nature—this time his own," puts patriarchy in its place.

Rank's emphasis on acknowledging the "irrational" (or more-than-rational, i.e., feeling, intuition, or even mysticism) pre-date Einstein's teaching that we've been given two gifts, the gift of the rational brain and the intuitive brain. The rational should serve the intuitive because values and ethics come not from the intellect but from intuition or "deep feeling"—which are the same thing. And Einstein criticized how the society we live in honors the rational and ignores the intuitive.

Rank knew this and that is why he celebrates what he calls "the irrational" and pits it against the rational, insisting that what killed the Roman Empire was excessive rationality. "For at bottom, life is irrational," Rank said of the fantastic mystery of creation itself.

Rank taught that when religion in the West lost its connection with the cosmos, with Oneness, all of society became neurotic. As an outcome, we had to invent psychology to deal with the neurosis.

Rank makes concrete the hope of our time in continuing to discover and uncover the mystery of the universe, which reveals a new creation story believable to our entire species.

This vast universe made our species possible after a 13.8 billion year journey that has birthed trillions of galaxies, each with hundreds of billions of stars. I think Rank, were he living today, would be overjoyed with the miracle of the Hubble and Webb Telescopes, which have brought into our living rooms and computer screens pictures of these "more-than-rational" triggers to awe. And with awe and wonder comes the possibility of wisdom.

This new cosmology contributes to recovering what Rank, in *Art and Artist*, calls the "potential *restoration* of a union with the Cosmos, which once existed and was then lost." In the prenatal condition, that "earliest stage of individualization, the child is not only factually one with the mother," he said, "but beyond that, one with the world, with a Cosmos in which present, past, and future are dissolved."

For Rank, the reunion of microcosm with macrocosm, our individual psyche with the cosmos, is something people still seek. Why? Because such reunion, no matter how fleeting, offers "an identity with the cosmic process," a "being one with the All." It allows us to feel "in tune with" the cosmos. Indeed, "psychology is searching for a substitute for the cosmic unity which the man of Antiquity enjoyed in life and expressed in his religion, but which modern man has lost," Rank said in *Beyond Psychology*, "a loss which accounts for the development of the neurotic type."

Robert Kramer shows how, in the 1920s, Rank launched the revolution in relationship and existential therapy carried forward by Carl Rogers and Rollo May in the 1950s and 1960s, and now extended worldwide by countless practitioners of social work, counseling, and psychotherapy.

After reading this book, you'll have no doubt that it was Rank who created the relationship principles of modern psychotherapy.

Moreover, Rank's many contributions to a 21st century spirituality render him a spiritual innovator as well, not just a psychotherapist. I recognize him as a spiritual genius of the Jewish lineage and, in his own way, a holy person who sought after truth, who honored the "image of God"—that is, the artist or creativity within all persons—and strove to bring it alive and remain healthy.

Rank used his gifts for the common good, for healing and truth-seeking and truth-telling and working for justice. And Rank possessed the courage to do all this on his own after breaking, painfully, with his mentor Freud.

His was a life well and fully lived. He was generous and joyful and courageous. He was true to his calling as a healer and leader of other healers. He remained free of bitterness even though he was so maltreated by his Freudian family. He sought the good. All these are signs of a deep spirituality.

And, as Robert shows in his Epilogue, and I have long maintained, he was a "creation-centered mystic" in touch with what he called the *unio mystica*.

Rank observed that "new personality types are created during social and spiritual crises of religious, political or economic origin." Was Rank himself such a new personality type? Medieval historian Pere Chenu, who named the creation spirituality tradition for me, and has been called the "father of liberation theology" as well, said that certain periods of history produce new meanings of holiness.

I believe that Otto Rank did exactly that, calling for a new meaning of holiness by moving "beyond Freud" and "beyond psychology" to a place where the trauma or "original wound" of separation from our mother might be healed. In such a place, the reunion of cosmos and psyche comes to life. He called this place the *unio mystica* of art and love, two experiences that were synonyms for Rank.

And by art he does not mean the "art project" or *objets d'art* but creativity itself, the will to create, to give birth, which is found in women and also in men once they move beyond the neurosis of control over, and fear of, women's life-giving power. Rank recognized signs of masculine self-destruction in Freud and what Adrienne Rich called the "fatalistic self-hatred" that invariably accompanies patriarchy.

In her *Diaries*, Anaïs Nin quotes Rank calling on us to create "in spite of our *mal de siècle*." While Rank was referring, of course, to the *mal de siècle* in the first part of the 20th century, we in the 21st century can surely recognize our times as something equally dark, even more disturbing. Global climate change, nuclear war, modern warfare, fascism, and autocracy on the rise—all of it calls on us, as it called Rank in his day, to welcome the emergence of "new personality types."

Rank to me was such a new personality type, who stayed grounded in joy and creativity, in a commitment and, indeed, vocation to heal, not by calling for all-knowing, charismatic or autocratic leaders but by calling for a quantum leap in the development of self-leaders, beginning with women—especially those practicing social work, counseling, and psychotherapy—and minorities of all kinds.

His plea was for all of us to learn how to enter into mutually empathic relationship with each other, with one's client if one is a social worker, counselor, or therapist, with our families and communities and our whole planet if we are not in the helping professions, engaging our capacity for love.

This is a relationship born of a cosmic history greater than our own species, born therefore of reverence and gratitude, awe, and respect. For him, deeply felt, genuine relationship was central to healing.

For Meister Eckhart, relationship was the key to existence: "Relation is the essence of everything that exists," he said. Isn't quantum physics saying the same thing? A student of science, not just a poet, cultural historian, psychologist, and philosopher, Rank was keenly aware of the physics of his day, of Planck, Heisenberg, Einstein, relativity and the rest. He said in a letter to Jessie Taft that his life project was to do for psychology what Einstein had done for physics.

This book, wonderfully composed and gathering testimony from so many and diverse subjects, is a feast—a banquet where, in the spirit of Rank himself, everyone is invited to the table. Deeply human and deeply hopeful, it dares talk about fear and death, cosmos and psyche, women and men, religion and science, the rational and the irrational, art and the *artiste manqué*, symbols and war, mysticism and healing, mothers and fathers, the "Beyond" and the "Now," indigenous wisdom and modern-day fascism.

Rank was a leader, a prophet, a lover, and a healer, one who "interfered" (Rabbi Heschel's naming of the prophetic calling) with what Rank called the overly rational "masculine ideology" and "immortality projects" that drive national empires and are today killing the earth, Mother Earth. Empire building by nation-states, corporate greed, and patriarchal religions have driven indigenous peoples almost to extinction.

But not fully so. They and their love of the Earth are on the rise and what Frederick Turner calls the "aboriginal mother love" that is their essence are still with us, bearing wisdom we are desperate for. All this Rank foresaw.

We thank Robert Kramer for this book and once again assisting Otto Rank to come alive in our times and providing us with both an overview and an in-depth understanding of his journey in birthing a new kind of psychology, one that takes us "beyond" and that begins with the poor as did Rank's ancestors, the Jewish prophets of old.

Robert's judiciously annotated bibliography is sure to assist those eager to research Rank more deeply.

Matthew Fox, PhD
Spiritual theologian, Episcopal priest, activist for
gender justice and eco-justice
Vallejo, CA
https://www.matthewfox.org

Preface

Today, millions of mental health professionals practice social work, counseling, and therapy worldwide. Who created modern psychotherapy—Sigmund Freud?

One of the most influential thinkers in history, Freud was "the greatest modern writer," said literary critic Harold Bloom (1986). Freud proposed that repressed thoughts and feelings exert a profound effect on our lives. Father of psychoanalysis, he made case histories into narrative works of art, even while insisting he was a scientist.

His writings continue to be studied by literary scholars, philosophers, cultural critics, and students of religion, cinema, and entertainment. His influence is ineradicable. But Freud did not create modern psychotherapy. What he invented was a new form of human interaction: the analytic hour.

I argue in this book that it was Otto Rank, Freud's closest associate in Vienna from 1906 until 1926, who created the principles of modern psychotherapy, which focus on the quality of the therapist-client relationship.

If the 20th century was the century of Freud, the 21st is shaping up to be that of Rank—"the brooding genius waiting in the wings," according to Irvin Yalom (1980:293). The "single most important lesson the psychotherapist must learn," insists Yalom, is that "it is the relationship that heals" (401).

Relationship is also at the core of the client-centered therapy of Carl Rogers, who "has had such a major influence on social work practice," writes Judith A. Lewis (1991), "that his principles and tenets could be viewed as almost synonymous with our own professional standards" (166). As I will show, Rogers learned relationship therapy directly from Rank during a weekend encounter in 1936, and, in the process, abandoned his earlier Freudian training.

Moreover, by stressing the value of short-term rather than endless therapy, Rank revolutionized the way mental health professionals practice their craft today. "Rank has triumphed over Freud in America," said psychoanalyst Ellie Ragland (2024). "Not only do psychiatrists use the short sessions Rank recommended, but psychotherapists do as well" (18).

❧

For almost twenty years, Freud and Rank were as close as father and son. By 1924, Freud had designated Rank, almost 30 years his junior, as "my heir" (Lieberman & Kramer 2012:225). Rank venerated his mentor, who, in turn, esteemed Rank above all his other colleagues in Vienna. Only the Hungarian psychoanalyst Sándor Ferenczi was as close emotionally to Freud as was Rank.

At the beginning of their conflict over *The Trauma of Birth*, published in 1924, neither Freud nor Rank expected they would break ties. Coining the term "pre-Oedipal," Rank's book focused on the role mothers play in our early psychic life. The problem was that by elevating the power of mother over that of father, Rank had undermined the significance of the "Oedipus complex," a discovery Freud believed had secured his place among the immortals of science—Copernicus, Galileo, Darwin.

The Trauma of Birth gave Freud "a shock of alarm," said Ernest Jones (1957), "lest the whole of his life's work on the etiology of the neuroses be dissolved" (59). Stricken with oral cancer in 1923, and given no more than five years to live, Freud was deeply unnerved by Rank's book, which challenged his status as the premier cartographer of the human psyche.

"I am boiling with rage," Freud finally erupted (Freud & Ferenczi 2000:178). Soon thereafter, he confided to Ferenczi that he was drafting a new manuscript to crush Rank's "anti-Oedipal" heresy. His mood toward Rank, he added darkly, was "an absolutism moderated by treacherous assassination" (222). Terrified of Freud's boiling rage, which could just as easily turn against him next, Ferenczi immediately aborted his own enthusiasm for *The Trauma of Birth*, and broke with Rank, then his best friend.

Published in February 1926, *Inhibitions, Symptoms and Anxiety* was Freud's first full-throated attack on *The Trauma of Birth*, which he had never before criticized in public, only in private letters exchanged with members of his inner circle. In *Inhibitions*, Freud (1926a) leveled a devastating critique of Rank: "[I]t becomes impossible to shut one's eyes any longer to the far-fetched character of [his] explanations" (136).

Wounded over being attacked in public, Rank accused Freud, to his face, of not having "any more insight than a small boy" (Jones 1957:172). Incensed by Rank's effrontery, which challenged the hard-won Oedipal insights of his self-analysis, Freud retorted that Rank was a *Hochstaplernatur* (Gay 1988:471), a con artist, an "imposter by nature."

In April 1926, Freud and Rank chose to part ways. They would never speak again. It was a tragic ending. Their collegial—indeed loving—relationship ultimately strained to the breaking point: unforeseen, unwanted, inevitable. Over 75 years later, Helene Rank-Veltfort (2002) wrote that the break between her father and Freud was "still not completely understood" (1443), even by family members. Neither Adler nor Jung had produced this level of rage in Freud, whose emotions were usually kept under tight control. Why did Freud erupt so explosively at Rank for *The Trauma of Birth*?

Drawing on letters between Freud and Rank, and other sources, I tell the unknown story of why Freud's "boiling rage" led to Rank's departure from the inner circle. It's a deeply personal, tragic story, a story that had great consequences for the future of psychoanalysis—and, in turn, for the development of social work, counseling, and psychotherapy.

After he left Vienna, Rank published over a dozen books and lectured regularly in America. Reticent about revealing what happened behind closed doors between him and Freud, Rank only hinted at the personal reasons for their break, although their theoretical differences were rehearsed countless times in their writings. "The whole history of psychoanalytic thought has to be written one day," Rank told a friend in 1933, "and I am afraid that I am the only one who can write it" (quoted in Lieberman 1985:317).

Both men died in 1939—Freud, aged 83 in September and Rank, 55, one month later. Rank did not live to write his history. A vendetta by Freudians against Rank would extend for the rest of the 20th century, long after Sigmund Freud's death. Following Freud's lead, psychoanalysts condemned, caricatured, or simply ignored Rank's subsequent books.

Yet the fundamentals of Rank's relationship approach to therapy can today be found everywhere in social work, counseling, and psychotherapy, even though few know how this approach emerged, and even fewer can practice it with his artistic flair—which led Rank to create a new theory and technique for each client.

"In each separate case," Rank (1936a) wrote in *Will Therapy*, "it is necessary to create, as it were, a theory and technique made for the occasion without trying to carry over this individual solution to the next case" (6). The first practitioner of therapy as an art form, Rank stressed difference rather than likeness, uniqueness rather than sameness. One size did not fit all. "It is in Rank's will psychology," said Esther Menaker (1995a), "that we find the first true expression of an interest in the uniqueness of the individual in psychoanalytic thought" (73).

Almost a century ago, Rank created a new psychotherapy for each patient, a commonplace idea today. "It has been only in the past 15 or 20 years that the quest for personalizing psychotherapy has been fully supported by solid research. The enshrined clinical lore of creating a new psychotherapy for each patient," write Norcross and Cooper (2021), "now rightfully carries the designation of *evidence-based* practice" (ix; italics in the original).

In this book, I bring together Rank's most brilliant ideas, with vignettes—in the words of his patients—of how he practiced his artistry as a therapist.

As early as 1914, with his book on *The Double*, Rank observed that each individual, although unique, can experience a different identity, many identities, at the same time. Generations before the term diversity entered our vocabulary, Rank called for a *psychology of difference.*

Jessie Taft and Virginia Robinson made Rank's psychology of difference a hallmark of the curriculum of the University of Pennsylvania School of Social Work. They taught generations of social work students how to discover the resilience and power of their own, unique life force—what Rank called the "creative will"—a resilience and power that could also be drawn out within the relationships they built with their clients.

In his history of American social work, John Ehrenreich (1985) credits Taft and Robinson with fostering the "functional school" of social work, which held that the task of the social worker was to promote the creativity and self-empowerment of clients, rather than diagnose their psyches according to the Freudian criteria then prevalent in casework.

Almost a century ago, Rank, Taft, and Robinson planted the seeds for what today is called the *strengths-based* approach to social work. The universally accepted rule in social work to "start where the client is" (Tropman 2020:147) was formulated by Rank in the mid-1920s and then adopted by Taft and Robinson.

While studying for her PhD at the University of Chicago, Taft was deeply influenced by the writings on the social self of George Herbert Mead. Applying Mead's pragmatic approach, she incorporated what she learned from Rank about the creative will into a new model for social work education: the Penn School would develop the capacity for *self-leadership* of social work students and their clientele, a capacity "whose scope expanded to the network of relationships that comprised the social self" (Reuland 2015:8).

Many chapters in Rank's books—he published 22 in his lifetime, most never translated into English—begin with an epigraph. You can get the gist of Rank merely by studying his epigraphs. Of his epigraphs, these are my favorites:

- *Feeling is all.* (Goethe)
- *I and fear are born twins.* (Hobbes)
- *You will learn from me not philosophy but to philosophize, not thought to be imitated but to think.* (Kant)
- *There are people who appear to think only with the brain, or with whatever may be the specific thinking organ; while others think with all the body and all the soul, with the blood, with the marrow of the bones, with the heart, with the lungs, with the belly, with the life.* (Unamuno)
- *Be what you are!* (Pindar)

- *This Atman ... that I have in my heart is smaller than a grain of rice, smaller than an oat, smaller than a mustard seed .... This Atman that I have in my heart is greater than the globe, greater than the expanse of air, greater than the heavens, greater than all the spaces of the universes. In it are all deeds, all scents, all tastes contained; it embraces all, it speaks not and cares for nought. This Atman that I have in my heart, it is this Brahman. With it I become One when I depart this life. He who has attained to this knowledge, for him verily there is no more doubt.* (Upanishads)
- *The individual becomes conscious of himself as being this particular individual ....* (Kierkegaard)
- *This above all: to thine own self be true.* (Shakespeare)

For my book, I chose an epigraph from Rank that he jotted on a scrap of paper in June 1939, while he was drafting *Beyond Psychology*, his last work: "I was born beyond psychology and I will die beyond it, but first and foremost I want to live beyond it—and formerly it has been in my way."

Perhaps because the remark was too autobiographical, Rank, always an intensely private person, decided not to include it in its original form in *Beyond Psychology*, the only book he ever wrote in English. Removing the personal pronoun—"I"—he wrote:

> Man is born beyond psychology and he dies beyond it but he can live beyond it only through vital experience of his own—in religious terms, through revelation, conversion or rebirth. My own life work is completed, the subjects of my former interest, the hero, the artist, the neurotic appear once more upon the stage, not only as participants in the eternal drama of life but after the curtain has gone down unmasked, undressed, unpretentious, not as punctured illusions but as human beings who require no interpreter. (Rank 1941a:16)

Four women, all of whom had been in therapy with Rank, penned the other epigraphs. They express gratitude to him for releasing their creative will from bondage to what, in *Beyond Psychology*, Rank (1941a) calls "masculine ideology" (235–270).

As I will show, Rank helped them surface and unlearn *Lebensangst*, the term he coined for "life fear"—fear of accepting your difference—a fear that all of us must surmount in order to create something new, unprecedented: our unique lives.

Lebensangst is the fear of self-actualization, of self-realization, of self-leadership—the fear of becoming and being yourself. Its counterpart, said Rank, is "death fear," *Todesangst*, which is not just the fear of death, but also the fear of union and merger—in essence, the loss of our dearly bought individuality. We oscillate from birth to death, according to Rank, between the poles of *Lebensangst* and *Todesangst*.

Appendix A is a chronology of Rank's life and work. Appendix B is an annotated bibliography of the most significant writings on Rank since 1953, when social worker Fay Karpf published the first book on Rank. It was two decades later, however, that Ernest Becker's Pulitzer Prize–winning *The Denial of Death*, which has sold over one million copies, would bring Rank back as a major figure in the human and social sciences.

Rank's formulation of *life fear* and *death fear*, which Becker develops at length in *The Denial of Death* (1973) and *Escape from Evil* (1975), can illuminate much that goes on outside the therapy room, in particular the underlying existential motives for the wars in Ukraine, Gaza, and elsewhere.

In 1985, E. James Lieberman published the first authoritative biography of Rank, based on dozens of interviews with family members, students, patients, and colleagues who knew Rank. Following the pioneering researches of Paul Roazen (1974), Lieberman uncovered a host of distortions in Ernest Jones's treatment of Rank in his Freud biography. Envious of Rank's leadership role in the inner circle and his intimacy with Freud, Jones was "an incorrigible fibber," said Loe Kann, his common-law wife (quoted in O'Mahony 2023:121n).

"[T]he truth about Rank himself can scarcely be found in print," concluded Lieberman (1985:xv), who was amazed at the abundance of errors he found concerning Rank's life and work in the writings of psychoanalysts.

What, exactly, did Rank mean when he wrote "I was born beyond psychology"? In a sense, this book is an extended meditation on Rank's enigmatic autobiography and the four epigraphs by his women clients. As I will show, Rank had his eye on "the Beyond" beginning with *The Trauma of Birth* and throughout his later writings on art and creativity.

For their generous support, I gratefully acknowledge E. James Lieberman, Esther Menaker, Matthew Fox, Paul Roazen, André Haynal, James MacGregor Burns, Edgar Schein, Marie Becker, Elizabeth Hostetler, Edit Trunko, Edit Szilvasy, Bill Van Buskirk, Kirk Schneider, Siebrecht Vanhooren, Robert H. Abzug, Will Wadlington, Cynthia M. Jackson, Bence Varga, John Reuland, Sandra Crewe, Eszter Láncos, Ernst Falzeder, and Ruhama Veltfort (Rank's granddaughter).

Robert Kramer, PhD
Visiting Professor of Public Leadership
Corvinus University of Budapest
robertkramer@gwu.edu
December 2024

1

Creating modern psychotherapy

A leader in psychoanalysis, Otto Rank discovered—and first taught—the principles of relationship therapy.

Catapulted out of Freud's orbit a decade earlier for *The Trauma of Birth*, Rank was lecturing in the mid-1930s at universities across America on how his model of relationship therapy differed from psychoanalysis. "Simply speaking," said Rank (1996) in his American lectures, "this is the definition of relationship: one individual is helping the other to develop and grow, without infringing too much on the other's personality" (271).

Paradoxically, it is relationship that allows individuality to emerge, that spawns the self-acceptance necessary for discovering—or, better, recovering— one's creative potential. Only by *willing to be oneself within relationship*, said Rank, by accepting one's own difference and having it accepted by another, can a person locate the courage and creativity to change oneself—to be "reborn" spiritually.

In *Will Therapy*, Rank (1936a) proposed that a "here and now" (55) relationship with an empathic therapist is more healing than interpretations of a client's unconscious. "Not only less theory, but less 'art of interpretation' is necessary" (9). Rank's advocacy of empathy in therapy was considered heresy at the time by Freudians. According to historian of psychoanalysis Aner Govrin (2016):

> Insight achieved through interpretation was [then] considered the most important process to be developed. Though it is true that Freud referred to empathy a number of times in his treatises on jokes (Freud 1905) and group psychology (Freud 1921), it was never thought by him to be a key tool of analysis. . . . Freud mostly adopts an intellectual attitude toward empathy because he was ambivalent about emotions and suspicious of their place within the analyst. (162)

Over the last 30 years, psychotherapy outcome research has shown conclusively that the quality of the therapist–client relationship is *the* crucial factor in healing (Wampold & Imel 2015; Norcross & Lambert 2019).

The Center for Compassion and Altruism in Research and Education at Stanford University School of Medicine publishes a list of organizations that research

Otto Rank and the Creation of Modern Psychotherapy. Robert Kramer, Oxford University Press.
© Robert Kramer (2025). DOI: 10.1093/9780197698303.003.0001

the healing effect of relationships.[1] Conducted for over 85 years, the Harvard Longitudinal Study has found that the quality of our relationships is the main determinant of human flourishing.[2]

Today there are three major forms of therapy: cognitive-behavioral (CBT), psychodynamic, and existential-humanistic. They're all effective to the extent that they focus on the relationship between therapist and client. Even advocates of CBT emphasize the quality of the relationship, although manualized procedures are still considered essential (Okamoto et al. 2019). Striving to integrate all effective therapies, practitioners and scholars are now exploring how to infuse the principles of existential-humanistic therapy into CBT and psychodynamic therapy (Heidenreich et al. 2021; Salamon 2019).

Recently, researchers in the burgeoning field of relational neuroscience have proposed the radical idea of facilitating nurturing relationships—from birth to death—not only for individuals, families, and communities, but for society as a whole (Mizen & Hook 2020). But this idea is not new. "*All living psychology is relationship psychology,*" Rank (1996) observed in his American lectures, adding:

> What we learned from the analysis and understanding of this therapeutic relationship seems to have a bearing on other forms and types of relationships— such as exist between parent and child, teacher and pupil, husband and wife, in friendship, and so forth. That is to say, in all these relationships there seems to be a therapeutic element, if we conceive of that term in the broadest sense of the word. (271; italics in the original)

By most accounts, Carl Rogers, not Otto Rank, is credited with creating modern psychotherapy. "With the publication of *Counseling and Psychotherapy* in 1942, [Rogers] established himself as a major figure in the field," said clinical psychologist Frank Tallis (2021). "Indeed, some argue that no single volume influenced the practice of psychotherapy in the United States more" (273).

But Rogers himself always pointed to Rank as his North Star—the one who led the way. Asked in an interview about who had been his teachers, Rogers (1983) answered: "Otto Rank and my clients."

Rogers became the second most cited clinician, after Freud, over the span of the 20th century (Haggbloom et al. 2002). Except for the writings of Freud, "it is hard to name another set of books that has had an impact on clinical practice equal [to those] of Rogers" (Kahn 1997:38).

Otto Rank's teachings on the healing possible within an authentic relationship would have their biggest impact only after World War II, with the vast expansion of psychotherapy in America initiated by Carl Rogers, who learned

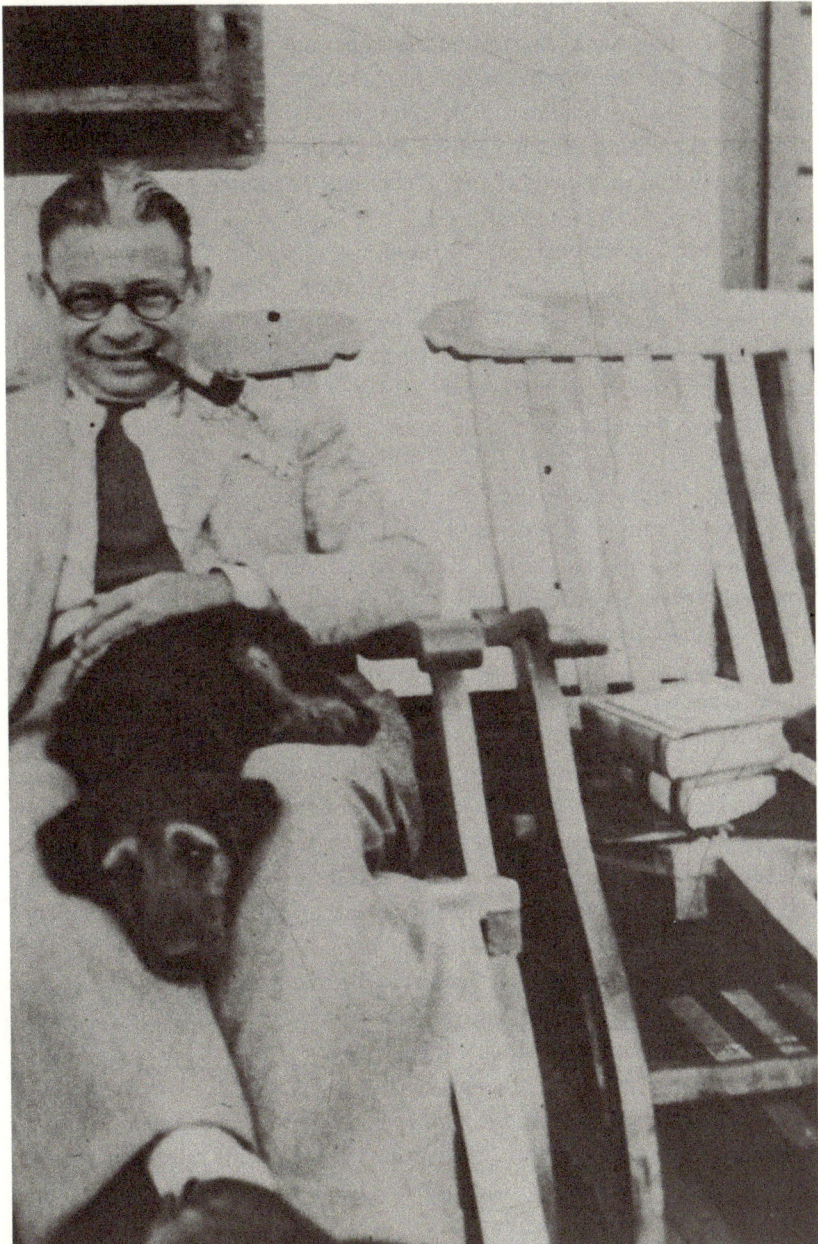

Figure 1.1 Rank with his dog Spooky
Credit: Ruhama Veltfort for the Estate of Otto Rank

the principles of relationship therapy from Rank—personally—over the course of a single weekend in 1936, as I recount later.

Before meeting Rank, Rogers had been offering interpretations, as psychoanalysts did, in order to provide "insight" to change the behavior of his clients. Afterwards, Rogers would devote the rest of his life, half a century, to releasing the innate actualizing tendency—what Rank called the "creative will"—*within* his clients so that they could change themselves, becoming self-empowered in the process.

"In my early professional years," writes Rogers (1961) in *On Becoming a Person*, "I was asking the question, How can I treat, or cure, or change this person? Now I would phrase the question in this way: How can I provide a relationship which this person may use for his own personal growth?" (32). Rogers describes "the curative force in psychotherapy [as] man's tendency to actualize himself, to become his potentialities" (350)—to become, what today would be called, a self-leader.

Although Rogers rarely used Rank's term "creative will," he increasingly focused on therapy as a process of promoting the self-empowerment of his clients, for the same reason that Rank gave. "Rogers discovered that a self-propelled process arises from inside," said Eugene Gendlin (1988:127), one of Rogers's closest colleagues. In 1929, at Yale University, Rank (1996) had pointed to "this *inner* self of the individual . . . that is not taken from without but grows somehow within" (242; italics in the original)—in other words, the capacity for self-leadership.

A prolific writer, Rogers published 16 books and over 200 scientific articles beginning in the late 1920s, when he started practicing therapy, until his death at age 85 in 1987. His writings have been translated into more than 60 languages.

"I became infected with Rankian ideas," said Rogers of his personal encounter with Rank in 1936, "and began to realize the possibilities of the individual being self-directing" (quoted in Kirschenbaum 1979:95). Promoting the self-empowerment of clients became central to the therapeutic practice of Rogers, and has been adopted by hundreds of thousands of social workers in the relationships they build with their clients.[3]

Today, relationship is at the heart of all social work, counseling, and psychotherapy. Summarizing the central message of client-centered therapy, Raskin, Rogers, and Witty (2019) write "that individuals are most able to access their own creative resources when provided a relationship offered by a genuine, congruent therapist who is experiencing unconditional positive regard and warm acceptance and is empathically receptive to the client's own perceived realities" (102).

The legacy of Carl Rogers extends far beyond psychotherapy. *Active listening*—a term coined by Rogers as a synonym for empathic understanding—is essential for building trust with others in such professions as teaching, medicine, nursing, hospice care, the ministry, coaching, conflict mediation, diplomacy, consulting, and organization development (Thorne & Sanders 2013).

Rogers spent much of the 1970s and 1980s facilitating dialogue in a wide variety of collective settings, from small encounter groups to large multicultural populations in conflict zones around the world (Kirschenbaum 2007).

"We think we listen, but very rarely do we listen with real understanding, true empathy," said Rogers (1980) in *A Way of Being*. "Yet listening, of this very special kind, is one of the most potent forces for change that I know" (116). The more one is able to practice empathic listening in relation to another, the more the other person is likely to be able to practice it in relation to you.

Rogers's view on empathy is not universally held. In *Against Empathy: The Case for Rational Compassion*, psychologist Paul Bloom (2016) argues that, rather than empathy, it is "much better to use reason and cost-benefit analysis, drawing on a more distanced compassion and kindness" (39). Bloom insists that "when it comes to certain interpersonal relationships, such as between doctor and patient, compassion is better than empathy" (50–51). But neither Rank nor Rogers saw a need to differentiate between empathy and compassion.

Recently, researchers (Yaden et al. 2024:112) have shown that compassion and empathy are highly correlated ($r = .53$, $p < .001$). By using regression analysis, they extracted measurements of compassion from those of the same person's empathy, concluding that empathic concern for others (controlling for compassion) is associated with "poor physical and mental health, missing workdays due to illness, and with greater perceived stress" (ibid.).

In my view, however, differentiating compassion from empathy is a well-intentioned—but misguided—attempt to address the long-standing crisis of emotional burnout in the helping professions, especially among social workers.

According to Rank and Rogers, empathy can be practiced in a conscious, thoughtful way that energizes the creative will of *both* parties in the relationship, without the helper experiencing emotional burnout. As I show later, one can "be with" a client, in deep spiritual communion, while being oneself—in other words, without burning out or losing one's sense of difference.

In the process of experiencing the healing within an empathic relationship, clients will also be learning how to feel empathy toward others and, perhaps most importantly, toward themselves—their own suffering. Empathic listening, said Rogers, is "a listening to oneself, as well as a listening love for the other" (Kirschenbaum & Henderson 1989a:78). According to Rogers, the optimal experience of empathy is mutual, a give-and-take between client and therapist that balances the need each has, simultaneously, for union and separation, connection and distance, likeness and difference.

In *Empathy: A History*, Susan Lanzoni (2018) identifies Rank as the most important influence on how Rogers practiced empathic listening in the therapeutic relationship. "Empathy depends on movement between the poles of similarity and difference, of distance and closeness, of immersion and alienation," writes Lanzoni. "Empathy marks a relation between the self and the other that draws a border but also builds a bridge," adds Lanzoni. "If at first we might see empathy as a sharing of similarities, empathy also hinges on difference" (17–18).

In her study of empathy, Lanzoni explores the work of Kenneth B. Clark, a prominent Black civil rights activist in the 1950s who advocated that people of different races learn mutual empathy as a way of overcoming racial division. In the wake of World War II, Black soldiers returned home to face segregation almost everywhere. Race riots broke out in cities across America. Empathy offered "new possibilities for connection, identification, and understanding that might improve social relations of all kinds," says Lanzoni (12).

In collaboration with Harvard professor Gordon Allport, a pioneer in the study of prejudice, Clark devised creative role-playing workshops to teach mutual empathy to racially mixed groups of police officers. For Clark and Allport, the cultivation of mutual empathy in an increasingly diverse society was the best means to come closer to achieving racial justice. Empathy, concludes Lanzoni, "comprises a complex, artful but also effortful practice that enrolls feeling, intellect, and imagination" (280)—what, since the mid-1990s, has come to be termed "emotional intelligence."

The heart of Carl Rogers's contribution to psychology is that to *listen with empathy* when in relationship with another is to facilitate the psychological growth of each participant in the never-completed process of becoming a fully-functioning human being, of accepting and being oneself, while remaining connected. The growth is mutual. Each person in the relationship will become more whole as a result of the deepening of *connection* and, at the same time, the affirmation of the other's *difference*.

A person's core tension, according to Rogers, is to be a self with others, to maintain a separate identity while simultaneously participating in the community, to deal with the dilemma of being one among many, utterly different from everyone else, yet related to the whole.

One of Rogers's closest students, Maureen O'Hara (2015) sums up Rogers's lasting contributions to the psychology of human growth and healing:

Rogers's profoundly humanizing psychology of human potential has been embraced by not only American culture but by much of the developed world.... Rogers's ideas are deeply embedded in all understanding of human behavior, and their revolutionary and fundamentally democratic implications have become part of our contemporary way of life.

The faith that relationships built on honesty, mutual respect, empathy, and the unconditional affirmation of a person's inherent tendency to move towards individual self-fulfillment and social harmony provide the essential substrate for all human growth and healing—once heresy within a mechanistic psychology with no faith in the resources of the human spirit—can now be found in every arena of life. . . .

From the speeches of presidents, to the leadership strategies of corporate executives who have come to respect employees as creative agents of change, to the work of parents and teachers who have learned to align with rather than stifle the child's inborn capacity for healthful growth, Rogers's simple, elegant and life-affirming values now permeate the culture. (n.p.)

Carl Rogers's greatness as a psychologist and therapist is universally acknowledged, but, as I will show, Otto Rank's impact on his way of being runs even deeper than is generally known. There are traces of Rank's ideas *throughout* Rogers's mature work, not only in the 1940s, at the birth of client-centered therapy, but also much later, in the 1970s, at the emergence of a profoundly spiritual Rogers. Like Rank, whose last book was entitled *Beyond Psychology*, Rogers (1986) concluded by the end of his life that there is an "other-wordly" realm "beyond" psychology, a realm he came to prize as "the transcendent, the indescribable, the spiritual" (199).

Like spirit itself, however, these traces of Rank in Rogers are barely visible. For those who have not studied Rank, the traces may in fact be invisible. In the course of developing his own original and powerful thinking, Rogers seems not to have been fully aware of just how much of Rank's vocabulary he was echoing.

Yet after reading them side by side, I cannot escape the uncanny feeling that the spirit of Rank is present, hovering in the white space between the lines of Rogers's text. And every now and then, if we pay close attention to the language Rogers favored—especially his *metaphors*—it rises to the surface and speaks in the voice of Otto Rank.

By teasing out Rogers's close affinity with Rank, however, I do not intend to diminish in the slightest the genius of Carl Rogers, whose contributions to the betterment of humanity are extraordinary. For me and countless others in the helping professions, Rogers remains, without exaggeration, "the most influential psychologist in American history" (Kirschenbaum & Henderson 1989b: xi).

Scholars have long noticed similarities between Rank and Rogers (Raskin 1948; Sollod 1978; Gendlin 1988). With the publication in 1996 of my compilation of Rank's American lectures, *A Psychology of Difference*, practitioners of the person-centered approach—as Rogers's client-centered therapy is called today—began to look more closely at what Rogers had learned from Rank (Barrett-Lennard 1998; deCarvalho 1999; Ellingham 2011; Vanhooren 2022; Vanhooren 2023).

Listening empathically to the feelings—the music—underneath a client's words was the main theme of Rank's teachings on relationship therapy at the University of Pennsylvania School of Social Work during the 1920s and 1930s (Cnaan et al. 2008).[4]

After scrutiny of the writings of Rank and Rogers, Ellingham (2011) concluded that the Rogerian approach, originally called non-directive therapy, "is essentially an evolved elaboration of Rankian relationship therapy" (181). Because listening to feelings is central to "the practice of non-directive therapy, no essential difference appears to exist between it and relationship therapy," said Ellingham (189).

In psychoanalysis, however, listening to the feelings of patients is a relatively recent phenomenon, which became acceptable to mainstream analysts only after the death of Anna Freud in 1982, and the subsequent rise of "relational psychoanalysis" (Mitchell 1988). "For the first time, the patient's feelings—not just the analyst's theoretical abilities—were recognized as being relevant to the therapy" (Govrin 2016:95).

Why did psychoanalysts take so long to recognize that listening to the feelings of patients is essential for healing? The answer can be traced back to a dramatic battle Otto Rank had with Sigmund Freud in the mid-1920s over *The Trauma of Birth*—a "David-and-Goliath" conflict that I recount in detail later in this book.

Around the world, millions of social workers, counselors, and psychotherapists now consider the creation of an authentic, respectful, and empathic relationship to be the principal healing element in therapy.

While Otto Rank did not form a separate school of therapy to teach his ideas, the person-centered ideas of Carl Rogers have been incorporated into about 200 research and training institutes worldwide (Kirschenbaum & Jourdan 2005). Half a dozen schools of therapy deriving from the person-centered approach trace their origins to Rogers (Sanders 2012). In Germany, about 4,300 clinicians belong to the person-centered professional society, in Britain about 1,000, and in the Netherlands about 850 (Cooper et al. 2013). Among Japanese counselors, Rogers is more highly regarded than any other Western therapist. "Counseling in Japan has always meant client-centered therapy" (Sakanaka 2015:157).

❦

In addition to formulating the principles of relationship therapy, Otto Rank pioneered in the practice of *existential therapy*, which helps clients encounter, as Rank (1936a) explains in *Will Therapy*, "the metaphysical problems of human existence" (180).

What makes it so hard for us to bear the burden of selfhood—of our uniqueness—for accepting and being ourselves, utterly different from anyone else? This was the existential question posed by Rank in *Will Therapy*. In *The Denial of Death*, Ernest Becker (1973) sums up Rank's question as "the basic problem of the child's life: whether he will be a passive object of fate, an appendage of others, a plaything of the world or whether he will be an active center within himself—whether he will control his own destiny with his own powers or not" (35–36).

At the core of existential suffering, according to Rank, is anguish, dread, or anxiety—*Angst* in Rank's German. Even with the kindest of parents, and the least violent of births, the tiny human being is born afraid, a shivering bundle of *Angst* cast adrift in an awesome and uncaring universe. "Here lies the truth," writes existential therapist Rollo May (1983), "of the symbol of the birth trauma as the prototype of all anxiety" (111).

In *Will Therapy*, Rank (1936a) suggests that *Angst* is "erected [at birth] as a dividing line between the [I] and the world, and vanishes only when both have become one, as parts of a greater whole" (278). Becoming part of a "greater whole," feeling a sense of Oneness, even if only for a short while, can heal the pain of separation that marks human existence from birth to death, the final separation. *The Trauma of Birth* "is really a great vision of the idea of separation governing the universe," Rank once told a friend (quoted in Lieberman 1985:317).

Emerging from a germ cell smaller than the period at the end of this sentence, the human being spends a lifetime trying to heal its sense of painful *Angst* and loneliness, its sheer difference. *Difference = suffering*. I = loneliness.

The onset of suffering in adults, proposes Rank (1936a) in *Will Therapy*, typically comes from the streaming together of two anxieties—the fear of living and the fear of dying.

A crisis "seems to break out at a certain age when the life fear [*Lebensangst*] which has restricted the [I's] development meets with the death fear [*Todesangst*] as it increases with growth and maturity," says Rank. "The individual then feels himself driven forward by regret for wasted life and the desire still to retrieve it" (265).

He adds: "But this forward driving fear is now death fear, the fear of dying without having lived, which, even so, is held in check by fear of life" (ibid.). The fear of dying correlates with "unused life, the unlived in us" (211). The more our life is "unlived," maintains Rank, the more we will fear dying.

Even the empathic listening at the heart of relationship therapy, according to Rank, is not sufficient to eliminate the universal suffering of human existence, although it can be attenuated considerably by the clinician's affirmation of the client's difference, uniqueness, and creative will.

In *Beyond Psychology*, Rank (1941a) writes of existential pain as "part of man's life on this earth. We are born in pain, we die in pain, and we should accept life-pain as unavoidable—indeed a necessary part of earthly existence, not merely the price we have to pay for pleasure" (16).

Only by giving and receiving love, together with the fullest expression of our creative will, insists Rank, can we hope to heal, but just temporarily, our brokenness, our anguish, our eternal loneliness.

As the first existential therapist in the world, Otto Rank revolutionized the thinking of Rollo May, one of the most prominent American psychotherapists and public intellectuals of the second half of the 20th century.[5]

Unlike Carl Rogers, who knew Rank personally, May never met Rank, but immersed himself in Rank's writings on love and will—and life fear and death fear—in the mid-1930s (Kramer 2023).

For the next 50 years, May would establish himself as the most influential existential therapist in America. In his practice of counseling and therapy, May's objective was to spark the creative will, the repressed capacity for self-leadership—the creative life force—of his clients.

Like Otto Rank and Carl Rogers, May (1953) defined self-leaders as "persons who can *be*, that is persons who have a center of strength within themselves. It is our task [as therapists] to find the sources of this inner strength" (80; italics in the original).

With deep empathy, May strove to heal the existential suffering of his clients by exploring, together with them, their fear of life and fear of death. He encouraged them to learn how to transcend anxiety, despair, and loneliness through the expression of their creative will and capacity to love others.

"I have long considered Otto Rank to be *the* great unacknowledged genius in Freud's circle," attests May (1996: xi; italics in the original) in his foreword to *A Psychology of Difference*, a collection of 22 lectures that Rank delivered from 1924–1938 at universities across America, including the New School for Social Research, Yale, the University of Minnesota, and, most frequently, at the University of Pennsylvania School of Social Work. Terming Rank's American lectures "dazzling," May adds:

> Decades ahead of his time, Rank speaks of neurosis as a failure in creativity and the suffering human being as an *artiste manqué*, a failed artist. In these lectures Rank explores in simple English the rich interplay between I and Thou, separation and union, the individual and the collective, will and love, creativity and guilt. (xi)

In the mid-1960s, Rollo May joined with Carl Rogers and Abraham Maslow to lead a *third force* in psychology after behaviorism and psychoanalysis, then the two dominant approaches to therapy. Unfortunately, Rank had died in 1939, otherwise he would certainly have spearheaded this movement in tandem with May, Rogers, and Maslow.

Maslow knew of Rank, and occasionally cites him, but there's no evidence that he applied Rank's ideas on the creative will to his theory of self-actualization, which was based, instead, on the writings of Kurt Goldstein (Kaufman 2020:86). On the other hand, Rogers and May always went out of their way to credit Rank as their greatest inspiration.

By the late 1920s, Rank had already "anticipated demands of post-1960 youth for self-creation," according to historian William M. Johnston (1983:261), long before Rogers, May, and Maslow published their major works.

Far ahead of his time, Rank was the first psychoanalyst to integrate existential and humanistic psychologies, opening up new horizons for social work, counseling, and psychotherapy.

Over the course of the first two decades of the 21st century, the existential-humanistic movement "has infiltrated not only the fortress of clinical psychology," report Shahar and Schiller (2016) in the *Journal of Psychotherapy Integration*, "but also mainstream academic psychology in general and has assumed a quiet, albeit steadfast, control" (1).

In recent years, research on ultimate human concerns has expanded by leaps and bounds. Despite the restrictions of manualized care and the limits of what health insurance will reimburse, many clients of social workers, counselors, and therapists are seeking to explore deeper, existential concerns rather than simply obtaining temporary "symptom relief."

Funded mainly by the John Templeton Foundation, the *International Society for the Science of Existential Psychology* (ISSEP), a network of psychologists and researchers committed to using experimental and other quantitative methods to study existential psychology, identifies these ultimate concerns as:

- Matters of life and death
- Culture and identity
- Freedom, responsibility, and the will
- Isolation, uncertainty, and shared reality
- Meaning and purpose
- Religion and spirituality
- Personal growth, physical health, and well-being[6]

All of these existential-humanistic concerns were probed by Rank, Rogers, May, and Maslow. Today, they are receiving increasing attention by researchers in mainstream psychology. On its website, ISSEP notes:

Around the world, researchers are using diverse methods—from controlled laboratory experiments to analyses of large data sets—to rigorously test ideas about the roles of various existential concerns. This trend is popping up in almost every domain of contemporary psychological science, including cognition and neuroscience, social and personality psychology, clinical and counseling psychology and more. A growing number of major peer-reviewed research journals such as *Personality and Social Psychology* (2010), *Religion, Brain & Behavior* (2016), *Review of General Psychology* (2018), and *Journal of Social and Clinical Psychology* (2020), have been hosting "special issues" focused exclusively on existential topics. (n.p.)

In one of his most striking contributions to existential psychology, Otto Rank describes the overly anxious human being as one whose courage and creative will are, essentially, on life-support, one who has refused the loan of life in order to escape the payment—death.

"I've always been intrigued with Otto Rank's formulation of going back and forth between the poles of life anxiety and death anxiety," said Irvin Yalom in an interview with Ruthellen Josselson (2008:114). Yalom's guide to Rank's thought was Rollo May, who served as Yalom's own therapist for many years (Abzug 2021).

In the German text of *Will Therapy*, Rank (1936a) merged the *Lebensangst* and *Todesangst* that human beings oscillate between during the interval between birth and death into a single, unforgettable term: *Urangst*—which Jessie Taft translated as "universal human primal fear" (189).

In later chapters, I show in more detail how Otto Rank's focus on relationship transformed the therapeutic thinking of Carl Rogers, whose ideas remain pre-eminent in the practice of social work, counseling, and psychotherapy today.

2
Self-leadership

More than just the first existential-humanistic therapist, Otto Rank introduced what today is called "leadership development" at the University of Pennsylvania School of Social Work, in close collaboration with pioneer feminists Jessie Taft and Virginia Robinson, two of the most influential voices in social work during the 20th century.[1]

"In the analytic situation," said Rank (1996) in his American lectures, "we can study the psychology of the love relationship and the leader relationship as well as the relationship to the educator" (198). Expressing the life force of one's creative will—self-leadership—is at core of all leadership, according to Rank.

"Leadership," adds Rank (1941a) in *Beyond Psychology*, "from the legendary hero who creates culture to the artist and scientist who enrich it, is necessary for the constant stimulation towards cultural achievements" (232).

The term "transforming leadership" was coined in 1978 by political scientist and historian James MacGregor Burns in *Leadership*—the seminal work in the field of leadership studies. According to Burns (1978), "the result of transforming leadership is a relationship of mutual stimulation and elevation that converts followers into leaders, and may convert leaders into moral agents" (4). Like Rank, Burns saw leadership as a *relationship*, not as an individual person issuing commands from on high.

Burns's thinking led to a change in the way we should view and practice leadership. Trans-*forming* occurs when the *frame* of reference people have—their mental framework or categories of understanding—undergoes a radical and discontinuous shift. By introducing the term "transforming leadership," Burns intended to radically shift our frame of knowing by questioning the taken-for-granted assumptions, the existing paradigms, of leadership theory and practice.

Drawing on the principles of existential-humanistic psychology, especially the writings of Abraham Maslow, Burns observes that a "leader's fundamental act is to induce people to be aware of or conscious of *what they feel*—to feel their true needs so strongly, to define their values so meaningfully, that they can move to purposeful action" (44; italics added). Listening empathically to feelings, according to Burns, is at the core of healthy relationships.

Otto Rank and the Creation of Modern Psychotherapy. Robert Kramer, Oxford University Press.
© Robert Kramer (2025). DOI: 10.1093/9780197698303.003.0002

An interdisciplinary thinker, Burns was the first scholar to make the study of leadership a legitimate academic field distinct from the study of management, which had always been a staple of business schools.

The word "management" derives from the Italian *maneggiare* ("to control a horse," from the Latin *manus* "hand"). Managers control the energy of others, like a rider controls the reins of a horse. Understanding management as a means of control was first theorized in 1911 by Frederic Taylor in his *Principles of Scientific Management* and remains a bedrock principle in all organizations. In contrast, "transforming leaders," said Burns, strive to release the creative will of others through building authentic relationships. The purpose of these relationships is to help followers *reframe* the meaning of their own capacity to lead.

Averse to expressing genuine feelings, except perhaps anger, managers typically conduct transactions with employees, who receive "contingent rewards," depending on task performance and outcome. Relationships are not the concern of most managers. "Leave your feelings at home," is their mantra. In contrast, said Burns, transforming leaders deploy their feelings as an instrument to help spark the creative will—and elevate the ethical aspirations—of followers, creating conditions for them to become leaders themselves. Unethical, manipulative leadership is not "transforming leadership, " which Burns defines as an interactive relationship in which "leaders and their followers raise one another to higher levels of morality and motivation" (20).

Although leaders manage and managers lead, these processes are not the same. Leadership is a relationship, argued Rank and Burns, not a single person. In this relationship, both leaders and followers are practicing "leadership." At times, practicing "leadership" means that followers lead and leaders follow (Kellerman 2024). For Rank, as for Burns, followership is active and ethical—not passive or morally neutral.

"The key distinctive role of leadership at the outset is that leaders take the initiative," said Burns (2003). "They address their creative insights to potential followers, seize their attention, spark further interaction. The first act is decisive because it breaks up a static situation and establishes a relationship. It is, in every sense, a *creative* act" (172; italics in the original).

Throughout all his writings on the creative will, Otto Rank saw leadership as an *art form*. While he did not use the term "transforming leadership," Rank spoke often in his lectures to students at the Penn School about the creativity essential for leading change by social workers.[2]

His 1909 book *The Myth of the Birth of the Hero* was the first cross-cultural study of leadership—for good or ill. In this internationally acclaimed work, written when Rank was 25, he framed leaders through the narratives of world mythology. "Here one may note an amusing example," wrote Rank in his expanded and updated edition of this book, "of the unconscious humor of children. A politician explained to his little son that a tyrant is a man who forces others to do his will without regard to their wishes. 'So,' said the boy, 'then you and Mama are also tyrants!'" (Rank 1922a:119n.37).

Rank understood the appeal of charismatic leaders who seduce others to follow their will as a way for people to escape the existential burden of their freedom—*Lebensangst*, the fear of life, the fear of accepting responsibility for one's self, and the fear of being one's own leader with the resilience, strength, and creativity to solve one's own problems.

In *Beyond Psychology*, Rank (1941a) observed: "There is always the larger group which will join the leader in order vicariously to share his power and the still larger group which wants to be led" (43). Pointing to the rise of Hitler and Mussolini, he noted the dangerous appeal of charismatic leadership. In *Will Therapy* Rank (1936a) described the price we pay for refusing to accept the burden of self-leadership: we will inevitably carry a high degree of existential guilt for "unused life, the unlived in us" (211).

Rank's paradigm shift for social work—leading clients to lead themselves—is virtually identical to Burns's definition of transforming leadership, which applies most clearly to leading large-scale movements for social justice.

জ্জ

Over many decades, the world has been torn by contradictory forces, according to Jean Lipman-Blumen (1996), author of *The Connective Edge: Leading in an Interdependent World*.

Diversity and interdependence pull in opposite directions. If leaders in coming generations try to use the same one-dimensional behaviors that they've used in the past—authoritarian, charismatic, ego-driven, or even naively collaborative—they are bound to fail.

As defined by Lipman-Blumen, "connective leadership" involves a paradoxical way of being, neither authoritarian nor simply participatory, neither command-and-control nor anarchic, neither arbitrary nor self-sacrificial. For leadership in an era of confusion, chaos, and war, when no one knows what to do and technology is ascendant, the dichotomy between interdependence and diversity, ally and competitor, friend and enemy, must be transcended. This, above all, is the role of the "connective leader," argues Lipman-Blumen, echoing Burns and Rank's theory of leadership as a relationship.

"Social workers have a great opportunity to become leaders in this area," writes Clay Graybeal (2001), "as strengths-based assessments exert influence well beyond the worker and client. They have the potential to change the perceptions of other current and future providers, and plant seeds for those providers to see clients as resources in their own process, whether that process is called treatment, therapy, recovery, personal growth, collaboration, or social work" (241).

"Will therapy" is virtually a synonym for leadership development. For Rank, the practice of will therapy meant releasing the power of the creative will of social workers and their clients, a will that had been buried, perhaps for decades, under the *external* restrictions of societal oppression and simultaneously repressed by *internal* inhibitions, which were largely self-created. In the language of his time, Rank called such internal inhibitions "neuroses," a term no longer in use by professionals in mental health.[3]

A deeply empathic person, Rank saw that oppression of the poor, minorities, and the disadvantaged existed everywhere—especially oppression of women—but so did a learned helplessness on their part, stemming from beliefs coming from society that resulted in various degrees of internalized self-disempowerment.

"Rank was preoccupied with social problems and felt individual therapy was not enough to solve our problems," said Anaïs Nin (1968). "He wanted it more widely and generally applied and concentrated its effectiveness through education and through the psychological training of social workers" (94–95).

From Jane Addams and Leymah Gbowee (both recipients of Nobel Peace prizes) to Secretary of Labor Francis Perkins and Senators Barbara Mikulski and Deborah Stabenow, social work has been a woman's profession with many prominent female leaders.

Decades ahead of his time, Rank made leadership development the aim of educating female social workers for their role as change agents in a democratic, highly technological society. In the field of social work, Rank was the first to see leading as a performing art, not as a practice of managing or controlling others.

At all levels of society, democratic leaders, argued Rank, must learn how to tap into their *own* passionate, creative wills, and then draw on their feelings as instruments to spark the repressed creativity of others, in order to transform them into ethical self-leaders who can determine themselves.[4]

Democratic leaders move themselves and others to committed action. For Rank, the mission of democratic leaders, first and foremost, is to grow other leaders. Adopted by Jessie Taft and Virginia Robinson, Rank's will psychology was the first strengths-based approach to leadership in social work.

In the therapeutic relationship, wrote Rank (1932b) in *Modern Education*, the therapist "must allow the patient the leadership [role] even when [he] imagines that he is directing the whole situation" (226).[5]

Although clients, feeling overwhelmed by the stress of their daily lives, may at first seek advice and problem-solving from social workers, Taft and Robinson taught their students that it was not their function to "diagnose" clients, and tell them what to do or how to behave. Rather, they should treat clients with respect and empathy, building authentic relationships with them and their families.

Clients have the creative will, maintained Taft and Robinson, to take the lead in solving their own problems. According to the Oxford bibliography on the strengths-based practice of social work:

> Prior to the advent of strengths-based perspectives and practices, the dominant ideology involved an "expert" practitioner diagnosing clients and determining what needed to be done. People were viewed largely in terms of their pathologies, weaknesses, limitations, and problems. In strengths-based models, in contrast, the helper, in collaboration with the client system, identifies and amplifies existing client system capacities to resolve problems and improve quality of life. Strengths-based approaches can be viewed as respectful toward and empowering of the oppressed and vulnerable people to which the field of social work traditionally has been committed.[6]

It was Rank's focus on developing the strengths of both social workers and their clients that Taft and Robinson adopted as their standard for the creative practice of social work.

According to historian William M. Johnston (1983), Rank became "Freud's most perceptive critic, propounding a psychology of creativity whose relevance for technological society has yet to be hailed" (258).

Promoted by business schools such as Harvard, Wharton, and the MIT Sloan School of Management, the development of leaders, with powerful wills tempered by empathic listening skills, is now considered essential for the progress of a highly technological society, especially with the rise of Artificial Intelligence, whose hidden algorithms, deepfakes, and capacity for spreading disinformation have already severely undermined democracy worldwide.

MIT Sloan School Professor Edgar Schein, founder of the study of organizational culture and a grandmaster of leadership development, says: "If we now ... are arguing for experientially based self-development and are accepting . . . of the importance of will in addition to brain and heart, perhaps it turns out that we are all Rankians" (quoted in Kramer 2017:344).

But Rank did not want the social workers he taught at the University of Pennsylvania to become "Rankians." As an existential psychologist, he urged them to become themselves, *fully alive* and energized as leaders, and simultaneously to feel awe and humility at the breathtaking fact that they *were alive*, recalling always that human beings are merely specks of dust in the vast, incomprehensible cosmos.

In spite of our Nothingness in the universe, Rank wanted all of us—social workers, counselors, psychotherapists, clients—to express the life force of our creative will to the fullest, accepting the existential burden of our difference, and, when necessary, step outside the ruling ideology of our own mindset when it blocks us from developing our creative potential.

The creative will, said Rank, isn't limited only to artists; every human being is creative, to a lesser or greater degree. He worked tirelessly to release the creativity innate to all human beings.

"By supporting the individual striving for self-realization," wrote Rank (1941a) in *Beyond Psychology*, "I freed the therapeutic process from the fetters of ideological prejudices and permitted it to be a growth process . . . instead of an educational training towards conformity" (49). Expelled from Freud's inner circle for his iconcoclasm, Rank was not interested in making people fit into the ruling political, economic, or social ideologies.

He urged social workers to develop empathy for the suffering of fellow human beings—especially the suffering of women, children, the poor, minorities, and the oppressed. In his American lectures, Rank (1996) called his teachings "a philosophy of suffering" (252).

Social workers, said Rank, need first to learn how to develop their own creative wills, and then, through empathic use of *self-in-relationship*, lead their clients to reach "higher levels of morality and motivation," in the words of James MacGregor Burns. The relationship between social worker and client is mutual, according to Rank. Both parties will be transformed in the process.

In the early decades of the 21st century, due to funding reductions, waves of mass migration, pandemics, and wars, social workers—often emotionally and physically exhausted by the overwhelming responsibilities they carry— feel deeply frustrated that they are unable to function according to this high standard, but it remains a noble ideal worth striving toward.

With the support of Jessie Taft and Virginia Robinson, Rank inspired generations of social workers to discover the power of their creative wills to foster innovation and healing in their communities. Today, no matter how challenging the practice of social work has become, this view of power is commonplace in social work.

Recently retired as president of California State University San Marcos, having also served as a social worker for many years, Karen S. Haynes (2014) writes:

Think about the power we have in knowledge and compassion, our systems perspective. Think about the power that comes with knowing that social work is both an avocation and a vocation. Think about the power that comes from understanding that service on behalf of others is the purpose of life. Think about the power that comes with knowing that we do not offer quick fixes but human dignity, inclusiveness, equality, and social justice. (n.p.)

It was Rank who introduced the term "power" into the vocabulary of the female-dominated profession of social work. "The real I, or self with its own power, the will, is left out" of psychoanalysis especially when it comes to the experience of women, suggested Rank (1936a) in *Will Therapy* (160). Paradoxically, even though Freud denied the existence of free will, he always granted men—but not women—the unlimited power and, indeed, freedom of will to lead the development of ethics, law, politics, religion, art, science, and civilization.

With respect to the origins of religion, wrote Freud (1939) in *Moses and Monotheism*, "[W]hat is sacred was originally nothing other than the prolongation of the will of the primal father; the father's will was . . . something one trembled before. . . . [W]hat seems to us grandiose about ethics, so mysterious and, in a mystical fashion, so self evident, owes these characteristics to its connection with religion, its origin from the will of the father" (121–122).

In Freud's model of the psyche, three competing forces battle inside every human being's psyche: id, ego, and super-ego. The sole source of ethical behavior in society, the super-ego is formed between ages 4 and 6 by internalization of the powerful will of the father. "The super-ego retains the character of the father," declared Freud (1923a) in *The Ego and the Id*, "the more powerful the Oedipus complex [is] . . . the stricter will be the domination of the super-ego over the ego later on" (34–35).

When Rank said that "The real I, or self with its own power, the will, is left out," he was not claiming that Freud had "left out" the will of men or fathers from psychoanalytic theory. Rank knew perfectly well that Freud, from beginning to end, sanctified the powerful will and leadership of men and fathers. During the earliest years of human society, and even up to the present, the "arbitrary will" of the father, said Freud (1930) in *Civilization and Its Discontents*, "was unrestricted" (100).

Psychoanalysis, Rank (1936b) wrote in *Truth and Reality*, "unveils to us the psychology of the strong man of will" (35). But what about women? Does psychoanalysis have a "psychology of the strong woman of will"? Do mothers have powerful wills of their own? Are women ethical? Can women become leaders? Not in Freud's Oedipal theory. Without a strong ethical sense, women are small, weak, helpless creatures, persons who constantly seek help, comfort, and leadership from men.

"One might point out," observed Rank (1932b) in *Modern Education*, "that Freud explained the concept of God as an exalted father image which he actually identified with the concept of leader-father" (121).

Freud's self-analysis in the late 1890s, as conducted in an exchange of letters with his friend Wilhelm Fliess, included, according to Didier Anzieu (2021), seeking and finding "*the way to stem the power of the female sex*" (478; italics added)—as Freud declared triumphantly to Fliess in a poem he penned to celebrate the birth of his friend's son, Conrad.

For Freud, a woman was always a failed man—*un homme manqué* (Hoffman 2017)—passive, powerless, without a moral center, never commanding authority, entirely without a will of her own. Not as ethical as men, women oppose social change, argued Freud, and, therefore, can add nothing to the advancement of civilization, law, or culture. Indeed, women, complained Freud (1930) in *Civilization and Its Discontents*, "soon came into opposition to civilization" (103).

For Rank, Freud's propositions about "stemming the power of the female sex" were intended to exclude women from political, economic, cultural, and societal leadership. Drawing on a lecture delivered by his wife Beata (Tola) Rank (1923) at the Vienna Psychoanalytic Society, which included a portrayal of the role played by Liberty, the "Goddess of Reason," in the French Revolution, Rank (1924) asserts in *The Trauma of Birth*:

> Through her sexual power woman is dangerous in the community, the social structure of which rests on the fear displaced to the father. Man depreciates her only consciously; in the Unconscious he fears her. On this account she is also desexualized and idealized in the French Revolution as Goddess of Reason. . . . The development of the paternal domination into an increasingly powerful state system administered by men is thus a continuance of the primal repression, which has as its purpose the ever wider exclusion of woman. (93–94)

By displacing the fear of the power of mothers onto fathers, Rank is suggesting that psychoanalysis had disempowered all women, desexualizing and idealizing them, which, in turn, had led to the exclusion of women from any leadership role in politics, culture, law, economics, or society.

In her Vienna Psychoanalytic Society lecture, Tola Rank proposed that women could be as strong-willed as men. She influenced Otto to adopt her view, according to Lina Magnone (2024), who recently published the first comprehensive study of Tola Rank's life and career. After the Rank family moved to Paris in 1926, Tola worked at the Bibliothèque nationale de France on "a large three-part study" on the subject of women in society, which, unfortunately, she did not complete, according to her daughter, Helene (Rank-Veltfort 2002:1443).

When the Rank family emigrated to the United States in 1935, Tola Rank became a leader in American psychoanalysis and was appointed "an honorary Professor of Psychiatry at Boston University School of Medicine, a consultant and supervisor at Judge Baker Guidance Center and, with Marian C. Putnam, co-founded and co-directed the James Jackson Putnam Children's Center in

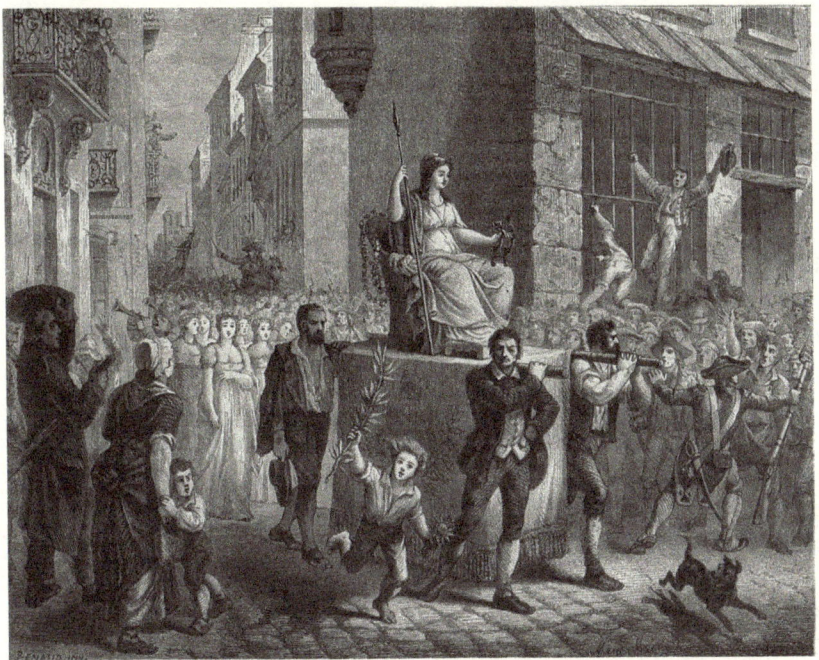

Figure 2.1 Goddess of Reason
Credit: Henri Renaud via Wikimedia Commons

1943. This center was a pioneering day-treatment for pre-school children and their parents" (1444). As a psychoanalyst, Tola Rank treated a number of well-known Harvard academics, including psychiatrist Robert J. Lifton and learning theorist Jerome A. Bruner (Roazen 1990:258).

A century ago, Otto Rank (1924), influenced by his wife, Tola, wrote in *The Trauma of Birth* that "paternal domination" had turned "into an increasingly powerful state system administered by men" (94). How much has changed since then?

According to the 2023 *World Economic Forum Global Gender Gap Report*, which has for many years measured the gap between the power and influence of men and women across 146 countries, at "the current rate of progress over the 2006–2023 span, it will take 162 years to close the Political Empowerment gender gap, 169 years for the Economic Participation and Opportunity gender gap, and 16 years for the Educational Attainment gender gap. The time to close the Health and Survival gender gap remains undefined" (Zahidi 2023:6).

Citing a McKinsey study, a recent report in the *New York Times* concludes that "true gender equality everywhere would raise the global gross domestic product by up to $28 trillion" (Thompson 2023).

When Freud dismissed a woman as a "failed man," Otto Rank saw that Freud had also dismissed the creative life force of all women. Rather than being denigrated as a "failed man," Freud's powerless woman should instead be considered a "failed artist"—an *artiste manqué*, in Rank's terms—whose creative will had been crushed by patriarchal ideology or repressed by herself, unconsciously, because of fear of life—*Lebensangst*—the fear of becoming and being herself, the fear of being different, unique, more than merely a daughter, mother, wife, or lover of powerful men.

Just as ethically grounded as men, women have the creative will, maintained Rank, to ignite transformational change to promote a more just society, advancing a beneficial civilization of women and men with the empathy to make the development of the most helpless among us, our children and our poor and our disadvantaged, their highest priority.

Rank first used the term "creative will" in a 1927 lecture (entitled "Social Adaptation and Creativity") that he gave to his mostly female students at the University of Pennsylvania School of Social Work (Rank 1996:190). As an outcome of his encounters with these students—and the female-dominated field of social work—Rank decided to focus his writing over the next few years on creating a psychology for women, and also for men, that would affirm their "creative will."

Facilitating the growth of female social workers as self-leaders spurred him to publish *Will Therapy*, which he wrote (originally in German) during 1929–1931 while lecturing at the Penn School. Through his teachings on the creative will, Rank was the first psychoanalyst to legitimize the exercise of power by women in leading change for gender, racial, economic, and social justice.

Rank's difference with Freud on the inherent power of women was at the core of their battle over *The Trauma of Birth*, as I shall recount later. From the beginning of his self-analysis in the 1890s to the end of his life in 1939, Freud virtually deified the will of men, never writing a word about the will of women.

In *Beyond Psychology*, Rank (1941a) observed that in Freud's "psychology of the male the masculine qualities appear exaggerated to the point of caricature in a libidinal superman" (287). On the other hand, women, incapable of acting powerfully, could never be leaders in or promote the ethical development of society, according to Freud.

In *Civilization and Its Discontents*, Freud (1930) argued that, in the course of evolution, "The work of civilization has become increasingly the business of men, it confronts them with ever more difficult tasks and compels them to carry out instinctual sublimations of which women are little capable" (103). The business of women is to take care of their families, and serve the will of their husbands.

In his writings after *The Trauma of Birth*, Rank opposed Freud on the question of women's capacity for exercising power. Coined by Charles Manz (1986), the term "self-leadership" captures the essence of Rank's thinking on the expression of creativity "as part of a broader and positively existential approach to self-influence," according to Manz (2015). "Ultimately, the most effective framing and practice of self-leadership will differ for each individual" (146)—an echo of Rank's psychology of difference.

Manz and Sims (1991) suggest that "The most appropriate leader is one who can lead others to lead themselves" (18). In this view, also held by Rank and Burns, leadership exists within each individual, and it is not confined to formally appointed leaders. Democratic leaders help others learn how to lead themselves.

Today, self-leadership in social work is becoming increasingly accepted as essential for the education of social workers (McKitterick 2015). In the late 1920s, Rank was the first to make this argument, an approach to developing the leadership capacity of women which was inculcated by Jessie Taft and Virginia Robinson at the Penn School—but without Rank, Taft, or Robinson ever using the term "self-leadership."

Women, taught Rank, were quite capable of being leaders—once their creative will was set free from bondage to "masculine ideology," a term Rank (1941a) used in *Beyond Psychology* to describe the disparagement of women by Freud and others who promoted patriarchy.

"In attempting to make conscious again the repressed primal memory of the birth trauma," wrote Rank (1924) in *The Trauma of Birth*, "we believe that we shall reinstate the high estimation of woman which was repressed simultaneously with the birth trauma, and we can do this by freeing her from the weight of the [masculine] curse on her genitals" (37).

Powerlessness, Rank said, is not a virtue. Through his writings on will therapy, he urged women to raise to consciousness and unlearn the deeply ingrained assumptions of their powerlessness in society, which they often had unconsciously adopted themselves, reject the "masculine ideology" that continually reinforced their expectations of powerlessness, and become, in Nietzsche's terms, "who they truly are."

Warren Bennis (1989), like James MacGregor Burns a seminal thinker in leadership studies, argues in *On Becoming a Leader* that "becoming a leader is synonymous with becoming yourself. It is precisely that simple, and it's also that difficult" (9). Becoming yourself—a lifelong process, not a single event—was the ultimate goal of Rank's will therapy, whether his therapeutic clients were women or men.

In a 1935 lecture before the New York Graduate School for Jewish Social Work, Rank spoke of the creative power of self-leadership as essential for *both* social workers and their clients:

> This was first and foremost achieved by the University of Pennsylvania School of Social Work, the leaders of which were, by virtue of their own approach, attracted to my philosophy. What they accepted from it was not only confirmation of their own activity as social workers, but the more essential and deeper meaning of the therapeutic process as an active—*almost creative*—experience on the patient's part. (Rank 1996:262; italics in the original)

For Rank, the practice of social work meant designing ecological settings that would foster authentic, respectful, and empathic relationships, resulting in the transformation of disadvantaged clients from patients to ethical agents, passive victims of social oppression to active self-leaders able to care for themselves, their families, and their communities (Furman 2002).

Jessie Taft was electrified by Rank's ideas on the development of self-leadership, a process that needed to begin as early as childhood, argued Rank, not adulthood: "The child, according to Rank," wrote Taft (1968) in a review of Rank's book, *Modern Education*, which contained a chapter on leadership, "is literally the future, the leader who is to construct out of himself, a new ideology. We have no other" (85).

In a stunning work entitled *The Role of the Baby in the Placement Process*, Taft (1946) proposed that the child, seen by Freudians of the era as completely subordinate to the powerful will of its father, take an "active part in his own placement and that the social worker not only can but must allow him to take the lead" (2). The idea of seeing *the child as leader* remains a breathtaking vision for educators even today, when leadership development for students is in the mission statement of almost every university in the United States.

Moreover, only as self-leaders could social work clients—mostly women—find the courage and creative will to lift themselves and their families out of poverty and despair *by themselves*. No psychoanalyst before Rank had ever made such a radical proposal.

The Freudians in social work were outraged by Rank's promotion of self-empowerment—i.e., self-leadership—for social workers and their impoverished clients. Rank's ideas on will therapy were "unscientific," they caviled, and therefore harmed the professional prestige of social workers as psychoanalytic authorities—based on Freud's "scientific" writings on the Oedipus complex—in the fields of child and adult guidance.

Jessie Taft (1958), on the other hand, felt "a revelation that lit up my whole way of thinking and working" (144) when she first heard Rank use the word "will." She grasped instantly what it meant for the future of her predominantly female profession and clientele.

In *The Challenge of Existential Social Work*, Mark Griffiths (2017) writes that Taft, one of the most gifted and far-sighted social workers of the 20th century, was strongly influenced by Rank's thought in *Art and Artist* (1932a) on the "immortalization" possible not just for artists but also for leaders in social work:

> Jessie Taft used the term "the immortal social worker" to refer to the professional social work self. It sounds very grandiose. Taft is applying Rank's view that the artist is seeking immortality through his or her creative endeavors. While this may apply to famous artists, Taft is suggesting that social workers are seeking a kind of immortality through their influence on others when they apply their creative skills to the practice of social work. Helping others has its own rewards. Most social work is anything but immortal, but Rank had a very wide definition of creative endeavor, which included institutional creation, the creation of new programs, and creative work done in social work practice. Rank regarded the creative person or artist as someone trying in their work to immortalize their mortal life. Taft applied many of Rank's therapeutic ideas about creativity to social casework. (25–26)

Rank's mission to develop the self-leadership and creative will of women— of social workers and the mostly female and minority clientele they served— flew in the face of everything Freud had written about the power of the will, which was, for Freud, entirely the province of men. Freud saw no trace of will in the psyches of women. They certainly could never become self-leaders, ethical change agents, or "immortal social workers" in society.

Two years before his death, Freud went even further—to repudiate women entirely. This is no exaggeration. "The repudiation of femininity," wrote Freud (1937), "can be nothing else than a biological fact, a part of the great riddle of sex" (252).

According to John Ehrenreich (1985), "at the time and in subsequent histories of the social work profession, the controversy was described as simply a difference between two schools of therapy, one based on the theories of Otto Rank, the other on the theories of Sigmund Freud, or as a dispute regarding techniques of casework" (135).

It was both. And it was also a dispute on just how "scientific" Freud's ideas were about the Oedipus complex, which, at its core, integrated three assumptions about human nature: (a) the powerful will of the father, (b) the origin of ethics through internalization of the father's will in each child's super-ego, and (c) the repudiation of femininity—a repudiation that began, as Didier Anzieu (2021) has shown, with Freud's self-analysis in the 1890s, which generated his theory of the Oedipus complex in the first place.

In the process of pointing out the absence in psychoanalysis of the will of women, Rank also strongly opposed the practice of Freudian diagnosis, which was based on "experts" analyzing the Oedipus complex of their clients, who were seen as weak and helpless.

According to Freudians, social workers themselves were supposed to be "passive," like psychoanalysts, not "active" like Rank. Thus these Freudian social workers focused most of their energies on diagnosing and analyzing the "transference" of Oedipal desires from the past, rather than listening deeply to the feelings of their patients in the present.

Only a social worker whose Oedipus complex had been analyzed could correctly diagnose—and deploy Freud's "scientific" knowledge of the unconscious to reduce—intrapsychic conflict, at the core of which was the Oedipus complex.

Otto Rank replaced Freudian diagnosis of the Oedipus complex with a person-to-person relationship in the "here and now," will therapy, and existential therapy. What helps in therapy, said Rank, is the human touch. "The making-good must be individual, personal, from the analyst as a person to the patient as a person," wrote Rank in *Will Therapy* (1936a:84).

Along with Jessie Taft and Virginia Robinson, he taught his social work students that it was their ethical responsibility to *draw out* the power, the creative life force, of clients, not *diminish* it by means of promoting transference—which Rank saw as a form of "power over" not "power with," as I show later.

"[The] creative will," said Anaïs Nin (1973), "was Rank's great contribution to the psychology of woman" (57), a psychology of self-leadership that, through the legacy of Taft and Robinson, lives on today in the values and practices of countless social workers worldwide.

3

The denial of death

Brutally attacked by orthodox analysts for abandoning Freud's Oedipal teachings, Otto Rank, according to more than one estimate, "will probably turn
out in the end to have been the best mind that psychoanalysis contributed to
intellectual history" (Jones 1960:219).

In recent years, there has been a remarkable renaissance of interest in Rank.
While profoundly transforming Carl Rogers, Rollo May, Jessie Taft, and Virginia
Robinson, Rank's thought also influenced an array of other prominent figures,
including:[1]

- Nobel laureate in literature Samuel Beckett;
- creator of modern dance Martha Graham;
- novelist of the Harlem Renaissance Nella Larsen, author of *Quicksand*
  and *Passing*;
- diarist and novelist Anaïs Nin;
- surrealist painter Salvador Dalí;
- modernist architect Richard Neutra;
- feminist Betty Friedan, author of *The Feminine Mystique*;
- novelist Henry Miller;
- founder of experiential family therapy Carl Whitaker;
- novelist Lawrence Durrell, author of the *Alexandria Quartet*;
- philosopher of the New Left Paul Goodman, co-creator of Gestalt
  therapy;
- professor of leadership Jean Lipmen-Blumen, theorist of "connective
  leadership" and "toxic leadership";
- theologian, feminist, and proponent of "Creation Spirituality" Matthew
  Fox;
- psychiatrist R.D. Laing;
- philosopher Peter Sloterdijk;
- psychoanalyst D.W. Winnicott;
- poet Sylvia Plath;
- psychoanalyst Jacques Lacan;
- curators at the National Gallery of Art who organized an exhibition in
  2022 in Washington, DC, entitled *The Double: Identity and Difference in
  Art Since 1900*; and, most importantly,

Otto Rank and the Creation of Modern Psychotherapy. Robert Kramer, Oxford University Press.
© Robert Kramer (2025). DOI: 10.1093/9780197698303.003.0003

- cultural anthropologist and philosopher Ernest Becker, who won the Pulitzer Prize for *The Denial of Death* (1973), a brilliant merger of the thought of Rank with that of Kierkegaard.

Since the publication of *The Denial of Death*, tributes to Becker's book have come from scores of well-known people, including Louise Glück, winner of the 2020 Nobel Prize in literature; filmmaker Woody Allen; author Don DeLillo; philosopher Cornel West; cosmologist Brian Greene; and President Bill Clinton. "Fifty years on," wrote the *New York Times* in 2023, "Ernest Becker's *The Denial of Death* remains an essential, surprisingly upbeat guide to our final act on Earth."[2]

Flight From Death: The Quest for Immortality, a film made in 2003 about Becker, received seven Best Documentary awards.[3] In 2020, *Lies of Heroism–Redefining the Anti-War Film*, also based on Becker, critiqued the cinematic description of war, showing how purportedly "anti-war films" often promote "heroic lies" justifying war as a patriotic way to transcend death.[4] In 2024, Terrence Malick and Robert Redford co-produced a third film on Becker, entitled *All Illusions Must Be Broken*.[5] In an ongoing series entitled *Lit Century: 100 Years, 100 Books*, the website https://lithub.com selected *The Denial of Death* as its choice for best book published in 1973.[6]

"There's no substitute for reading Rank," argued Becker (1973) in *The Denial of Death*. "[H]e is a mine for years of insights and pondering." He added: "You cannot merely praise much of his work because in its stunning brilliance it is often fantastic, gratuitous, superlative; the insights seem like a gift, beyond what is necessary" (xx).

More than any other psychoanalyst, Rank's thought is interdisciplinary. Steeped in cultural anthropology, world literature, and the history of art, myth, religion, philosophy, psychoanalysis, and leadership, Rank presents a formidable challenge to students of social work, counseling, or psychotherapy with little or no exposure to these disciplines.

What makes reading Rank so challenging? The main reason is that his "thought always spanned several fields of knowledge," Becker (1973) observed. "[W]hen he talked about, say, anthropological data and you expected anthropological insight, you got something else, something more. Living as we do in an area of hyperspecialization we have lost the expectation of this kind of delight" (ibid).

As one example, if you were to pick up Rank's 1930 book *Psychology and the Soul*, assuming that it's just an anthropological study of "belief in the soul" as its German title (*Seelenglaube*) indicates, you'd be flabbergasted to discover that Rank's last chapter summarizes the most recent findings of quantum physics.

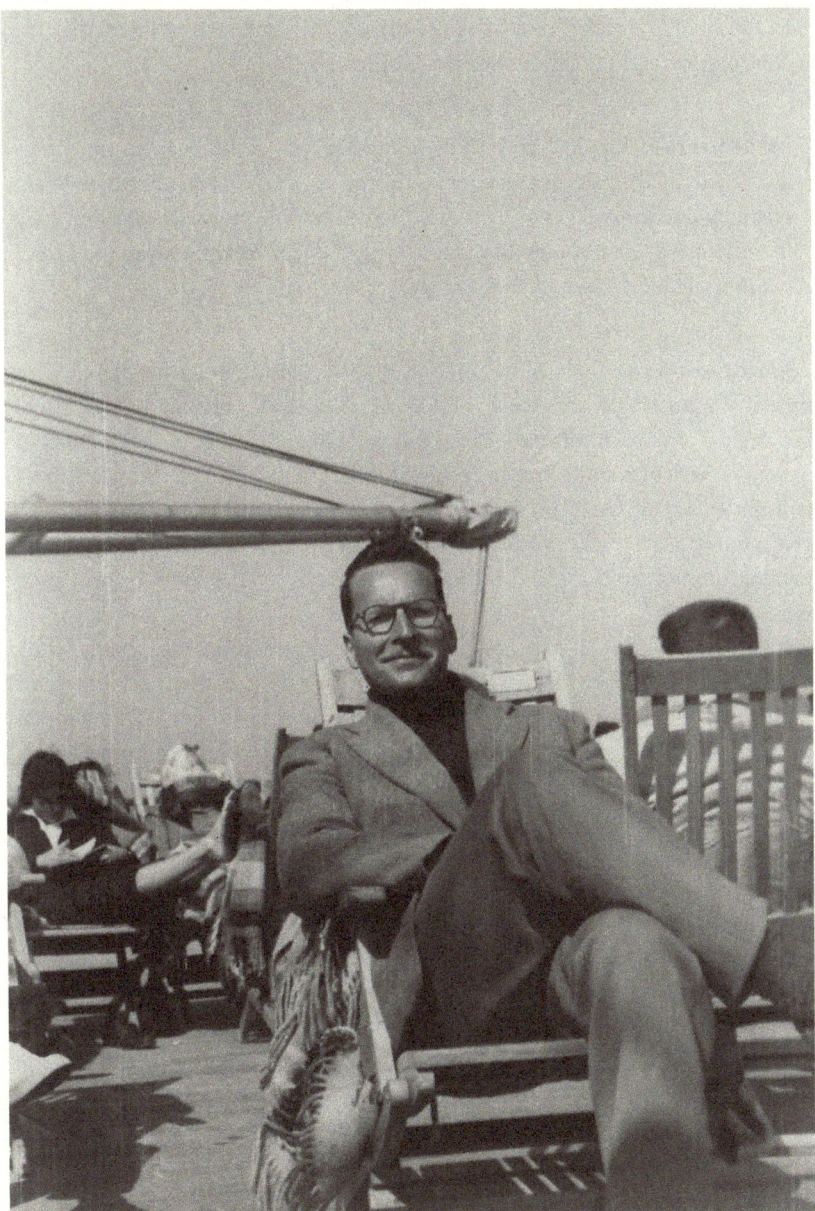

Figure 3.1 Ernest Becker

Credit: Marie Becker for the Estate of Ernest Becker

Criticizing Freud's philosophy of science, which divorced observer from observed—analyst from patient—Rank argued in 1930 that physicists were no longer studying separate objects but their *relations*.[7]

In *Psychology and the Soul*, Rank (1930) asserts that his stress on relationship had revolutionized the practice of psychotherapy:

> I jolted [Freud] by analyzing the *relationship* . . . in the analytic situation itself. This relativistic orientation led in my more recent publications to a relativity-based psychology, in which there is no longer a fixed position for the [therapist] . . . but only the moment-to-moment dynamic relation of the twosome. (113; italics in the original)

Freud's concept of causality, notes Rank, is Newtonian, and "explains the present in terms of the past" (116), by means of transference of Oedipal desires from childhood. But "the effective therapeutic experience is present experience, not historical understanding" (ibid.). Psychotherapy in the here-and-now can only be "a science of relationships" (128), insists Rank, who argues that quantum physics has proven that the human being lies beyond predictability and cannot be explained by the causal theories of psychoanalysts.

Past traumas provide the context for current suffering; thus Rank would always help his clients sort through the painful rubble of their earliest years, spending as much time on the past as the situation demanded. But therapeutic healing of suffering occurs only in the here-and-now, in the moment-to-moment, person-to-person relationship between the twosome.

According to Rank, offering interpretations in the context of a trusting, respectful relationship has the potential to help clients construct fresh meanings of their lives. It was not an "either-or" choice: *either* interpretation *or* relationship.

What was helpful for one client might not help another. Similarly, what was helpful at one moment might not be helpful for the same client at another moment. For Rank, an authentic relationship establishes the context in which more freedom is present for clients to explore their most painful thoughts, feelings, and actions. But *without* an empathic relationship, he insisted, interpretations can be harmful.

Not focused merely on therapy for the individual, Rank was the first systems thinker in psychoanalysis. "If you treat a patient you also affect the lives of other members of the family," said Rank, anticipating family systems therapy by decades. "With individual therapy you may be helping or hurting people you never see" (quoted in Lieberman 1985:377). Today, Rank's systems thinking is the hallmark of family therapy and social work:

In the physical world, the world of Newton, it makes sense to talk of causality in linear terms: A causes B, which acts upon C, causing D. In human relationships, however, the "billiard ball" model, which proposes that a force moves in one direction only and affects objects in its path, rarely—if ever—applies. Consequently, *any search for the "real" or ultimate cause of any interpersonal event is pointless.* A does not cause B, nor does B cause A; both cause each other. Explanations cannot be found in the actions of the parts but in the system as a whole—its communication patterns, complex relationships, and mutual influences. (Goldenberg et al. 2017:21; italics in the original)

In Rank's thought, relationship can be visualized metaphorically as a latticework of crossed strips, interweaving the warp and woof of part and whole, separation and union, difference and likeness—a latticework in which the whole infuses each of the parts, and the parts themselves might be able, with the help of the therapist, to feel more whole.

Dorothy Hankins, a student of Rank's at the Penn School, served as chief social worker at the Philadelphia Child Guidance Clinic for over three decades, working for many years under the directorship of Salvador Minuchin, the renowned family therapist. Rank's influence on the development of family systems therapy lasted over the course of Hankins's thirty years of work in the field (Lieberman 1985:377), and was extended by Carl Whitaker, who "affirmed Rank's notion of the therapist as 'creative artist'" (Neill & Kinskern 1982:4) when Whitaker worked at the Louisville Child Guidance Clinic.

The founder of experiential family therapy, Whitaker—co-author in 1953 of a landmark work, *The Roots of Psychotherapy*—was transformed by his encounter with Rank's systems thinking. In a striking phrase, Whitaker writes that "there is no such thing as a person, that a person is merely the fragment of a family" (quoted in Goldenberg et al. 2017:228).[8]

Pointing to the mutuality within relationship therapy, "Whitaker took the audacious position, never before espoused in family therapy, that each participant in therapy is to some degree simultaneously patient and therapist to the other. . . . Both invest emotion in the process, both are vulnerable, both regress, both grow as individuals as a result of the experience. Both expose themselves to the risks of change" (227).

This was Rank's view of how relationship helps promote growth and development. The relationship therapy that Rank created and taught others violated the most sacred rule Freud had mandated his students to follow—a technique of emotional distancing now abandoned by most analysts, but prevalent during the better part of the 20th century. "I cannot advise my colleagues too strongly," urged Freud (1912), to model themselves during the psychoanalytic treatment on the surgeon, *who puts aside all feelings,* even his human sympathy, and concentrates his mental forces on the single aim of performing the operation as skillfully as possible.... The justification for requiring this *emotional coldness* in the analyst is that it creates ... for the doctor a desirable protection for his own emotional life and for the patient the largest amount of help we can give him today. (115; italics added)

Aware of the perils of "emotional burnout"—a term coined only in the 1970s—Rank nevertheless maintained that Freud's mandate for analysts to be "unfeeling" and "emotionally cold" in order to protect their own emotional lives while conducting their sessions would be re-traumatizing to patients, already feeling severely traumatized by the emotional suffering that had brought them to therapy in the first place.

"What helps is not *intellectual knowledge* but human understanding," Rank said in his American lectures, "which is *emotional* and hence cannot be schematized" (Rank 1996:221; italics in the original). By intellectual knowledge, Rank meant the giving of interpretations without connecting emotionally to the suffering and feelings of clients. Empathic listening—human understanding—was at the core of his relationship therapy.

In *Psychology and the Soul*, Rank (1930) found support for his relationship approach by pointing to the latest discoveries in quantum physics—even going so far as to explain the implications for psychotherapy of Einstein's theory of relativity, Bohr's theory of complementarity, and Heisenberg's Uncertainty Principle in two long footnotes (114n).

Rank's main purpose in *Psychology and the Soul*, which he dedicated to his wife, Tola, was to explore the historical evolution of the "psyche"—a term derived from the Greek *psykhē*, "the soul, mind, spirit, life." In a letter to Jessie Taft (1958), Rank summed up his book:

[O]ur scientific psychology grew out of the belief in the Soul (Immortality) and still represents for us the same although it denies the existence of the soul. In one word, psychology [is] our religion. This idea is carried through all the stages of human development from the magic world view of the primitive to psychoanalysis and of course to my own concepts. (143)

In *Will Therapy* Rank (1936a) writes of the "soul life of feeling and willing" (231)—equating feeling and willing with "the soul," which, he asserts, is an expression of the creative life force of each human being. Relationships are constituted of feelings.

As I show later, the act of willing, according to Rank, is always relational: we are all connected. "Classical physics," wrote Heisenberg (1958), "can be considered an idealization in which we speak about the world as entirely separated from ourselves" (106). But in the world discovered by quantum physics, there is no objective observer, only relationship. Henry P. Stapp, a mathematical physicist at the Berkeley-Livermore Laboratory, who worked with Heisenberg in the 1960s on quantum mechanics, admires *Psychology and the Soul* for championing the creative will and relationship. Now over 95 years old, Stapp (2017) regrets that the word "soul" has vanished from academic discourse in psychology (65).

"Does the word soul have a place in modern psychology?," asks Robert Kugelmann (2023) in *The Soul in Soulless Psychology*. "Apparently not," he answers.

> Yet the soul has survived. Everything has a soul—an essence, heart, central purpose, deepest meaning. Soul can be searched, murdered, lost, and found. Everything, science, new machines, corporations, music, food, and activities of all kinds, can have a soul. There are battles for the soul of science, of Western culture, of America, of Canada, of capitalism. Everything, that is, except living beings. (1)

In *Psychology and the Soul*, Rank (1930) asserts: "The soul, an ideology born of belief in immortality, produces new ideologies in order to maintain soul-belief. In this way the soul is *creative*" (61; italics in the original).

Freud read Rank's *Psychology and the Soul*, but dismissed Rank's ideas on relationship in a talk at the Vienna Psychoanalytic Society he gave in 1930. He lambasted Rank for using "the theory of relativity, the quantum theory, and the principle of indeterminism to express doubts about psychic causality, so that there is nothing left except soul and free will. But psychoanalysis cannot possibly be an illusion," insisted Freud (quoted in Sterba 1982: 116).[9]

Although claiming to be a scientist, Freud always objected to experimental testing of his theories. Said Freud: "The wealth of reliable observations on which [my] assertions rest make them independent of experimental verification" (quoted in Wallerstein 2002:376).

Reflecting Freud's disdain for scientific verification, few of the 12,000 members of the International Psychoanalytical Association, or the 3,000 members of the American Psychoanalytic Association, are today interested in experimental testing of their theories. The vast majority are uneasy with—or even oppose—research on the effectiveness of psychoanalysis as a therapy, claiming it's unnecessary or impossible.[10]

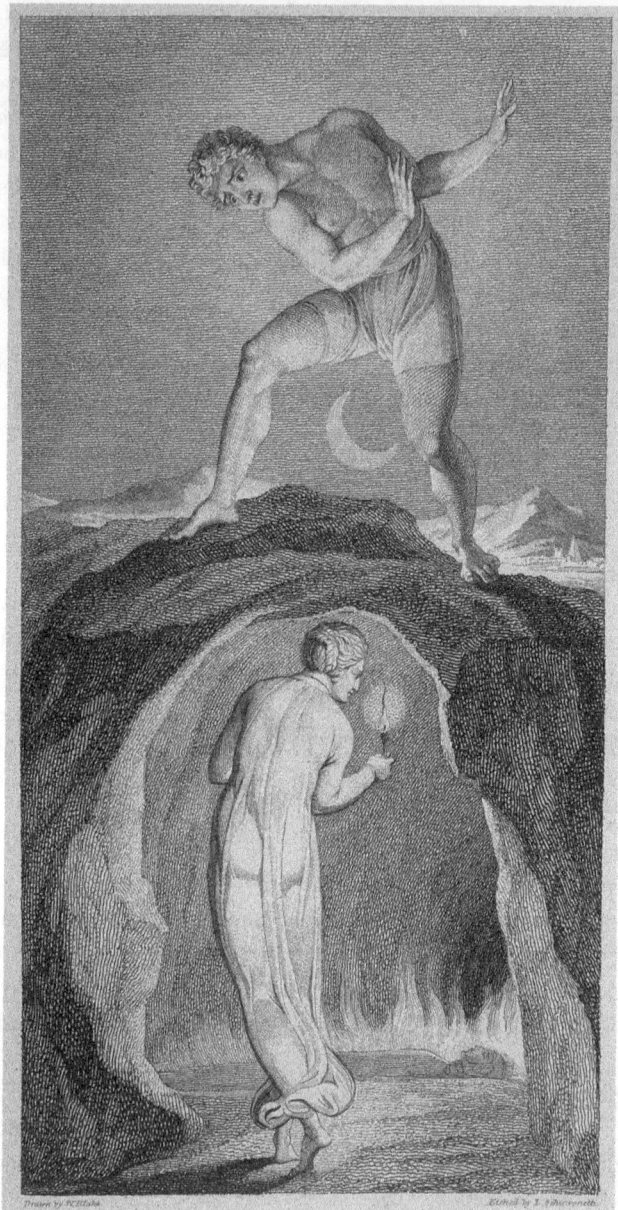

Figure 3.2 The soul exploring the recesses of the grave
Credit: Harris Brisbane Dick Fund, 1917, Metropolitan Museum of Art

"At my graduation from psychoanalytic training, a supervising analyst said to me, 'Your analysis will cure you of the need to do research,'" Andrew Gerber, the president of a psychiatric treatment center in Connecticut recently told the *New York Times* (Dominus 2023).

On the other hand, Otto Rank's approach to relationship, as elaborated by Carl Rogers and his students, has now been researched extensively. In fact, no psychoanalyst's hypotheses have ever been tested, with as much scientific rigor, and across so many different populations, as those of Rank.

Influenced by *The Denial of Death*, scores of researchers at universities worldwide are now testing Rank's propositions on how the *fear of life* and *fear of death* contribute to men's continuing oppression of women and, by extension, to hatred and scapegoating of "the other," to racism, and to war.

How did Rank come up with these propositions? During his studies of cultural anthropology Rank observed a widespread fear of "difference," a fear that he believed had originated in the difference between men and women. For man, Rank writes (1941a) in *Beyond Psychology*, "fear of woman . . . is *the fear of difference*" (223; italics added). About the mindset of Freud and other defenders of patriarchy, Rank asks,

> [W]hy does woman always come into the class of the evil, dangerous, and less valuable? This, as I have explained [in *Art and Artist*], arises from man's urge to eternalize himself personally, an urge threatened by sexual propagation, of which woman is the representative; and so woman passes into what I have called the Not-I class. . . . Man divided the visible universe, as it were, into two categories, the "I" and the "not-I." . . . [Woman] automatically became identified with the not-I class. (246–247)

Over the last four decades, experimental social psychologists studying "terror management theory" (TMT) have published a tsunami of research on one of Rank's most compelling hypotheses, which Ernest Becker (1975) placed at the core of *Escape from Evil*.[11]

"The death fear of the [I] is lessened by the killing, the sacrifice, of the other," argued Rank (1936a) in *Will Therapy*. "Through the death of the other, one buys oneself free from the penalty of dying, of being killed" (183).

After quoting the same sentence in *Existential Psychotherapy*, Irvin Yalom (1980) adds: "Obviously Rank refers to more than literal killing: more subtle forms of aggression—including domination, exploitation, or 'soul murder,' as Ibsen puts it—serve the same purpose" (127).

To date, across dozens of different cultures, over 1,500 experimental findings have shown that we tend, unconsciously, to project our fear of death onto what Rank calls "the other"—those who are *different* from us.

Much of man's disparaging, hateful, and evil behavior toward women, said Rank, is deeply rooted in fear at the prospect of his own death, a fear that men project onto "the other," the one who is different from them. In *Otto Rank: A Rediscovered Legacy*, Esther Menaker (1982), who studied with Taft and Robinson at the Penn School, explains:

> It is clear that, for a long time, both individually and collectively a masculine way of life has been imposed upon women. Rank attributes this in large mea-sure to man's attempt to *blot out his mother-origin in order to deny his mortal nature*. For to be born of woman is to share one's fate with all other living crea-tures whose birth inaugurates the inevitability of death. Mythology, religion, art, and social organization reflect the attempt ... to prove man's supernatural origins and therefore his immortality. (89; italics added)

Afraid of difference, men, according to Rank, will often seek to denigrate, dominate, exploit, humiliate, physically attack, or even kill "the other," thereby justifying acts of injustice *firstly* against women—the original "not-I" who gives them birth and death—and then *extending* the "not-I" category to justify racial hatred, homophobia, scapegoating, war and, in its most extreme form, genocide.[12]

Before the Great War, about 2 million Christian Armenians lived in the Mus-lim Ottoman Empire. By 1922, however, only about 400,000 remained. The others—some 1.6 million—were murdered because of their different religion and ethnicity in what historians today call the first genocide of the 20th century.

As a professor of social work committed, like Taft and Robinson, to gender, racial, economic, and social justice, Otto Rank was deeply troubled by human evil.

In the spring of 1938, as war clouds hung over Europe, Rank designed a new course for the Penn School. He intended to help his social work students under-stand the existential reasons for the coming war. Over a decade earlier, Hitler had already made crystal clear in *Mein Kampf* his intention to eradicate all the Jews of Europe.

Entitled *Symbols of Government*, Rank's course showcased the range of his intellectual interests. He required students to read Thurmon Arnold's recently published book of the same title, as well as two others from a list of thirty. On that list were works by some of the leading intellectuals of the day, includ-ing Mortimer Adler, Kenneth Burke, Stuart Chase, J.H. Denison (*Emotion as the Basis of Civilization*), Carl Jung (*Psychology and Religion*), Alfred Korzyb-ski, C.K. Ogden, Vilfredo Pareto, Talcott Parsons, William Sumner, Thorstein Veblen, and Alfred North Whitehead (Lieberman 1985:381).

Rank selected *Symbols of Government* as the main reading for his course because he was attracted to Thurmon Arnold's dry wit, and even tried, unsuc-cessfully, to get Arnold, then an assistant attorney general in the FDR adminis-tration, to guest lecture. "The penalty for retiring from the dance of life," quipped Arnold (1935) in *Symbols*, "is death" (244).

An iconoclast, Thurmon Arnold skewered the uniformity—the *likeness*—of the overly "rationalistic" jurisprudence of his time. Arnold saw too much like-ness in judicial theorizing during the early years of the New Deal, when the U.S. Supreme Court uniformly rejected FDR's boldest initiatives. In *Symbols*, Arnold termed this conformity a "shining but unfulfilled dream of a world governed by reason" (58).

In June 1937, dedicating a copy of Arnold's book to Jessie Taft, Rank wrote on the flyleaf: "No 'Symbols' and no 'Government' attached to this simple gift for your birthday." In the endpaper margins of her gift, Taft jotted: "The better therapy (Rank) you do—the less likeness you produce. <u>He</u> [i.e., the client] is the change."[13]

In this 1938 course, and other courses he taught at the Penn School, Rank crit-icized Freud's *Civilization and Its Discontents*, the first chapter of which had been published by Freud in a German journal called *Psychoanalytische Bewegung*, November-December 1929, and the rest in 1930.

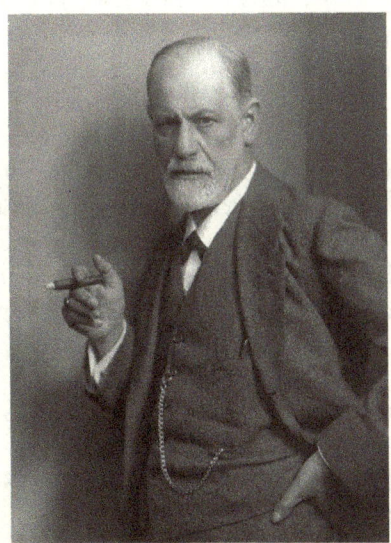

Figure 3.3 Sigmund Freud, c. 1921

Credit: Max Halberstadt, via Wikimedia Commons

Partly in response to *Civilization and Its Discontents*, but mainly to develop the creative will of his female social work students and their clients, Rank had written two books in German, one published in 1929 and the second in 1931, both of which would later form the body of *Will Therapy*, translated into English by Jessie Taft in 1936.

In *Will Therapy*, Rank offers an alternative to the death drive (*Todestrieb*)—which Freud had argued in *Civilization and Its Discontents* was a universal, innate biological drive to aggression, self-destruction, and war: in short, to committing human evil.

First formulated by Freud in 1920 in *Beyond the Pleasure Principle*, the *Todestrieb* was deployed by Freud as his explanation for war, masochism, and suicide. In *Civilization and Its Discontents*, Freud even went so far as to use the *Todestrieb* to explain "resistance" by patients to accepting his Oedipal interpretations (Green 2023)—a suicidal act in Freud's view.

The "negative therapeutic reaction"—a euphemism for patients not accepting the interpretations of their analysts—is due, at bottom, to the universal, demonic force of the *Todestrieb*, according to Freud.

Resisting interpretations offered by analysts, according to Freud, meant that "people don't *want* to get better" (Menand 2012:205; italics in the original). In contrast, Rank believed that people resisted analysts who wielded denigrating terms like *Todestrieb* or "innate death drive" as weapons against them. In other words, people *want* to get better, if only they're permitted to do so by their analyst.

"The idea of an unconscious demonic principle driving the psyche to distraction," insists literary critic Jacqueline Rose, justifying Freud's therapeutic pessimism, "could be said to sabotage once and for all the vision of man in control of his mind" (quoted in Sehgal 2023:18). As an "impossible profession," the psychoanalysis that Freud created at the turn of the 20th century had no theory of cure, other than providing transference interpretations of the Oedipal unconscious. Today, most psychoanalysts no longer accept the *Todestrieb*, even if a number of scholars in the humanities, like Rose, still do.

But not the slightest evidence exists for a biological "drive" inside human beings to commit evil. There is no *Todestrieb*, said Rank, only *Todesangst*—a word Rank coined in *Will Therapy* to counter Freud's promotion of the *Todestrieb* as the explanation for evil.

Todesangst was translated into English by Jessie Taft as "death fear," but the German word *Angst* suggests something much more profound, much darker, and more unsettling than merely "fear" of an object. The *Angst* attached to mortality connotes a deep dread of the void, the Nothingness of nonbeing, that Kierkegaard pointed to in *Fear and Trembling* and Heidegger in *Being and Time*.[14]

As Nancy Seif (1984) observes, Rank was "particularly distressed by what he saw as Freud's pedagogical, moral use of the Oedipus myth, whereby Freud taught his students and patients about the inescapable evil [i.e., death drive] within them" (374)—an evil drive called *Todestrieb* that could never be tamed by social work, counseling, therapy, or by any other means.

In *Art and Artist*, Rank (1932a) elaborates on his motives for writing *Psychology and the Soul*. Venturing far beyond art into the realms of politics and nationalism, Rank, in his typically interdisciplinary way, shows how the quest for immortality is a basic driving force in human history and serves as the origin of collective ideologies, such as the nation-state:

I made [in *Psychology and the Soul*] the first attempt to find, on social-psychological lines, a common spiritual root for the meaning and origin of collective ideologies. This root I conceived to be the belief in immortality, and this belief I regarded (if one can say so of any one belief) as *the* original ideology, out of which, as it became increasingly untenable, there arose various others, more securely anchored in reality, but always animated by the same immortalization tendency. In religion this is of course obvious, but in the social ideologies too, with their political form and their national content, the tendency towards a collective conception of immortality is easily recognizable. (xxvi; italics in the original)

In a footnote to this passage, Rank adds that he was not the first to see the connection between belief in immortality and the creation of the nation-state: "Burke, for instance, in his famous *Reflections on the Revolution in France*, conceives of the state as a concretized immortality. Fichte, too, emphasized the immortality of national ideologies in his [*Addresses to the German Nation*]" (ibid.).

If immortality is the ideological quest of the nation-state, then how does the nation-state promote evil?

4

Immortality

"By projecting our nemesis, death, upon another whom we can kill," explains E. James Lieberman in his introduction to *Psychology and the Soul*, "we symbolically annihilate death" (Rank 1930:xii).

The worst form of evil committed by the nation-state—murdering others—argues Rank, is grounded in our ideological need to believe in the immortality of the group to which we belong and with which we identify. "The psychological creed of mankind," insists Rank (1930) in *Psychology and the Soul*, "is immortality" (128).

Pursuing his life-long study of leadership, a project that began with *The Myth of the Birth of the Hero*, Rank (1932a) notes in *Art and Artist*: "Every group, however small or great, has, as such, an 'individual' impulse for eternalization, which manifests itself in the creation of and care for national, religious, and artistic heroes" (411).

Drawing on Rank's *Todesangst*, rather than Freud's *Todestrieb*, Ernest Becker (1975) maintains in *Escape from Evil* that, by projecting our terror of death onto "the other," we justify war and genocide to save *belief in our own group's immortality*—not because we have a biological drive to murder others or for economic exploitation as Marxists claim, although the accumulation of money is often a surrogate for achieving immortality.

"The individual gives himself to the group," argues Becker (1975), "because of *his desire* to share in its immortality; we must say, even, that he is willing to die in order *not* to die" (139; italics in the original).

Echoing Becker and similar arguments made by Chris Hedges (2002) in *War Is a Force That Gives Us Meaning*, political theorist Jean Bethke Elshtain (2015), author of *Women and War*, observes that, in wartime, "the 'I' passes into a 'we,' and human longings for community with others find a field for realization." She adds:

> Communal ecstasy explains a willingness to sacrifice and gives *dying for others a mystical quality*. . . . Nor are women exempt from the sacralizing of sacrifice. There are hundreds of hair-raising tales of bellicose mothers, wives and girl-friends writing to the combat soldier and requesting the death of the enemy as a tribute, or gift, to her. (n.p.; italics added)

Otto Rank and the Creation of Modern Psychotherapy. Robert Kramer, Oxford University Press.
© Robert Kramer (2025). DOI: 10.1093/9780197698303.003.0004

Dying in the name of the nation-state, maintains Elshtain, is a *mystical* act—an act, one might say, of "dying-centered" mysticism. Believers in the immortality of the nation-state are, indeed, mystics. "The mystic chords of memory," Abraham Lincoln famously said in his First Inaugural Address, harmonize the heroism and patriotic graves of Union soldiers.

"Since the main task of human life is to become heroic and transcend death," writes philosopher Sam Keen in his foreword to *The Denial of Death*, "every culture must provide its members with an intricate symbolic system that is covertly religious. This means that ideological conflicts between cultures are essentially battles between immortality projects, holy wars" (Becker 1973:xiii).

The tragedy is that human action would be impossible if we didn't deny our fundamental impotence and insignificance in the vast, unfathomable cosmos. We deny our Nothingness, according to Rank and Becker, through the creation of symbolic, imaginary constructs like the nation-state.

"The nation," points out Becker (1975), "offers immortality to all its members" (160), male or female, but it is mostly men who fight, kill, and die in war. Man's primordial fear of woman—of difference, of "the other"—and its perpetuation in sexism, racism, scapegoating, war, and genocide derive from Rank's *Todesangst* not from Freud's *Todestrieb*, concluded Becker.

If our vulnerability to the terror of death could be treated by society's leaders and educators with empathy rather than transmuted by the mystifications of politicians into worship of flags, military uniforms, and national anthems, then there's a sliver of hope that human beings might, someday, be able to overcome the most murderous forms of evil.

"If men kill out of animal fears, then conceivably fears can always be examined and calmed," proposes Becker (1975) in *Escape from Evil*, "but if men kill out of [the *Todestrieb*], then butchery is a fatality for all time. The writer Elie Wiesel, who survived a Nazi concentration camp, summed it all up in a wistful remark during a TV interview: 'Man is not human'" (169).

During the inhumanity shown in war, argue Rank and Becker, we kill those different from us because we have an unceasing, irrepressible urge to merge our lonely, separate selves into *a larger whole*—like a political ideology, a religion, or a nation-state—whose members we want to be as like us as possible. By doing so, we unconsciously transcend our innate fear of death and existential loneliness.

"[T]he problem of loneliness," writes Becker (1974), "is compounded by a paradox that results from what we must call *the basic ontological motives of the human condition*." He continues:

> These motives are the familiar ones of Agape vs. Eros, the strivings of man in two different directions. Otto Rank summed them up for psychology by designating them as the universal problem of *sameness* vs. *difference*. . . . Under the

impulsion of Agape, or sameness, man wants to merge with the larger human group, come under its sway entirely, be exactly like everyone else. The person feels lonely when he is different or apart, feels guilty for sticking out. We may remember that as children we often tried to infect others with our contagious disease because we could not stand the stigma of difference and separateness. Under the impulsion of Eros, or difference, on the other hand, the person wants to affirm his own uniqueness, his particular identity, his special talent. He wants to stick out of nature as much as possible, be as unlike others as he can. He then becomes lonely when he is merged in the group, feeling estranged from his own true self. This is the cause of the guilt that results from failing to develop oneself. Hence, the paradox which cannot be straightforwardly resolved. To fulfill the Agape motive plunges one into the loneliness of non-individuation. To fulfill the Eros motive plunges one into the loneliness of separation. . . . In sum, there can be no cure for a problem that goes this deep into the human condition. (quoted in Liechty 2005:232; italics in the original)

Today, as vulnerable, confused, and increasingly lonely human beings huddle together behind the fortresses of their nation-states, with their bristling displays of military might, the awesome power of the nation-state assuages our existential loneliness and allows us to feel more secure, under the illusion that we're protected from death by the symbols of the immortal hero systems and cultures that envelop us.

"Being aware of their mortality," explains political theorist Yael Tamir (2019) in *Why Nationalism*, "individuals would like to believe their deeds survive them—nationalism offers them an effective tool of transgenerational presence" (61). Quoting from Milan Kundera's *The Book of Laughter and Forgetting* and Anthony Smith's *National Identity*, Tamir continues:

"A man knows that he is mortal, but he takes it for granted that his nation possesses a kind of eternal life" [Kundera]. These words sum up the message communicated by nationalism: nations are here to stay; they can therefore transcend the momentary, shifting finite experience from the sphere of the mundane and the contingent to the eternal. This notion of continuity is of particular importance in a modern era, when identification with the nation is "the surest way to surmount the finality of death and ensure a measure of personal immortality" [Smith]. (63)

In *Psychology and the Soul* (1930) and *Art and Artist* (1932a), Rank asserts that in our never-ending quest for assurance of eternal survival, we create symbols of culture—like the nation-state—in order to sustain belief in our group's immortality.

"Driven by his fear of extinction," adds Rank (1941a) in *Beyond Psychology*, writing at a time when Hitler was promoting his theory of *Lebensraum*, the continual expansion of the amount of living space Germany claimed it needed to survive, "man precipitates war against his fellowmen with the admitted or tacit slogan of nationalism—the conception that only one people has the right and the room to survive" (262). "Fear of extinction" and *Lebensraum* are outcomes of *Todesangst*—not *Todestrieb*.

In constructing "hero mythologies"—each an imaginary narrative of leadership tailored for a specific nation—we create the symbols of our immortality, with which we can identify and achieve a heroic self-image for ourselves and the nation to which we belong.

By submitting to the charisma of an all-powerful national leader, who is virtually always male, we partake of the leader's self-declared greatness. What was the appeal for millions of ordinary Germans, Russians, and Chinese of larger-than-life leaders like Hitler, Stalin, and Mao? In *The Denial of Death*, Becker (1973) quotes Alan Harrington's explanation of the fatal attraction: "I am making a deeper impression on the cosmos because I know this famous person. When the ark sails I will be on it" (148).

"[M]an's innate and all-encompassing fear of death drives him to attempt to transcend death through culturally standardized hero systems and symbols," argues Becker (1975) in *Escape from Evil*. "In this book," he adds, "I attempt to show that man's natural and inevitable urge to deny mortality and achieve a heroic self-image are the root causes of human evil. This book also completes my confrontation of the work of Otto Rank and my attempt to transcribe its relevance for a general science of man" (xvii).

The central mission of mortals on the planet Earth, Becker (1973) writes in *The Denial of Death*, is the overcoming of death. At the turn of the 20th century, when Rank published *The Myth of the Birth of the Hero*—comparing the leadership narratives of such "immortal heroes" as Gilgamesh, Sargon, Oedipus, Romulus, Julius Caesar, Moses, and Jesus—William James was making the same point as Rank: "Mankind's common instinct for reality," proposed James in *The Varieties of Religious Experience*, "has always held the world to be essentially a theater for heroism" (quoted in Becker 1973:1).[1]

William James, Otto Rank, and Ernest Becker understood that mortals, throughout the ages, have always sought to deny death by means of "heroic" acts of one kind or another. We can "prove" our heroism, and deny death, by sacrificing our lives for *a larger whole*, symbolized by the group—whether it be a group-sponsored collective ideology such as communism, fascism, or American democracy, or the family, tribe, religion, or nation-state.

For example, Islamist suicide bombers—wouldn't it be more accurate to call them *homicide* bombers?—have shown that preserving their belief in group immortality is more important than preserving their lives. Some of these suicide bombers are female. This is what Rank meant by immortality being the creed of humanity, for women as well as for men. Whether or not this creed is true is irrelevant; it's a belief system or ideology deeply embedded in our psyches, often beginning in childhood, and very difficult to question without suffering painful consequences such as being shunned by, or excommunicated from, the group of true believers.

Usually acting in the name of some nationalist or religious cause, homicide bombers are not "cowards," as Western politicians always make a point of denigrating them, wanting us to feel morally superior. In their own minds, and the minds of those who celebrate their ultimate sacrifice, homicide bombers are the most glorious of "heroes," whose noble actions will land them a berth in Heaven next to God, just as their followers will be blessed—mystically!—with eternal life if they identify with their heroism.

The *denial of death,* explains Becker (1975) in *Escape from Evil,* is actually "an expression of *the will to live,* the burning desire of the creature to count, to make a difference on the planet because he has lived, has emerged on it, and has worked, suffered, and died" (3; italics added). In contradiction to Freud's *Todestrieb,* which argues for a universal biological drive to commit murder and suicide, homicide bombers have a will to live—forever. They seek immortality, not death.

Deep down, wonders Becker (1973) in *The Denial of Death,* don't even the ordinary masses of mediocre men—he doesn't mention women in this regard—also want to be recognized by society for their heroic deeds, even if it's just surviving every day and earning enough to feed their families, no matter how much they might disguise their heroic inclinations? Many poor single women with families would surely count themselves in this group.

"In the more passive masses of mediocre men," Becker writes, "it is disguised as they humbly and complainingly follow out the roles that society provides for their heroics and try to earn their promotions within the system: wearing the standard uniforms—but allowing themselves to stick out, but ever so little and so safely, with a little ribbon or a red boutonniere, but not with head and shoulders" (6).

"The goal of politics," according to Louis Menand (2021), citing Hannah Arendt, Machiavelli, and the ancient Greeks, "is glory (*kleos*). In the arena of life on this planet, the only things that become immortal are great deeds," says Menand. "They are ends in themselves" (112).

Human beings have an almost limitless craving for the perpetuation of their group, reaching toward the dream of immortality, an immortality provided most readily today by the seductive blandishments of religion and the nation-state. The basic motive of humanity, argue Otto Rank and Ernest Becker—against Freud—is *existential*, not *murderous*.

Today, the nation-state is a universal symbol of group immortality—a mystical, "dying-centered" ideology held by countless people around the world, male and female. Each of the 193 member-states of the United Nations promises permanent safety, meaning, dignity, and heroism for its citizens.

Apparent in every war fought since the 1648 Treaty of Westphalia, the nation-state's desire to achieve immortality has again erupted on the world stage, just as it did in the 1930s with Hitler's "Thousand Year" Reich.

Russia's 2022 attack on Ukraine represents Vladimir Putin's second salvo in an existential struggle with the West, the first being the annexation of Crimea in 2014. In a blistering speech justifying the latest Russian invasion, Putin announced to the world: "For our country, it is a matter of life and death, a matter of our historical future as a nation. . . . It is not only a very real threat to our interests but to the very existence of our state" (Fisher 2022).

No clearer statement of Rank's insight that the existential terror of death—not Freud's biologically-based death drive—underlies the state-sponsored bloodletting of war has ever been uttered by a nation-state's leader.

Since 2022, Putin has been fighting a *holy war* against the West, not merely a war to return Ukraine to what he insists, indignantly, is its Russian origins. This is the meaning of his oft-repeated claim that the death of the Soviet Union was the "greatest geopolitical catastrophe" of the 20th century.

The theory of "toxic leadership," a term coined by leadership scholar Jean Lipman-Blumen (2005), explains why Russians, men and women, young and old, follow murderous leaders like Putin:

> Our existential anxiety and hankering for a life of meaning render us supremely vulnerable to leaders who insist that they can make us safe, instill our lives with significance, and ensure our eternal life either physically here or in another world, or symbolically, in the memory of generations yet unborn. As their followers, we work endlessly on what Otto Rank called our "immortality projects." (3)

A messianic leader, Putin dreams of being the great Slavic hero who saves the God-fearing Russian people from impending death at the hands of the decadent West, a West dominated by ungodly LGBTQ+ advocates, a West that had better be ready to have its cities go up in the flames of nuclear war if it attempts to interfere in the cause of Russia's immortality project.

"I would now like to say something very important for those who may be tempted to interfere in these developments from the outside," Putin warned in a speech at the outset of his sacred war. "No matter who tries to stand in our way, or all the more so creates threats for our country and our people, they must know that Russia will respond immediately, and the consequences will be such as you have never seen in your entire history" (Fisher 2022).

Putin is saying that he's willing to fight to the last Russian for the sake of Russia's immortality, willing to sacrifice countless bodies of his own country's youth, on top of murdering hundreds of thousands of Ukrainian civilians, for his glorious dream of the undying Russian nation-state.

"And the more blood the better," observes philosopher Sam Keen (2006) in *The Future of Evil*, "because the larger the heap of bodies the greater the testimony to [his] willingness to make a heroic sacrifice for the right cause, the divine plan, the destiny toward which history is moving" (7).

This is no exaggeration. Recently, Putin ordered a new nationwide, "dying-centered" curriculum for primary schools. In *The Moscow Times*, Jade McGlynn (2023) writes: "Russian soldiers lay down their lives to safeguard the value of high-quality patriotic education, and yet the highest measure of that education's success lies in producing future soldiers who are willing to die for its defense. It is hard to escape the impression that the new curriculum is bringing up children for the purpose of death" (n.p.).

But before we congratulate ourselves for being so superior ethically to the murderous goons in the Kremlin, let's not forget that the democratically elected leaders of the United States, the United Kingdom, and the European Union, all (except Trump) avowed foes of Putin's war—which Yale's Timothy Snyder observes, rightly, amounts to genocide of the Ukrainian people—share the same "dying-centered" imaginary of nation-state immortality.

As philosopher A.C. Grayling (2000) argues, all nation-states "are artificial constructs, their boundaries drawn in the blood of past wars. . . . [The nation-state] is an evil with its roots in xenophobia and racism".

In 2022 the nation-states of the world spent over two trillion dollars on preparing for war, a 4% increase in real terms over 2021, according to the Stockholm International Peace Research Institute.[2]

"Each nation-state imagines itself to be unique," writes Michael Billig (2017), who coined the term "banal nationalism" to characterize the imaginary nature of national uniqueness. All nation-states claim to be exceptional, with the supremacy of American "exceptionalism" perhaps the most ballyhooed in the world. "And in imagining itself to be unique, the particular nation is just like all other nations, imagining themselves to be unique" (322).

But only individual human beings are unique, not the 193 nation-states, whose culturally different hero systems are identical in the sacred pursuit of their uniform ideology of undying nationalism above all else.

We have met the enemy, Pogo said, *and he is us.* According to Rank and Becker, every nation-state constructs the sacrosanct symbols of national culture—flags, emotionally-stirring national anthems, military heroes, Founding Fathers, and timeless marble monuments—to give its citizens the illusion that their lives have meaning, that something permanent will outlast the decay and disappearance of their bodies.

"Unfortunately, the love of 'us' has an ugly cousin, the fear and suspicion of 'them': a paranoid nationalism that works against tolerant values such as openness to unfamiliar people and new ideas," writes the *Economist* (2023) in a cover story entitled "How Paranoid Nationalism Corrupts" (7).

Nation-states are super-families with a myth of common ancestry, a myth associated with a specific piece of territory on a tiny fraction of the landmass of the planet Earth, which is itself but a speck of dust in the vast universe.

After NASA photographed the planet Earth (shown as the circled dot in Figure 4.1) from a satellite 6.4 billion kilometers away, astronomer

Figure 4.1 The planet Earth
Credit: NASA/JPL-Caltech

Carl Sagan observed: "Think of the rivers of blood spilled by all those generals and emperors so that in glory and triumph they could become the momentary masters of a fraction of a dot."[3]

Yael Tamir and other political theorists who justify the emotional comfort offered by the mystique and mysticism of nationalist ideology tend to equate the nation-state with the metaphor of "home." What could be more anxiety-relieving, more heart-warming, to forlorn, lonely human beings than "going home"?

According to Tamir (2019), the nation-state's "sense of connectedness turns a place into a home, and this homely feeling makes people care about the state and wish to participate in its making" (36).

A glance at NASA's photograph of Earth shows how devastating Carl Sagan's response to Tamir's arguments would be. We live, said Sagan, on a "pale blue dot, the only home we've ever known."

We are ephemeral gnats who wander on a tiny portion of a minuscule planet in a vast, unfathomable, frightening universe that cares nothing for human beings, who, within a flash, will vanish into the void from which they emerged.

What happens to forlorn, lonely human beings when the imaginary fortress of the nation-state cracks open, as it did when the 9/11 homicide bombers knocked down the World Trade Centers and blew gaping holes in the Pentagon—the two most visible symbols of America's dream of immortality: unlimited financial and military power?

As a public relations strategy to reduce the ensuing daily panic of *Todesangst*—9/11, 24/7—the U.S. government rushed to create the Department of "Homeland" Security, and instituted security theater at all airports. The war in Iraq, which killed hundreds of thousands, was launched by President George W. Bush as "a force that gives us meaning" (Hedges 2002), seducing us into feeling the security of being safe at home. The United States, he proclaimed, is willing to sacrifice its young soldiers, male and female, to fight a "global war on terror" overseas, while vigilantly protecting the "homeland" from being attacked.

But, even as the gigantic statue of Saddam collapsed, the terror of falling into the void of Nothingness continued to overwhelm Americans with existential dread—the terror of death—as it once again has during the recent years of worldwide plague, no respecter of imaginary national boundaries, just as the devastation of global climate change respects no national flags.

Yael Tamir is right, of course: the ideology of nationalism *does* provide a feeling of "homeland" security, of warmth, dignity, and safety, but existential terror rumbles, unspoken, under the fluttering of the flag of stars and stripes to which American children pledge allegiance each morning at school.

"This is the terror," said Becker (1973) in *The Denial of Death*, "to have emerged from nothing, to have a name, consciousness of self, deep inner feelings, an excruciating yearning for life and self-expression—and with all this yet to die" (87).

The denial of death is so strong that, although over seven million died from COVID-19, the world today remains in emotional lockdown. Grief, sadness, depression, and mourning are covered over, left unfelt, by news of increases in national GDP, booming stock markets, and developments in Artificial Intelligence.

We are born to die, Freud said in *Beyond the Pleasure Principle*. Yet the expression of our creativity, argues Ernest Becker, drawing on Rank's writings on art, love, and the creative will, can allow us to transcend death—through the construction of time-defying monuments of music, philosophy, architecture, poetry, literature, and art, whose symbols provide human meaning in a terrifying cosmos, helping us transcend death in a much healthier, more creative, way than projecting our terror onto "the other" and killing off those different from us.

Often criticized for his dark pessimism, Becker, in fact, found great hope and inspiration reading Rank's *Art and Artist* (1932a) on how our individual psyches can reconnect with the wonder and awe of the cosmos through the experience of art and love—no matter how terrifying it is to live for just a fraction of a moment on a "pale blue dot."[4]

"Having been under the sway of the more misanthropic insights of Marx and Freud," says Becker's biographer, Jack Martin (2014), "Rank's emphasis on the power of art and love to heal the brokenness of man and woman lifted Becker's sights to a higher place of cosmic creativity and joy. Infused with the exhilarating positive life force of Rank's creative will, Becker was now able to set alongside the terror of extinction an ode of joy, the kingdom of death in balance with the kingdom of life" (68).

Even as he lay dying from cancer in late 1972, Becker remained devoted to extending Rank's legacy for the human and social sciences.

"In death and in life," writes Martin, "Becker echoed Otto Rank's heartbreaking, beautiful plea to all humanity; the 'volitional affirmation of the obligatory.' Let us learn, at long last, to say Yes to the Must by willingly accepting the obligation of death as deeply and freely as we accept the gift of life" (111n).

In the face of the No of death, according to Rank, we must learn how to say Yes to life—deliberately, joyfully—letting go of all that blocks us from fully expressing the vital power of our creative will and our capacity for loving others, especially those different from us.

In the choice between Freud's *Todestrieb*—which offers no possibility to reduce evil in the world—and Rank's *Todesangst*, Becker pleaded with his readers to turn to Rank. Perhaps, he writes at the end of *Escape from Evil*, Rank's existential thought, "when it is finally assimilated in its tragic and true meanings ... will introduce just that minute measure of reason to balance destruction" (170).

The "home-like" appeal of the nation-state will not vanish any time soon. Forced into exile by the Nazis, and left homeless, the Jewish philosopher Jean Améry saw the grim paradox of human beings dying for the immortality of nation-states, oblivious to their geographical location's insignificant place in the cosmos: "One must have a home in order not to need it," said Amery ruefully (1999:46).

The nation-state, for good or evil, is here to stay, and many more will sacrifice their lives for its seductive, but illusory, dream of immortality. In Arthur Koestler's view, "man is less driven by adrenalin than he is drugged by symbols, by cultural belief systems, by abstractions like flags and anthems. 'Wars are fought for words ...'" (quoted in Becker 1975:134).

In addition to the war in Ukraine, over 100 other wars are being fought today, according to the Geneva Academy of International Humanitarian Law and Human Rights, and at least a dozen are genocidal.[5]

In late 2023, at the outbreak of the most recent life-and-death struggle between Israel and Hamas, a Palestinian poet and clinical psychologist declared: "We exist, and our existence presents an existential affront. As long as we exist, we challenge several falsehoods, not the least of which is that, for some, we never existed at all" (Alyan 2023).

Rooted in the terror of death—two different existences, fighting each other like scorpions in a bottle—this holy war has been going on for decades, with no end in sight, and with empathy for "the other" in short supply.

"The consequence is a psychological chasm so deep that Palestinians are invisible as individuals to Israeli Jews, and vice versa. There are exceptions, of course: Some Israelis and Palestinians have dedicated themselves to bridging that divide. But generally, the narratives of the two sides diverge, burying any perception of shared humanity" (Cohen 2023).

When seeking to be "the momentary masters of a fraction of a dot," political leaders of all stripes and religions are toxic, promoting a "dying-centered" mysticism that seduces people into believing in the immortality of the nation-state. "Who has the power to mystify, how did he get it, and how does he keep it?," asks Ernest Becker in *Escape from Evil* (1975:49), referring to the three most horrific genocidal leaders of the 20th century—Stalin, Hitler, and Mao.

Influenced by the thought of Rank and Becker, Jean Lipman-Blumen (2007) alerts us to toxic leaders "who manipulate their followers' ordinary human needs and exploit their existential circumstances. They do this by creating illusions designed to allay the fears and address the human conditions to which we are all heir" (3), most acutely the terror of death.

We must find the courage to question and challenge these "political plague-mongers," urges Becker (1975), who spent his entire life trying to decipher "*exactly what cripples the autonomy of the individual*" (126; italics in the original) in confronting evil leaders.

In *Will Therapy*, Rank (1936a), who understood the consequences of toxic leadership, makes clear that it is *Lebensangst* and *Todesangst*—life fear and death fear—that cripples the autonomy of individuals, making them susceptible to the extravagant promises of charismatic political leaders offering the illusion of national immortality.

For Rank, the only way of *not* falling under the spell cast by toxic leaders is by promoting the capacity of individuals for self-leadership—the autonomy, strength, courage, and self-empowerment that comes with release of the creative will—especially for "powerless" women who have been oppressed for millenia by the toxic leadership of "all-powerful" men (Lipman-Blumen 2006).

On a collective level, Ukrainians, in the simplest sense, are declaring their right to exist and be different from Russians, just as Palestinians are declaring their right to exist and be different from Israelis. But what, exactly, is the *existential* meaning of difference?

5

Difference versus likeness

In 1996, I entitled my collection of Rank's American lectures *A Psychology of Difference*, a title I drew from a striking passage in *Beyond Psychology*, written by Rank in the late 1930s:

> That Freud's psychology, being an interpretation rather than an explanation of human nature, was not valid for all races, Jung pointed out; that it did not apply to different social environments, Adler emphasized; but that it did not even permit individuals of the same race and social background to deviate from the accepted type led me *beyond these differences in psychologies to a psychology of difference*. (Rank 1941a:29; italics in the original)

Rank often made a point of comparing his "psychology of difference" with Freud's "psychology of likeness." *Difference* versus *likeness* constitutes the basic paradox of being human, said Rank, a tension that must be lived with permanently, and can never be resolved once and for all.

In *Beyond Psychology*, Rank (1941a) argued that "it is not merely [a] question of seeing the two sides or accepting them intellectually which seems to be so difficult, but an experiencing of them in *actual living*" (22; italics added). Creativity, according to Rank, emerges when we are able to balance difference and likeness.

Freud (1937) always insisted that the difference between male and female was "biological bedrock." Although not disputing the force of biology or the sex difference, Rank peered *below* biological bedrock to confront the ontological, or better the pre-ontological, mystery of Being itself: that is, the awesome difference—the ineffable difference—between nonexistence and existence.

"The mere fact of difference," said Rank (1936a) in *Will Therapy*, "in other words, the existence of our own will as opposite, unlike, is the basis for the condemnation which manifests itself as inferiority or guilt-feeling" (79). To fully experience difference at its deepest level, observed Rank, is to feel the anguish, suffering, and guilt of existential loneliness, which only the mutuality of an authentic relationship can relieve, even if only temporarily.

Rank never minimized the enormous significance of the anatomical difference between the sexes. This difference, however, is the second most important difference the child confronts.

Otto Rank and the Creation of Modern Psychotherapy. Robert Kramer, Oxford University Press.
© Robert Kramer (2025). DOI: 10.1093/9780197698303.003.0005

"First, comes the perception of difference from others as a consequence of becoming conscious of self . . . then interpretation of this difference as inferiority . . . finally association of this psychological conflict with the biological sexual problem, the difference of the sexes" (78).

The difference between nonexistence and existence precedes and colors all other difference—whether it be the difference of gender, age, ethnicity, class, sexual orientation, religion, race, or nationality. Existence comes first.

"Human beings share a species membership; in that sense, we are all alike," writes Louis Menand (2021) in his history of art and thought during the Cold War. "But a condition of membership in our species is that each human being is different from every other human being who has ever lived" (112).

Everyone's life is different. "The only certainty we have," Nobel laureate Sir John Eccles (1992) affirms, "is that we exist as unique self-conscious beings, each unique, never-to-be-repeated" (163). No person is the same as anyone else. There is only difference.

This conclusion, however, Freud was never willing to accept. He always insisted that *all human beings are alike*—reducible to their most basic sexual and destructive desires, which, he claimed, were universal, as was the Oedipus complex.[1]

Because of Freud's claims about the universality of his theories, psychoanalysis could only ever be "a psychology of likeness," said Rank, never a "psychology of difference." Yes, we're all alike, Rank countered Freud, but only because we're all different. Accepting difference, our own and that of others, is the most difficult challenge any human being can face, according to Rank.

"Will people ever learn," asked Rank (1941a) poignantly in *Beyond Psychology*, written as Hitler was on the verge of murdering the Jews of Europe, including four of Freud's sisters, "that there is no other equality possible than the equal right of every individual to become and to be himself, which actually means to accept his own difference and have it accepted by others?" (267).

Today, the field of psychoanalysis is seeing a renewed appeal for a psychology of difference. A critique of Freud's psychology of likeness has gained traction among Black analysts and other minorities. Let me offer a few examples. About a decade ago, in a video posted on the *Psychoanalytic Electronic Publishing* (PEP) website, Black analysts bitterly lamented their struggles in getting White analysts who had trained and still supervise them to recognize their difference.

Here are some quotes from the PEP video, which was posted on the website in 2014 and quickly became its most downloaded item:

KIRKLAND VAUGHANS: "I had an analyst who was exceptionally bright, exceptionally on. But when it came to the issue of race, he was thoroughly blocked.

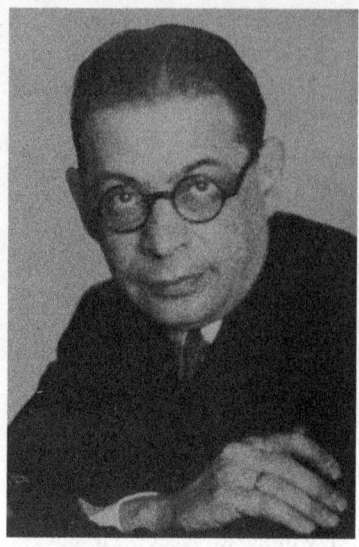

Figure 5.1 Otto Rank, c. 1930
Credit: Ruhama Veltfort for the Estate of Otto Rank

He said to me in his career, he had treated one Negro. That was his word—one Negro, [at] which I smiled. He told me, he said, 'the treatment didn't go well, because all the guy wanted to do was talk about race. I couldn't get him off race, OK?' I smiled again."

KATHLEEN WHITE: "One of my teachers was one of those old White guys who could not hear the word 'race.' He used his cane and beat the table."

ANNIE LEE JONES: "There has been near violent reactions to the things I say about the way racism, culture, and economic inequality affects my life and my work with patients. I presented in London at the Freud Museum, and I talked about race. One psychiatrist grabbed me by my arm and wouldn't let me go up the steps."

CLEONIE JAMES: "People sometimes say to me, 'No, but I don't think of you as Black. You're Cleonie.' What, then, do you think? And why is it necessary for you not to see my 'difference'? I was born in Jamaica, West Indies. I began to think about the way theories are written. Freudian theory, it's all about the internal world. And it's a structural theory, and everybody's the same. And so culture, and race, and class, and difference have no place in our thinking about personality, about development, about modes of attachment, about identity."

CHERYL THOMPSON: "I think psychoanalysis struggles from many misperceptions, one of which is the fantasy that people are all the same."[2]

In a talk delivered in 2021 at Berlin's International Psychoanalytic University, a Canadian analyst observed that the "systemic racism" of European psychoanalysts was "written into the heart of psychoanalysis, which was an inherently racist and colonial viewpoint that contrasted the superior rational and white European mind with the savage and primitive non-white other" (Frie 2021).

Unlike Freud, Rank (1941a) did not accept the inferiority of "primitive" cultures: "In order to appreciate primitive tradition as a different and not inferior order of culture," he wrote in *Beyond Psychology*, "we have to take into account the dualistic tendencies simultaneously striving towards permanency and change, in psychological terms, towards likeness and difference, respectively" (87).

"Likeness" still reigns in much of psychoanalysis. Beverly Stoute, a Black psychiatrist and psychoanalyst in Atlanta, Georgia, estimates that, out of a total of 3,000 psychoanalysts in the United States, only about 40 to 50 are Black (Bernstein 2023).

As an embodiment of "difference," a psychoanalyst named Carter J. Carter, who identifies himself as "part Afghan, among many other parts—WASP parts, Jewish parts, Portuguese parts, American parts," charged in a newsletter published in 2023 by the American Psychological Association that the problem of likeness remains intractable, with minimal progress being made on accepting difference due to "the Whiteness of professional psychoanalysis." Because of "systemic racism," his fellow psychoanalysts cannot see that the whole of his humanity infuses each of his parts, and, therefore, Carter's parts, because they are not being respected unconditionally, do not feel whole. As Carter (2023) writes:

> If psychoanalysis cannot fully countenance its own investment in Whiteness, it will die. Its most luminous insights are those that shed light on dynamics of abuse, hatred, shame, and persecution. These insights are most relevant to those of us with considerable personal experience with such things—people of color, queer people, poor people, disabled people, people at all kinds of margins and those who come near the margins to love us. The Whiteness of professional psychoanalysis is absolutely noxious to us. We might be the new life blood of this field, if Whiteness does not insist on segregating us out of the profession by being unsurvivably hostile to us. (n.p.)

Echoing Carter's critique, and that of the Black analysts quoted earlier, Orna Guralnik (2023), who teaches in New York University's postdoctoral program on psychoanalysis, said recently: "Coming to see the working of implicit biases on us, grasping that our views are contingent on, let's say, our gender, class background or skin color, is a humbling lesson. It pushes us beyond assuming sameness."

Because of the complaints in the PEP video by Black analysts, the American Psychoanalytic Association chartered a high-profile commission in 2020 to investigate systemic racism within its analytic training institutes. This commission produced a scathing report in 2023, concluding that:

> Systemic and structural racism is ubiquitous within psychoanalysis. Racism appears within psychoanalytic institutions including leadership, administration, and faculty, and throughout training. Racism is embedded in teaching, curricula, and supervisory and candidate experiences. Its psychosocial existence is so entrenched and seamless in its representation that it is often only in the presence of a minoritized people or Black, Indigenous, and People of Color (BIPOC) that racism is revealed, often within an enactment.
>
> Simultaneously the poor representation or absence of minoritized people at the institutional and national organizational leadership level is a stark demonstration of the effects of systemic and structural racism. While many more white candidates and faculty are becoming aware of and speaking to these systemic and structural problems, there continues to be an active preservation of the racist status quo. (American Psychoanalytic Association 2023: 44)

This conclusion, however, has been contested by many White training and supervising analysts, who continue to deny that systemic racism is embedded in the leadership and training institutes of psychoanalysis. "At every step," writes J. Oliver Conroy (2023) in the *Guardian* about another recent brouhaha in the Freudian house, "psychoanalysis seems to have failed its practitioners. The two main camps accuse each other of bigotry, stifling free expression, condoning violence and betraying the creeds of their profession." This story has been repeated many times throughout the history of psychoanalysis from its very beginnings.

In May 2023, Harriet Wolfe, President of the International Psychoanalytical Association (IPA), wrote to her 12,000 members about the IPA's continuing difficulties in tolerating difference:

> Given recent expressions of dismay in each of the IPA Regions, we will be thinking about these questions: Why do we sometimes behave as if one or another level of our psychoanalytic organizations is the enemy rather than our potential psychoanalytic ally? What can the IPA contribute to tolerance of difference, to healing and reconciliation? (Wolfe 2023).

There are no statistics available from the IPA on the number of its members who are Black, indigenous, people of color, or minority. However many such members there might be, almost certainly they have felt problems like those reported by Black analysts in the United States who continue to struggle to have their difference seen by White colleagues at training institutes.

In his writings on *The Double*, which first appeared in 1914, Otto Rank emphasized the ways in which each individual, although unique, can create a different identity—many identities—all at the same time. This is how he conceptualized and taught his psychology of difference at the University of Pennsylvania School of Social Work—anticipating what today is called intersectional identities (Yamada et al. 2015).

The double, or *Doppelgänger*, carried a host of meanings for Rank, all of which were existential. The double means multiple, simultaneously created, identities; the "I's" conflicted relationship to its own self and that of others; the immortal soul; a protective or pursuing spirit; the shadow; split-off parts of the self; the narcissistic self; an alter-ego.

The double is an essential trope not only in art, photography, and movies but also in fiction, representing a fundamental dualism in every human being's psyche—likeness versus difference—as well as division and fragmentation of the self into many identities.[3]

Rank revisited his 1914 thesis in *The Double* often, the last time in an essay entitled "The Double as Immortal Self," published as a chapter in *Beyond Psychology* (1941a). According to Harry Tucker (1971), who translated a 1925 edition of Rank's work, "the double points up... 'man's eternal conflict with himself and others, the struggle between his need for likeness and his desire for difference'. . . . a conflict which leads to the creation of a spiritual double in favor of self-perpetuation and in abnegation of the physical double which signifies mortality" (xvi).

About a decade before Rank published his work on the double, the Harlem Renaissance began with W.E.B. Du Bois's writings on Black "double consciousness," an idea that Du Bois first formulated in *The Souls of Black Folk*. "One ever feels his two-ness," wrote Du Bois (1903a), "an American, and a Negro; two souls, two thoughts, two unreconciled strivings; two warring ideals in one dark body, whose dogged strength alone keeps it from being torn asunder" (11).

Double consciousness strongly attracted Rank, whose favorite book was Mark Twain's *Huckleberry Finn*, a gift from Jessie Taft. Delighted that Samuel Langhorne Clemens had chosen the pen name "Twain," an archaic word for "the two"—the double—Rank frequently signed his letters to Taft as "Huck," whom he considered his roguish alter-ego.

When Huck Finn and Tom Sawyer debated how to free "Nigger Jim," the runaway slave, Huck improvised, wanting simply to cut Jim loose and set him free, while Tom had a highly intellectualized strategy that, according to Rank, did not take into account Jim's feelings of humiliation and will to be freed immediately. "Both Hucks," writes E. James Lieberman (1985), pointing to Rank's spontaneity as a therapist, "would improvise in order to free an enslaved soul. In doing so, each used his art and will to change some hallowed man-made laws of human nature" (412).

Although there's no evidence that Rank read Du Bois's *The Souls of Black Folk*, or that Du Bois read Rank's *The Double*, the two writers would most likely have found each other's way of thinking congenial. Like Rank, Du Bois maintained that the tension between likeness and difference must be held in balance, never resolved straightforwardly, in order for Black writers and artists to allow their creative wills—their "dogged strength"—to emerge and be exercised to the fullest.

Among the novels which *The Souls of Black Folk* inspired, Henry Louis Gates Jr. (1989) names James Weldon Johnson's *The Autobiography of an Ex-Colored Man* (1912), Zora Neale Hurston's *Their Eyes Were Watching God* (1937), Richard Wright's *Black Boy* (1945), and Ralph Ellison's *Invisible Man* (1952).[4]

In *Sex and Race in the Black Atlantic: Mulatto Devils and Multiracial Messiahs*, Daniel McNeil (2010) interprets the writings of W.E.B. Du Bois and Frantz Fanon, who created anti-colonial existential psychiatry, through the lens of Rank's ideas in *The Double* (21–34). Forced to become double by the racist gaze, the black subject splits into a private self and a public self.

In the mid-1930s, Anaïs Nin (1967) took Rank dancing in Harlem, where, as she records in her diary, they witnessed "[h]alf white people, half black, beautiful women, well-dressed men, and jazz" (32). She adds: "Rank could not forget Harlem. He was eager to return to it. He could hardly wait to come to the end of his hard day's work. He said: 'I am tempted to prescribe it to my patients. Go to Harlem!'" (6).

As Badia Sahar Ahad (2010) observes in *Freud Upside Down: African-American Literature and Psychoanalytic Culture*:

> Though Rank never mentions the black subject in his own work, his response to the Harlem scene intimates that, like Nin, he believed that 'negroes are natural and possess the secret of joy. That is why they can endure the suffering inflicted upon them. The world maltreats them but among themselves they are deeply alive, physically and emotionally.' . . . Though Rank was apparently oblivious to the Harlem scene in the 1920s and 1930s, he appealed to a number of [Harlem] Renaissance artists in the 1920s and 1930s because he theorized that artists were able to find relief from [fear of death, *Todesangst*] by immortalizing themselves in the creation of their works. (39)

Rank's *The Trauma of Birth* and writings on art were read and discussed in Harlem during the 1920s and 1930s in the racially and sexually mixed circles around Carl Van Vechten, literary executor of Gertrude Stein. "Rank's theories were of particular interest to the New York artistic community," according to Ahad, "precisely because he thought the artistic mind mastered anxiety by inserting the self into a creative product that would long outlive the subject" (46).

When he wrote *The Trauma of Birth*, notes Rank (1936b) in *Truth and Reality*, he had referred to "the creation of the individual himself, not merely physically, but also [spiritually] in the sense of the 'rebirth experience,' which I understood psychologically as the actual creative act of the human being" (5). A creature made of matter, born out of a mother's womb, "the human being," continues Rank, "moves from creature to creator, in the ideal case, creator of himself, his own personality" (ibid.).

Among the Black writers most strongly attracted to Rank's ideas on self-creation was Nella Larsen, author in 1928 of *Quicksand*. A major figure in the Harlem Renaissance, Larsen is today considered to be an outstanding exemplar of American modernism.

The protagonist of *Quicksand* is Helga Crane, a bi-racial woman. "She was different," writes Larsen (1928). "She felt it. It wasn't merely a matter of color. It was something broader, deeper, that made folks kin. And now she was free" (353). Interpreting *Quicksand*, Ahad (2010) observes:

> Helga Crane follows, in a rather paradigmatic fashion, the various processes that Rank theorizes the subject undergoes in order to relieve himself or herself from the anxiety of birth, specifically "symbolic adaptation," "religious sublimation," "artistic idealization," "sexual gratification," and "neurotic reproduction." (40–41)
>
> . . . Perhaps Larsen found Rank's call for the subject to simply learn to exist with ambivalence both an affirmation and a model for the expression of her unique racial composition and her then-progressive notions of a woman's role. In many respects, Rank's model successfully captured the psychic split that Larsen articulated through Helga's struggle to locate a distinct subjectivity against racial and gendered limitations. (59)

Nella Larsen wanted to portray women as subjects in their own right—*absolutely different*—not merely as sexual appendages to men, Black, White, or any mixture thereof. She found in Rank that at least one psychoanalyst was insisting that women had powerful wills of their own, a radical idea that Freud had dismissed as "penis envy."

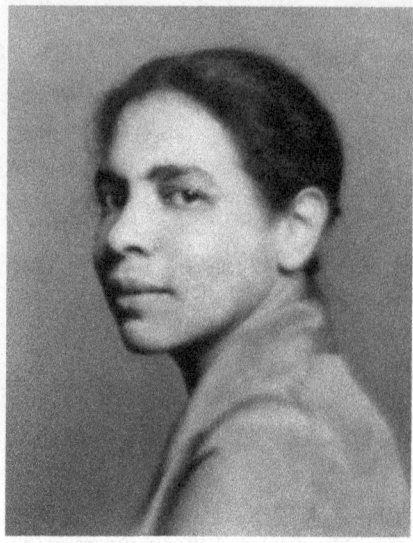

Figure 5.2 Nella Larsen, 37, in 1928
Credit: James Allen, via Wikimedia Commons

How much do we know about the "real" Nella Larsen? Very little. In an early biography, *Nella Larsen, Novelist of the Harlem Renaissance: A Woman's Life Unveiled*, Thadious Davis (1994) concludes that "not all of the pressing questions about the 'real Nella Larsen'... can be answered definitively because Nella Larsen was not only an invented name, a public and private pseudonym, but also a self-created persona" (xix).

In a more recent biography, based on a study of all extant documents, George Hutchinson (2006) writes that, "like her most important fictional characters, she nearly always inhabited the space between black and white, by necessity and by choice. ... That space, her fiction itself testifies, is hidden" (9). In Rank's terms, Larsen's liminal space—her "betweenness"—represents the struggle between her need for likeness and her desire for difference, a tension that is unresolvable but could be addressed creatively.

According to Rank, artists are self-appointed. By creating multiple representations of her own identity, Larsen corresponds almost exactly to Rank's artist in *Art and Art*: "The creative artistic personality is thus the first work of the artist," Rank (1932a) argues in *Art and Artist*, "and remains fundamentally his chief work" (28).

Rank defines the process of creativity as a form of separation or unlearning—a "liberation of creative force from the chains of old ideologies" (429). Creating one's life as an artwork is a lifelong process. By the late-1920s, long before the writings of Melanie Klein, Donald W. Fairbairn or Donald Winnicott, Rank had already invented psychoanalytic object relations theory and therapy (Rudnytsky 1991).

Unlearning necessarily involves separating from one's *own* self-concepts, as they have been culturally conditioned to conform to familial, group, religious, occupational, organizational, or national allegiances (Kramer 2012).

In *Art and Artist*, Rank (1932a) asserts that unlearning one's own self-concepts is "a separation which is so hard, not only because it involves persons and ideas that one reveres, but because the victory is always, at bottom and in some form, won over a part of one's own ego" (375).

A continual capacity to separate from "mental objects" or "mindsets"—the internalized restrictions or narratives of parents, teachers, religious authorities, political leaders, social conformity, and received wisdom—is the *sine qua non* for life-long creativity, said Rank.

Like other Harlem Renaissance writers of the 1920s and 1930s, Nella Larsen found Rank's ideas helped inspire her to be reborn as the artistic creator of her own life, a self-leader, in the face of the intense racial discrimination and oppression that she, and all other Blacks, then faced in America. "But even with Rank's neat paradigm, Larsen could not reconcile the predicament of her interracial female subject" (Ahad 2010: 59).

Larsen's attraction to Rank's thought in the late 1920s contrasts with Black analysts's current strong dissatisfaction with the psychology of likeness promoted for decades by psychoanalysis—a dissatisfaction that has a surprising patrimony.

Although not widely known, Freud had a habit of calling his patients "negroes," a reflection of his disdain for patients and for the practice of psychotherapy in general. "This strange appellation," which Freud began to use in the early years of his practice, when his consultation hour started at noon, "came from a cartoon in the *Fliegende Blätter* depicting a yawning lion muttering 'Twelve o'clock and no negro'" (Jones 1953:151).

As late as 1924, according to Ernest Jones, Freud was still using the appellation "negro" for American patients (ibid.). In *Beyond Psychology*, Rank (1941a) criticizes Freud for likening psychoanalytic treatment, which Freud considered an impossible profession, to "the white-washing of a negro" (272) – i.e., nothing would change as a result of treatment.

To Rank, Freud wrote in 1924 while Rank was on his first lecture tour in America: "It often seemed to me that analysis suits Americans like a white shirt suits a raven" (Lieberman & Kramer 2012:202). Freud closed his letter to Rank: "Give my greetings to all the squirrels"—his former American patients, "negroes" all—"and feed them for me with nuts for the monkeys. The only zoo worth visiting is in the Bronx" (ibid.).

Freud compared psychoanalytic treatment with the "white-washing of a negro" more than once: for example, in *Studies on Hysteria* (1895) and in correspondence with Karl Abraham. "The expression," writes historian of psychoanalysis Ernst Falzeder (1998), "was omitted in the *Standard Edition*, and in the English edition of the Freud/Abraham correspondence was euphemistically translated as 'cleaning up neurotics'" (136).

Reflecting the Central European prejudices of his age, Freud did nothing to question or combat racism, and never had a Black patient, although he was a staunch opponent of anti-Semitism. "[P]sychoanalysis offers no clear and immediate path to greater freedom and justice," according to Black literary scholar Claudia Tate (1996), compared to "demonstrations, sit-ins, and legal battles" (53)—the lifeblood of political activists and social workers who spend their lives promoting racial, economic, gender, and social justice.

"I have made it a point not to teach about Freud because of his toxic assessment of women," writes Sandra Crewe, Dean of the Howard University School of Social Work, which pioneered in teaching sociocultural competence decades before other schools did. "[Rank's] work is one that I would use because it presents a view compatible with our Black perspective at Howard.... Rank's self-leadership is inextricably linked to black liberation" (personal communication).

Sandra Crewe is following in the footsteps of W.E.B. Du Bois (1903b), who advocated for Black leadership by "The Talented Tenth," and Inabel Burns Lindsay, the founding dean of the Howard University School of Social Work, who "displayed tenacity and provided the leadership needed to build the institution during a time of blatant racial and gender oppression" (Crewe et al. 2008:375).

Sadly, an argument can be made that Freud's unsavory attitude toward "negroes" was passed on, consciously or unconsciously, to White analysts trained at psychoanalytic institutes during the 20th century. Moreover, analytic institutes in the United States and Europe continue to cater almost exclusively to Whites, "thereby condoning a social system that privileges the wealthy and the middle class" (Safran & Kriss 2014:47).

While considerable progress is clearly being made, psychoanalysts around the world, principally because many cling to a psychology of likeness, still lag behind social workers who long ago adopted a psychology of difference, even if they do not know its origins in the teachings of Rank, Taft, and Robinson at the University of Pennsylvania School of Social Work almost a century ago.

In a 2023 webinar talk at the International Psychoanalytical Association entitled "Racism: The Elephant in the Consulting Room," a Peruvian psychoanalyst laments: "We were often reluctant to see racism as a fundamental characteristic of our intimate exchanges, so we could not admit its pregnancy in transference and countertransference. We can't continue working in such huge denial" (Bruce 2023).

And there was yet another "elephant in the consulting room" hiding in plain sight for decades. Just like the existence of systemic racism in institutional psychoanalysis, Freud "could not admit its pregnancy in transference and countertransference."

Sundering the relationship between Freud and Rank, this "huge denial" was about the meaning of "pregnancy" and "transference"—and, relatedly, about Freud's refusal to see the powerful will of mothers.

6
"David and Goliath"

Modern psychotherapy was born of Otto Rank's struggle with Sigmund Freud a century ago over a question that no one would even consider arguable today: *Who is more powerful in our earliest mental life, mother or father?*

At first half-receptive, Freud came vehemently to oppose Rank's arguments in *The Trauma of Birth* (1924) that the child's relationship to its mother takes precedence, insisting, instead, that the father's role was the primary one.

Rank fought a gigantic battle with Freud over this question for two years. The consequences of this conflict for the future of psychoanalytic theory and practice would prove to be momentous.

Before the battle was joined, however, Freud and Rank had co-led the psychoanalytic movement for almost 20 years from Freud's smoke-filled study at *Berggasse 19*, watching it grow into an intellectual, social, and cultural force throughout much of the world.

Virtually an adopted son, Rank dined with Freud and his family each Wednesday, before meetings of the Vienna Psychoanalytic Society, over which he often presided in Freud's frequent absences. Closer emotionally to Freud than any of

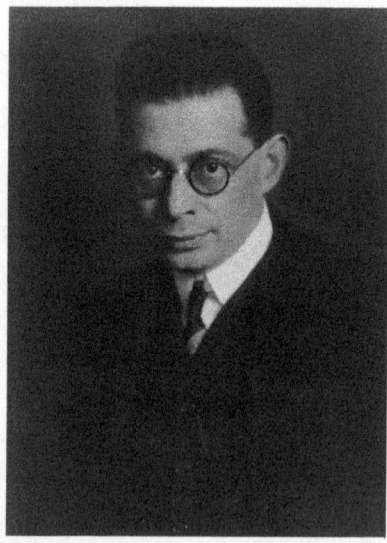

Figure 6.1 Otto Rank, in the early 1920s

Credit: Ruhama Veltfort for the Estate of Otto Rank

Otto Rank and the Creation of Modern Psychotherapy. Robert Kramer, Oxford University Press.
© Robert Kramer (2025). DOI: 10.1093/9780197698303.003.0006

the other Viennese analysts, Rank (1907) published the first book in psycho-analysis not written by Freud, *The Artist*, which used the word "artist" in as comprehensive a sense as Freud had used the word "*sexuality*."

"[H]is independence of me is greater than it appears," Freud told Jung in 1907; "very young, he has a good head and is thoroughly honest and open" (quoted in Lieberman 1985:98).

In 1909, Rank, at age 25, published *The Myth of the Birth of the Hero*, his cross-cultural study of leadership narratives over the ages, gifting a copy to Freud with the inscription: "Dedicated to the father of this book in thanks from—the mother."[1]

Immersed in the richness of the arts and humanities, Rank had little expe-rience with patients before the Great War, during which he served as an army news editor in Krakow, Poland, and where he met his future wife, Tola.

Freud always marveled at Rank's analytical skills and encouraged him, early on, to become the first lay (nonmedical) analyst. At 26, Rank (1910) published "A Dream That Interprets Itself," an interpretation so penetrating that Freud could not praise it too highly.

"Perhaps the best example of the interpretation of a dream," rejoiced Freud (1916–1917) in his *Introductory Lectures*, "is the one reported by Otto Rank con-sisting of two interrelated dreams dreamt by a young girl, which occupy about two pages of print: but their analysis extends to seventy-six pages. So I should need something like a whole term to conduct you through [it]" (185).

For every edition of *The Interpretation of Dreams* since 1911, Rank had helped Freud revise, word by word, each line of his masterpiece of self-analysis. "I am of intention," Freud confided to Ernest Jones in 1911, "to make him a partner in the coming edition of the *Traumdeutung*" (Paskauskas 1993:92).

Other than Freud, no one had plumbed the hidden levels of meaning in Freud's dreams more deeply than "little Rank" (150), who knew passages from the *Dreambook* virtually by heart.

In 1912, Rank published *The Incest Theme in Literature and Legend: Funda-mentals of a Psychology of Literary Creation*, a masterful 685-page study of the incest theme as it appeared throughout world literature, Western and Eastern.

Freud was so impressed by Rank's erudition that he invited his protégé to contribute two essays, on poetry and myth, in 1914 to *The Interpretation of Dreams*; thereafter, Rank's name would appear under Freud's on the title page of the foundational text of psychoanalysis for the next fifteen years.

In 1914, Rank also published *The Double*, which he regularly updated. Over a century later, Rank's work (only the 1925 edition has been translated into English) is his most cited book in literary and cultural studies.

"He is doing all the work," Freud reported to Ernest Jones in 1919, "perform-ing the possible and impossible alike, I dare say, you know him for what he is, the truest, most reliable, most charming of helpers, the column, which is bearing the edifice" (Paskauskas 1993:353).

In 1924, Fritz Wittels, an early acolyte, published the first biography of Freud, identifying Rank as Freud's closest associate, his right-hand man. "Freud's Eckermann," wrote Wittels (1924), referring to Goethe's colleague, "has had quite exceptional opportunities for conversations with Freud." Wittels hoped that Rank was keeping "careful notes" of his talks with the master (133).

By 1924, at only 39, Rank had become virtually indispensable to Freud, then approaching 70. Even before being diagnosed in 1923 with oral cancer Freud had already officially designated Rank as "my heir" (Lieberman & Kramer 2012:225).

Occupying a host of leadership positions, Rank was vice president of the Vienna Psychoanalytic Society; the most prolific author in psychoanalysis after Freud; managing director of Freud's publishing house, the *Verlag*; and editor of the two major psychoanalytic journals, *Imago* and *Zeitschrift*. Along with Freud, he was the gatekeeper for new ideas in psychoanalysis.

Everyone in the small psychoanalytic world knew that Rank was Freud's most trusted colleague, his designated "heir," a powerful leader in his own right. In 1924 there were 263 members of the International Psychoanalytical Association (Lieberman 1985:227), with Rank occupying the No. 2 position in the organizational hierarchy.

How Rank managed all his leadership responsibilities, in addition to being a practicing psychoanalyst, husband, and father, is attributable to his boundless emotional energy, intellect, and, above all, to his creative will.

After Freud, Rank was the most influential member of the Secret Committee—the Politburo of six men formed around Freud after the defection of Jung to serve as the final arbiter of psychoanalytic theory and practice. None of the other analysts in the world knew of the existence of this political body, which was not revealed until decades later by Hanns Sachs (1944).

In the only photo of the Secret Committee ever taken, Rank is seen with his right arm draped casually over the throne-like chair of Freud. "I was in the deepest of all," Rank told Jessie Taft (1958:xvi). Examining the photo closely, one notices that only Freud and Rank are looking in the same direction. "The future [leader] of the psycho-analytical movement might come out of this small but select circle of men," said Freud (Jones 1955:154).

After many defections from psychoanalysis, including those of Adler and Jung, the British sexologist Havelock Ellis (1923) acclaimed Rank as "perhaps the most brilliant and clairvoyant of the young investigators who still stand by the master's side" (102). By 1924, Rank had become "the one-man training institute of Vienna," recalls psychoanalyst Franz Alexander (Lieberman 1979:13). Hanns Sachs (1944) dubbed him, simply, "Lord Everything Else" (60).

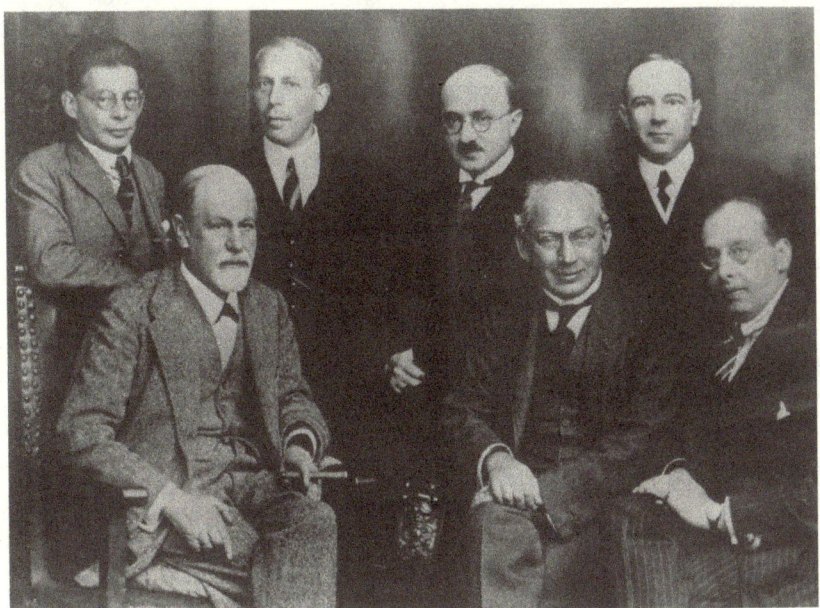

Figure 6.2 The Secret Committee, 1922
Credit: Archive Sigmund Freud Foundation, Vienna

The youngest and freshest of the Committee's members, he held a unique position in the nucleus of the secret ring: Freud cosigned Rank's circular letters to the Committee, giving them an imprimatur the others did not enjoy (Grosskurth 1991).

But when Rank's only ally on the Committee, Sándor Ferenczi, abandoned him in 1925, Rank lost his battle with Freud over who is more powerful in our earliest mental life, mother or father.

Unwilling to renounce his new idea, Rank, after many surprising twists and turns, chose to leave Vienna in 1926, wrenching himself out of the orbit of Freud, and becoming independent.

"Once the most orthodox of Freudians," writes Peter Gay dismissively (1988), "he became a Rankian" (471). Against the will of Freud, Rank had chosen to become himself. Ever since 1926, to be called a "Rankian" has been a term of derision among psychoanalysts. Gay, an orthodox Freudian, is no exception.

Rank moved to Paris with his wife, Tola, and their small child, Helene, but traveled often to the United States to deliver lectures, most often at the University of Pennsylvania School of Social Work, and to see patients. "Let him err and be original," a bitter Freud told Max Eitingon, a member of the Secret

Committee (Jones 1957:77). To Sachs (1944), Freud said: "Now after I have forgiven everything, I am through with him" (149).

But Freud had neither forgiven nor was he through with Rank. At Freud's instigation, the analytic establishment in America and Europe waged war against Rank, condemning all his writings on relationship, existential, and will therapy as "anti-Oedipal" heresy. Once recognized throughout the tiny psychoanalytic world as Freud's heir, Rank was now *persona non grata*. The American psychiatrists he had trained in Vienna were required to be re-analyzed by Freudians to retain their official credentials as analysts (Lieberman 2012).

"I wonder how [Rank's new idea] will work out, and believe it won't be easy," Anna Freud wrote Eitingon. "The [Vienna Psychoanalytic] Society has forgotten him so quickly and completely. . . . Not one person took the opportunity to ask what's going on with Rank. . . . But it was he himself who kicked himself out with such energy" (quoted in Lieberman & Kramer 2012:246).[2]

Anna replaced Rank as her father's heir. Rank became an invisible ghost haunting psychoanalysis. His writings were excluded from psychoanalytic training programs, unread, caricatured, or simply forgotten.

"Since 1926, Rank was silenced to death—'totgeschweigen,' in German—no respectable analyst could mention his name without attaching the diagnosis 'mentally ill' or 'psychotic,'" said Esther Menaker (personal communication). He was a victim of psychoanalytic cancel culture.[3]

Why the lasting bitterness toward Rank? The Freudians, suggests Ernest Becker (1973) in *The Denial of Death*, "never forgave Rank for turning away from Freud, and so diminishing their own immortality symbol (to use Rank's way of understanding their bitterness and pettiness)" (xxi).

In a rare mention of his departure from the inner circle, Rank (1932b) comments in *Modern Education*: "Psychoanalysis is as conservative as it appeared revolutionary; for its founder is a rebellious son who defends the paternal authority, a revolutionary who, from fear of his own rebellious son-ego, took refuge in the security of the father position" (191–192).

Mainstream psychoanalytic theory and therapy would remain patriarchal for another fifty years—until after Anna Freud's death in 1982.

What, exactly, led to the break between Sigmund Freud and Otto Rank? In 1924 Karl Abraham, a member of the Secret Committee, gravely warned Freud that Rank's thesis in *The Trauma of Birth* was "a question of life and death" for psychoanalysis (quoted in Chertok & Strengers 1992:87).

Abraham was not exaggerating. A monumental "David and Goliath" battle, amounting to a leadership succession crisis, had erupted between Rank and Freud, the two most brilliant minds in the psychoanalytic movement.

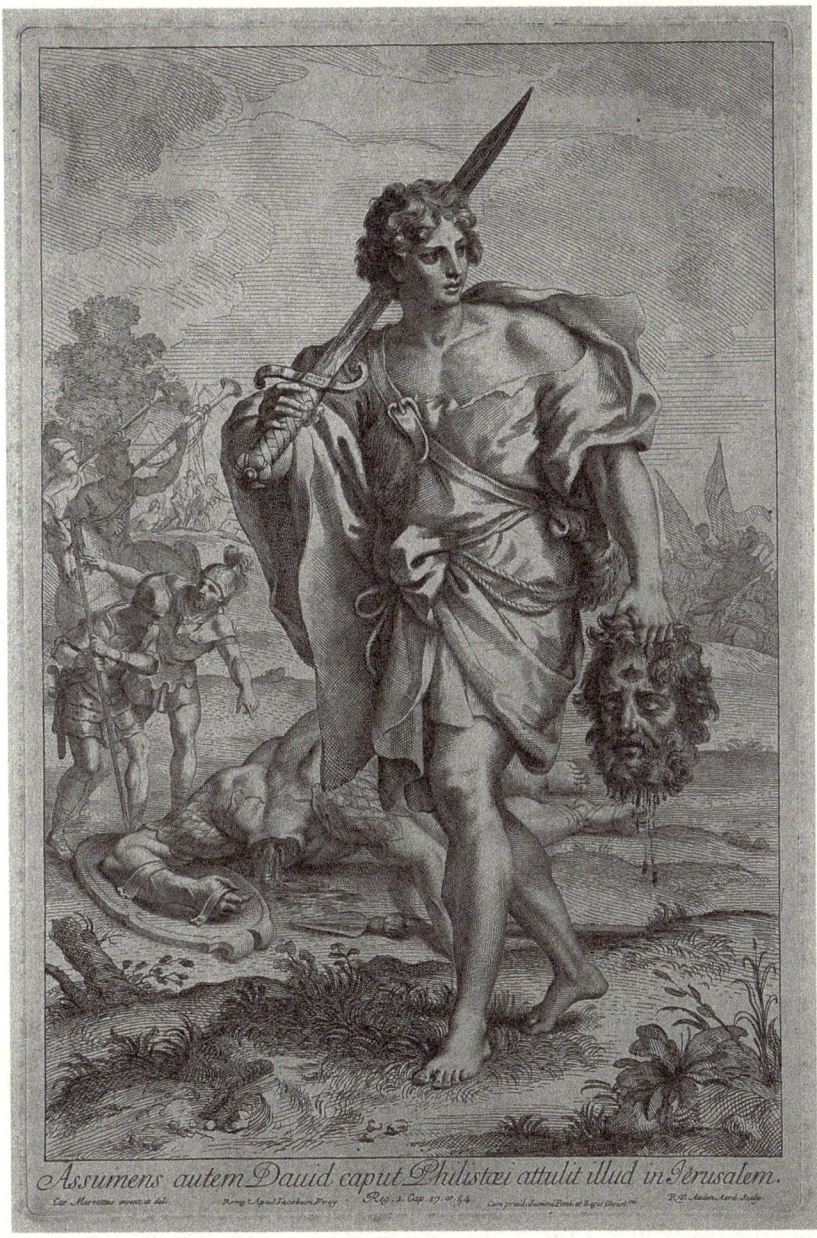

Figure 6.3 David holding the head of Goliath

Line engraving by R. van Audenaerd after Carlo Maratta, 1625–1713

Credit: Wellcome Collection, London, U.K.

In mid-April 1923, while Rank was composing *The Trauma of Birth*, Dr. Felix Deutsch examined Freud's mouth. He saw a cancerous growth. "If the disease is malignant," Freud told Deutsch, his long-time personal physician, "then I will have to see how one can disappear from this world with decorum. The matter has only one catch. You won't know I have a mother; she is 87. It will be difficult to do that to the old woman" (Freud & Ferenczi 2000:103n.1).

Few sentences ever uttered by Freud are more puzzling than these cryptic remarks to Dr. Deutsch. What was Freud referring to when he said, "It will be difficult to do that to the old woman"? *Do what?* And why, exactly, did Freud conjure up his mother, Amalia, then in robust health, rather than his wife, Martha, or their children at such an ominous time?

A few weeks later, on May 6, 1923, as a gift for Freud's sixty-seventh birthday, Rank presented the father of psychoanalysis with his new manuscript: *Das Trauma der Geburt*.

In the process of birth, asserts Rank, each new arrival on the planet finds its first object, mother, only promptly to lose her again: the primal catastrophe. For the tiny creature, this trauma is a loss beyond words, a harbinger of life's incalculable suffering, and takes precedence over the Oedipus complex.

Although biologically based, the trauma of birth is also a symbol of the "I's" startling discovery of itself and its anxiety-soaked separation from its first object, mother.

Analogizing to the analytic hour, Rank suggests that the relationship between mother and fetus—the unborn—forms a template for the encounter between therapist and patient, who unite in deep sharing, paradoxically, only for the patient to learn how to bear the trauma of separation with less anxiety than before.

But there is joy as well as pain in separation. In the healing relationship, therapist and patient merge into a larger whole, like Plato's mythical half-beings striving to reunite, in order to re-emerge at the end phase of therapy in their singular individuality, enriched, and spiritually renewed.

At bottom, suggests Rank, perhaps the birth trauma is nothing but the painful consciousness of living, in other words, consciousness itself, the dim perception of one's *difference* as a consequence of becoming conscious of life.

"One could formulate the [neurosis]," observes Rank (1924) in *The Trauma of Birth*, "as a cry 'Away from the [mother]!'" (52). Inevitably, the anxiety of the newborn is attached to its powerful mother, a primal object, who, when internalized in the psyche, becomes "the nucleus of every neurotic disturbance" (46).

For each trembling, vulnerable new arrival on the planet Earth, its first experience of anxiety is correlated with discovery of the existence of its mother.

Only later is the "fear of her caused ultimately by the birth trauma" (90), the wound of unspeakable loss, displaced onto the Oedipal father.

On first hearing of Rank's proposition about the primal anxiety attached at birth to the mother, Freud told Ferenczi, then Rank's best friend: "I don't know whether 66 or 33 percent of it is true, but in any case it is the most important progress since the discovery of psychoanalysis" (Jones 1957:59). But Freud's uneasiness also showed, since he joked, "Anyone else would have used such a discovery to make himself independent" (ibid.).

Ferenczi was hailing Rank's manuscript on the birth trauma, which included chapters on art, symbolism, religion, philosophy, and myth, as well as on therapy, even more strongly than had Freud. "Your presentation of the ideal Greek human being and his detachment from the ancient primal mother [Urmutter] in art is one of the most brilliant parts of your work," Ferenczi congratulated Rank. "I shall be glad when your book will finally be published, without it I am actually hindered in my own production, since all future work must be based on the trauma point of view" (quoted in Rank 1996:12–13).

Rank's celebration of the ideal Greek's "detachment from the ancient primal mother" is a direct quote by Ferenczi from the chapter on art by Rank (1924) in The Trauma of Birth (155). Going further, Rank had argued that the anxiety attached to the Urmutter is the "primal repression" (215), a repression more consequential for our psychic life than repression of the Oedipus complex.

For Freud, anxiety concerning infantile sexuality was at the repressed core of the Oedipus complex. In contrast, Rank was now suggesting that fear of maternal power is repressed to a deeper level than even infantile sexuality. It is "primal."

If not addressed, the primal repression, writes Rank, would block mature psychological growth and development. "Should not then the removal, by analysis, of the primal repression," asks Rank, ". . . be sufficient to make the neurotic grow up to the same limited degree as that reached by the ordinary civilized human being, who even today is only in the [infantile] stage?" (216). No matter how anxiety-provoking, separation from the powerful mother who is internalized in each of us at birth, as our first object, is essential for emotional maturity as an adult, argues Rank.

But whether 100, 66, or 33 percent of The Trauma of Birth were true, Freud had far more on his mind at this time, no matter how important Rank's revolutionary new focus on the Urmutter was for the future of psychoanalytic theory and therapy.

In October and November 1923, Freud underwent two major surgeries to excise cancer from his jaw and palate. By mid-October The Trauma of Birth was already printed but not yet published by the Verlag, the psychoanalytic publishing house directed by Rank.

On November 17, while convalescing from the second surgery, Freud requested a voluntary operation on his testicles to ligate the *vas deferens*, a duct that carries sperm to the seminal vesicle.

Then in vogue even among reputable physicians, this mysterious procedure, which Freud surely understood as a kind of self-castration, was supposed to improve vision, heighten intellectual insight, and halt, or even reverse, cancer (Romm 1983:73–85).

"[D]o not talk about it—not as long as I am alive," Freud admonished a physician attending him (84). Known today as a vasectomy, the "ligation allegedly promoted increased activity of the hormone-producing cells of the testes" (73). Freud had been given no more than five years to live by his surgeons.

❧

Three days after Freud's vasectomy, on November 20, 1923, Otto Rank paid a visit to Freud in his hospital room at the *Sanitorium Auersperg* in Vienna. At 11 o'clock that night, after returning home, Rank wrote a letter to Freud about an interpretation that had just occurred to him of "the 'witty dream' you told me today" (Lieberman & Kramer 2012: 176).

In the dream David Lloyd George, a great orator and former British prime minister, was delivering a lecture on *Das Ich und das Es*, Freud's latest book— *The Ego and the Id*—just published in April 1923, the same month in which Rank had drafted *The Trauma of Birth*.

The dream portrayed David Lloyd George speaking in English but mangling the meaning of Freud's new book, which was introducing to psychoanalysis a seminal concept: *das Über-Ich*, the "above-I" or super-ego, the shadow of the object that falls, after internalization of the powerful father's castration threat, on *das Ich*, the "I."

As director of Freud's publishing house, Rank was responsible for reviewing the manuscript of *The Ego and the Id* before publication. Curiously, although *The Ego and the Id* introduced a new term, the super-ego, *das Über-Ich*, into psychoanalytic theory, Freud had chosen not to put this word in the title of his book. While he was reading the pre-publication copy of *Das Ich und das Es*— literally *The I and the It*—Rank must have wondered about the absence of *das Über-Ich* from the title.

According to Freud's new theory, the super-ego is a derivative of the will of the powerful father, who is located in the nucleus of the unconscious. The super-ego is the child's first internal object. Virtually a synonym for the Oedipus complex, the *Über-Ich* is the source of all anxiety and guilt—and undergirds religion, law, society, ethics and, indeed, all of civilization.

With utmost cruelty the "above-I"—the will of the powerful father—rages against the "I," said Freud in his new book, as if it had taken possession of all of one's sadism, a self-destructive expression of the biological drive toward death, the *Todestrieb*.

Since the beginning of his self-analysis in the 1890s, for almost three decades, Freud had been investigating the Oedipus complex, an investigation that was confirmed repeatedly in every patient's analysis. No analysis by Freud had ever revealed anything but the Oedipus complex, and the super-ego was always there, hidden in the core, but not named as such. Now Freud had named it. This new term, Freud made clear, represented unconscious fear of castration by the powerful will of the father.

On November 20, 1923, while Rank was consoling Freud as he recovered from his surgeries at the *Sanitorium Auersperg*, Freud had shared with Rank his dream about David Lloyd George's lecture in English on the "above-I," *das Über-Ich*. Freud invited Rank to offer an interpretation of the dream.

Such an invitation was not unusual. During a session in 1909 of the Vienna Psychoanalytic Society, "Rank had the audacity to analyze Freud," according to E. James Lieberman (1985). "Later evidence indicates that he analyzed Freud's dreams from time to time over the years, to Freud's great delight" (113).

In 1905, even before meeting Freud, Rank had written the master a long letter, analyzing one of the dreams Freud had published in *The Interpretation of Dreams* (Lieberman & Kramer 2012:315–322). "The book is a defense," the 21-year-old Rank boldly told Freud, "playing itself out in the unconscious, against the fear that you may be a neurotic" (320). In the last lines of his letter, Rank added: "I could also explain to you why I had to be the one to 'discover' all of this, but—! Anyway, perhaps you'll guess the reason yourself" (322).

Rank's fearless interpretations of Freud's dreams endeared him to the master, who had the highest regard for Rank's skills in dream interpretation, which is why he had allowed him to edit *The Interpretation of Dreams* and add two new essays to it. Rank's name now appeared under his own on the title page of the Dreambook, Freud's greatest work.

How would Rank interpret Freud's new dream? On November 21, 1923, Rank penned a pun-filled letter, as masterful and subtle a dream interpretation as he had ever attempted, worthy of being read slowly in order to absorb its deepest meanings:

> I've been silent long enough . . . and now I want to return to public life and my work—which, however, means to speak, and indeed to speak English (conducting analyses), in which the pronunciation is harder for us German speakers. Yet you know English as well as the great English orator. You even make jokes and puns in English.

... This means: "It's high time I [Freud] return to work, and speak, for others do not understand me [*verstehen mich ja doch nicht*], but 'translate,' i.e., interpret me badly (<u>the I and the It</u> [written by Rank in English, and underlined by him]), and misuse psychoanalysis for their personal interests. The others understand *nichts* (<u>nothing</u>) or less than *nichts* (<u>over-nothing</u>) [a pun on *Über-Ich* since *übernichts* means "over-nothing" or less than nothing; Rank's underlining]." (This is reminiscent of the progression: *nix-nix aber schon garnix!* [nothing, nothing, nothing at all!].) Here, though, one notices that the "pun" relates to German: the *Ich* and the *N-Ich-T*, which presumably signifies the doubt: Will I be able to speak in English or not; will the others "understand" me or not?

... I hope the deeper layers will reveal as decisive a will to heal [*Genesungswillen*] as the ego-layer's will to work [*Arbeitswillen*]. (176–177)

What did this highly convoluted interpretation signify? While Freud related his dream, Rank had been listening empathically for clues to determine if Freud's "will to heal" (*Genesungswillen*) from his surgeries was as strong as his "will to work" (*Arbeitswillen*).

Somehow, Rank sensed that the "will" was implicated in Freud's recovery. But how? In the *Ego and the Id*, Freud (1923a) had written that the Id "cannot say what it wants; it has achieved no unified will. Eros and the death instinct [*Todestrieb*] struggle within it" (59).

On November 26, 1923, while still on his hospital sickbed, Freud responded to Rank's puns regarding *das Über-Ich*, and came to a startling conclusion about Rank's own intent in writing *The Trauma of Birth*, a letter that, because of its own complex word plays, also needs to be read slowly:

It's been a long time since you tried to interpret one of my dreams in an unusual, powerful analytical way. Since then much has changed; you have grown immensely and you know so much more about me and the result is different. Your work gives me the opportunity to ... focus on the interesting question of the standing of the *Über-Ich*. I can't confirm everything you write... but also have nothing to contradict.

... the joke was actually conceived in German: I-nothing-over-nothing. [*Ich nichts, über-nichts.*] In the dm. [*Tr.*, short for *Traum*, dream; but also a pun on the title of Rank's book, *Trauma*], in fact, only the <u>nothing</u> was clear, the <u>over-nothing</u> was just interpolation [Freud's underlining].

Now comes the question: Against whom is the dm. [dream or *Trauma*] directed [*Gegen wer richtet sich der Tr.*]?

... And the question about the super-ego [*Über-Ich*]? Does it act so force-fully too, showing such a brutal will to recovery [*Genesungswillen*]? Oh no, that would not be its way at all. ...

So this means: Watch out! The young man and the old interchanged. You [Freud] are not David [*nicht du bist der David*], you're the boast-ful giant Goliath, who another, a young David, will slay. And now every-thing falls into place, that you [*Sie*, i.e., Rank] are the dreaded David who, with a *Trauma of Birth*, succeeds in devaluing my work. . . . (177–179)

In the wake of his bout with cancer, Freud's association to David murdering Goliath (or perhaps it was the other way around), even if only in jest, must have startled Rank. Was Rank David or was Rank Goliath? Was the anxiety at sep-arating from the powerful *Urmutter* that Rank had declared in *The Trauma of Birth* to be critical to attaining adult maturity implicated, in some fantastic way, to Freud's cancer of the mouth? To his will to recover (*Genesungswillen*) from his surgeries?

And who or what, exactly, was responsible for the guilt-feeling that seemed to be haunting the "boasting giant Goliath," a guilt-feeling so dark and unspeakable that it was now threatening, literally, to shut his mouth, forcing the golem to remain silent?

Could Freud ever show the "will to heal" solicited by Rank in his interpreta-tion of Freud's dream? More ominously, did the "dreaded David's" new idea, which emphasized the powerful will of mother at the expense of that of the father—making her, rather than father, the primary source of the *Über-Ich*—reduce the value of psychoanalysis to *Nichts*—nothing? To *übernichts*—less than nothing?

As a close reading of this exchange of letters suggests, both Rank and Freud understood, at some dim level of awareness, that they were enmeshed in a conflict over the origins of the super-ego. Was *father* or *mother* its original source?

Insisting on the priority of the child's relationship to its father, Freud had always treated mothers only as passive objects of male sexual desire. He had given no importance in his theory or therapy to the emotional quality of the mother-child relationship.

Moreover, in none of his case histories did he see the mother's powerful will or her vital role in promoting the child's ethical development. "Mothers were not perceived [by Freud] as persons with whom the infant interacted emotionally," according to psychoanalyst Anthony Storr (1989:21).

With his theory of the fear of maternal power, Rank, in *The Trauma of Birth*, had undermined Freud's assertion, based on his self-analysis, that the Oedipus complex was at the core of the unconscious.

A few days after receiving Freud's "David and Goliath" letter, Rank personally delivered to Freud one of the first printed copies of *The Trauma of Birth*. On December 1, 1923, Freud sent a warm note to Rank, who had dedicated his birthday gift to the "Explorer of the Unconscious, Creator of Psychoanalysis."

In a tone far different from his earlier letter, Freud brushed aside any reservations he may have had, and was very generous toward Rank's work. He accepted the dedication, but modestly declined the grandiose title "Explorer of the Unconscious, Creator of Psychoanalysis." Yet, as if still unsure about the effect of Rank's work on him, he mentioned the immortality he expected Rank's new idea to bring him: "I gladly accept your dedication with the assurance of my most cordial thanks. If you could put it more modestly, it would be all right with me. Handicapped as I am, I enjoy enormously your admirable productivity. That means for me too: '*Non omnis moriar*' ['I shall not completely die,' from the Roman poet Horace]" (Lieberman & Kramer 2012:179–180).

On publication of *The Trauma of Birth*, the members of the Secret Committee, the Politburo of psychoanalysis, recognized immediately that Rank had attacked the centrality of the Oedipus complex. Inexplicably, Rank was dethroning the powerful father from his place in the deepest core of everyone's unconscious.

In the battle emerging between "David and Goliath," each member of the Secret Committee chose sides: only Sándor Ferenczi allied himself with Rank's new idea; the others remained loyal to Freud's Oedipal theory, with Ernest Jones and Karl Abraham lining up most stridently against Rank.

"Clinically it followed," observed Jones (1957) with alarm, "that all mental conflicts concerned the relation of the child to its mother, and that what might appear to be conflicts with the father, including the Oedipus complex, were but a mask for the essential ones concerning birth" (58). Was psychoanalytic theory a "mask" hiding something deeper than Oedipus, the nucleus of the neurosis?

After many twists and turns, Freud eventually directed Ferenczi to choose between himself and his best friend, Otto Rank. Terrified at the prospect of losing Freud's love, Ferenczi aborted his enthusiasm for *The Trauma of Birth* and denounced Rank. "He was my best friend," Rank told Jessie Taft (1958) ruefully, "and he refused to speak to me" (xvi).[4]

Looking back, we can see that Freud and Rank were engaging in a battle over a question that remains hotly contested even today: to what extent are women able—or allowed by the restrictions of patriarchy, sexism, and their own fear of life or *Lebensangst*—to exercise their wills in a world still ruled by the will of men?

The word "will," which was central to the vocabulary of William James, can hardly be found in the writings of modern psychologists, having been replaced by such terms as "motives," "goals," "self-efficacy," or "agency." In my view, all these words are synonyms. They all point to the capacity of human beings to exercise the power of their will.

Entailing the first-person experience of "*I am*," the word "will" distinguishes the agency of persons from their behavior. An agent—from Latin *agere* "to act, to do"—acts with intent.

To will is to be a cause of one's actions, whatever the neuronal underpinnings of willing in the brain might be. "The explication of motives without the recognition of the complicity of the will," writes psychoanalyst Stephen Mitchell (1988), co-founder of the field of relational psychoanalysis, "leaves *the person* out of the explanation, and hence encourages a self-serving and obfuscating bad faith" (250; italics in the original).

It goes without saying that neither Freud nor Rank would have employed the vocabulary of "motivation," "goal-setting," "self-efficacy" or "agency" in their battle over whether women have powerful wills of their own. The language they were immersed in reflected that of Nietzsche, the pre-eminent philosopher of the will in their era.

In the wake of the Second World War, the word "will" fell out of favor in psychology, being linked to Hitler. It was in the title of Leni Riefenstahl's 1935 *Triumph of the Will*, one of the most hideous propaganda films ever made.

In psychology, it was Rollo May who re-introduced "will" in 1969 with his huge bestseller *Love and Will* and, in 1980, Irvin Yalom made the word central to his widely acclaimed textbook, *Existential Psychotherapy*. "I gasped at his prescience when reading [Rank's] works," wrote Yalom (1980), "especially his books *Will Therapy* and *Truth and Reality*" (293). Both May and Yalom acknowledged borrowing the word "will" from Rank's *Will Therapy*.

In their "David and Goliath" conflict, within a short time after publication of *The Trauma of Birth*, Freud and Rank understood that they were battling each other over a fundamental question: Whose will is more powerful in our earliest mental life—that of father or that of mother?

7

The will of the father

Over the course of the 20th century, Sigmund Freud changed the way we speak and think about the psyche. He invented a new form of human interaction: the analytic hour. A mental alchemist, he transformed myth into scientific theory.

Drawing on Greek mythology and his daily self-analysis, Freud coined the term "Oedipus complex" to characterize the buried content in the deepest core of everyone's unconscious. "Freud told me he never ceased to analyze himself, devoting the last half hour of his day," reports Ernest Jones (1953). "One more example of his flawless integrity" (327).

Beginning in 1900, with the publication of *The Interpretation of Dreams*, Freud offered "Oedipus" as his fully drawn mental map of the human territory, a universal narrative of infantile sexual desire and its repression by the fearsome threat of paternal castration.

Subsequently, the father's will was lodged in our unconscious psyches as the super-ego, said Freud, and became the source of all morality and ethics, explaining the discontents inherent in the civilizing of ourselves.

Throughout his life, Freud (1905) was uncompromising on the centrality of the Oedipus complex, as he explained in a 1920 footnote added to *Three Essays on the Theory of Sexuality*:

> It has justly been said that the Oedipus complex is the nuclear complex of the neuroses, and constitutes the essential part of their content. It represents the peak of infantile sexuality, which, through its after-effects, exercises a decisive influence on the sexuality of adults. Every new arrival on this planet is faced by the task of mastering the Oedipus complex; anyone who fails to do so falls a victim to neurosis. With the progress of psycho-analytic studies the importance of the Oedipus complex has become more and more clearly evident; its recognition has become a shibboleth that distinguishes the adherents of psycho-analysis from its opponents. (226n.)

Through ever-deeper research into the unconscious of his patients, Freud believed that he would learn how to expand his discovery of the Oedipus complex into the realms of education, law, society, art, politics, religion, and leadership. Attempting a revaluation of all ethics through his Oedipal lens, Freud had "the mind of a moralist," said sociologist Philip Rieff (1959).

Otto Rank and the Creation of Modern Psychotherapy. Robert Kramer, Oxford University Press.
© Robert Kramer (2025). DOI: 10.1093/9780197698303.003.0007

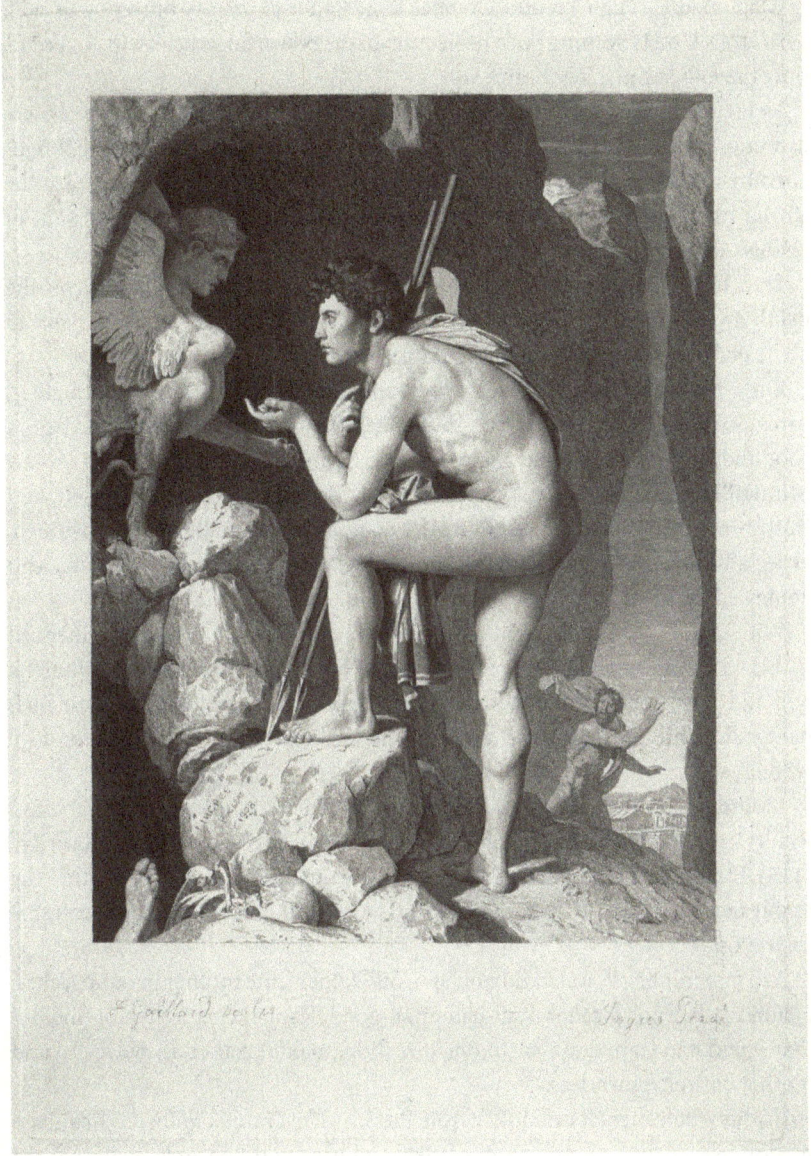

Figure 7.1 Oedipus and the Sphinx (after Ingres)
Credit: Claude-Ferdinand Gaillard, Metropolitan Museum of Art

In his Oedipal theory, Freud promoted an ethics commanded by the power-ful father, an ethics internalized into the psyche as *das Über-ich*, the "above-I," which watches, silently, like a secret agent in the mind, punishing us with anxiety and guilt for sexual transgressions, real or imagined.

Magnified through Freud's Oedipal lens, father expresses omnipotent will. Writ large, God is nothing but a projection of the powerful father's will. To Freud, only the father could symbolize will.

In Freud's view, women had no will or source of personal power of their own. Moreover, they were ethically inferior to men since women could not be threatened by castration. They were, therefore, unable to develop an "above-I" in the strong masculine sense. Deceptive and manipulative, women are resistant to change, declared Freud.

Due to the unconscious, self-destructive workings of the *Todestrieb*—the death drive—women refused interpretations by their analysts, did not *want* to be healed and suffered from an incurable "penis envy."

On a personal level, however, Freud encouraged women like his daughter, Anna, to become psychoanalysts—but only if they accepted his Oedipal theory, root and branch. Freud had many women friends, including his sister-in-law Minna Bernays, Lou Andreas-Salomé, Marie Bonaparte, Helene Deutsch, and Ruth Mack Brunswick. He enjoyed the company of sexually alluring women, especially narcissistic ones. But he fiercely attacked anyone, male or female, who contested his Oedipal theory.

With the publication in 1924 of *The Trauma of Birth*, Otto Rank, influenced by his wife, Tola, was the first psychoanalyst to recognize the power of women's will and their contributions to the ethical development not only of their husbands and children, but also to that of the larger society and civilization as a whole.

Mother is at once loving and fearsome, "capable of the deepest sympathy," Rank (1924) explained in *The Trauma of Birth*, "but also of the greatest severity" (115). Ethical development for both men and women originates from within the ambivalent matrix of the mother-child relationship, not from fear of paternal castration.

As a father himself, Rank did not "split off" father from mother in our psyches. Neither father nor mother is all-bad or all-good. Rank was merely pointing out that Freud had leaned too far in one direction, making father all-powerful and mother entirely powerless.

"[O]ur whole mental outlook," wrote Rank in *The Trauma of Birth*, "has given predominance to the man's point of view and has almost entirely neglected the woman's" (36).

Inevitably, said Rank, mother's will comes first in our psyches, father's second. "[M]y wife—ideal mother, i.e., almost no mother, since she commands!," Rank joked to Freud about Tola, mother of their young child, Helene (Lieberman & Kramer 2012:245).

In *The Trauma of Birth*, Rank suggested that women are invested with wills and ethical principles of their own. Mother, not father, is the earliest source of the "above-I" for both sexes, while internalization of the father's will comes afterwards.

Love and fear of the powerful mother precedes and grounds the Oedipus complex. The "primal repression [is] clinging to the mother," Rank (1924) asserted in *The Trauma of Birth* (215).

"Analytically expressed," concluded Rank, drawing on copious evidence from the history of art, mythology, religion, and philosophy, "this is the phase *before* the Oedipus complex" (216; italics in the original).

But there was no such phase in psychoanalysis. The term "pre-Oedipal" did not exist before Rank penned *The Trauma of Birth*.

"The elimination of the father in your theory strikes me as revealing too much the influence of personal factors in your life," Freud reproached Rank in July 1924 (Lieberman & Kramer 2012:208).

"That's not so, of course, and cannot be," Rank retorted, denying that he had eliminated the will of the father, "it would be nonsense. I've only attempted to assign him the correct place" (209). In the child's psyche, mother's will comes first, then father's will.

In August 1924, unsure that he would live much longer, the cancer-ridden Freud dangled the possibility that he was open to changing his mind, as long as Rank was open to changing his:

> In the course of time, if there is still enough time, either you'll convince and correct me, or you'll correct yourself, separating what is a permanent new acquisition from what the bias of the discoverer has done to it. I know you're not lacking praise for your innovation, but you must consider also how few people are capable of judging, and how strong are the efforts in most of them to be rid of the Oedipus complex where a path presents itself. (213)

But Freud was on the verge of concluding that Rank, by elevating the role of the powerful mother over that of the father, had undermined the significance of the Oedipus complex, a discovery Freud believed had secured his place among the immortals of science—Copernicus, Galileo, Darwin. In September 1924 Freud erupted to Ferenczi: "I am boiling with rage" (Freud & Ferenczi 2000:178).

A gigantic conflict was exploding within the Secret Committee as Ernest Jones and Karl Abraham allied to denounce Rank for his anti-Oedipal heresy. Although angered by the campaign being mounted against him by Jones and Abraham, Rank still revered Freud as his teacher and mentor, but, at the same time, was feeling sorely disappointed that Freud had turned against him.

For a while, Rank considered resigning from all his leadership positions, and moving with his family to Paris. "I saw he couldn't make himself go away," said Tola, his wife. "He wanted to and couldn't. . . . And this was the time he went to the Professor and told him about his conflict. And the Professor saw him" (quoted in Lieberman 1985:247).

In conversations with Freud, Rank never held back his true feelings. But he knew that Freud had been hurt by two strongly-worded letters Rank, while lecturing in America, had sent him, defending *The Trauma of Birth* as an advance in psychoanalytic theory and therapy. Yet Rank did not want this conflict between him and Freud to sunder their long-time relationship.

"Not a rebellion," according to E. James Lieberman (1985), "the new work was a tribute, accepted by Freud as the greatest progress since the beginning of psychoanalysis. Freud's gradual withdrawal of support forced Rank to either recant or fight back, perhaps for the first time in his life" (225).

Depressed by the vicious fighting inside the Politburo, and shaken by Freud's mortal cancer, Rank was still willing to reach out to rivals like Jones and Abraham, who wanted to expel him immediately from all his leadership positions.

At the urging of Freud, Rank sent a conciliatory letter in December 1924 to the Secret Committee, declaring that he was suffering from an "Oedipal neurosis" and accepting responsibility for creating a schism inside the Politburo—but refusing to abandon his new pre-Oedipal idea, in theory or therapy. Not a sentence in this letter, often interpreted as if written "on bended knee" (248), shows a willingness to recant anything in *The Trauma of Birth*.

In this carefully worded letter, Rank used the only language Jones and Abraham might have accepted as an apology—Rank had undergone an "Oedipal" crisis: in other words, a rupture in his personal relationship with Freud and his "brothers" on the Secret Committee.

"From analytical discussions with the Professor," Rank informed the Secret Committee, "in which I could explain my reactions in detail in terms of emotional factors, I can hope I've succeeded, first of all, in clearing up my personal situation, since the Professor found my explanations satisfactory and has forgiven me personally" (Lieberman & Kramer 2012:228).

Although wary of the enmity shown him by Jones and Abraham, Rank's letter ended on a hopeful note: "I'd be glad to hear that my explanations have found the same analytic understanding among you as they have with the Professor, and that they will also give you the satisfaction I hope will be taken as the prerequisite for recommencing our collaboration in the not too distant future" (229).

Demonstrating that his December 1924 letter of apology to the Secret Committee was not a retraction of his ideas in *The Trauma of Birth*, Rank reiterated during a January 1925 talk at the New York Psychoanalytic Society: "The only real new viewpoint in [my] contribution [is] the concept of the pre-Oedipus level" (Rank 1996:35).

During the first half of 1925, Freud and Rank met often in Freud's study at *Berggasse 19* to reconcile their differences. In long letters to Freud, Rank shared his dreams, including a remarkable one in which Freud appears as a maternal symbol: "your role as the caring mother, whom I feared losing due to your illness" (Lieberman & Kramer 2012:245).

In a 1924 lecture Rank had given while in America, he called Freud "a tender and loving foster mother" who had "reared the neglected and misunderstood being," psychoanalysis, throughout its travails (Lieberman 1985:xxvii). "Freud has been called many things, but only his foster son called him a mother! Otto Rank could not have done so unaware of its symbolic meaning" (ibid.).

In 1925, over the course of many months, Freud and Rank explored and debated every nuance of their differences on psychoanalytic theory and therapy. "The only measure is and remains whether one can be true to oneself," Rank had written Freud forthrightly in September 1924 (Lieberman & Kramer 2012:218). With Freud, Rank held his ground and stayed connected, unlike Ferenczi, whose will collapsed in the face of Freud's growing opposition to Rank.

"[T]horoughly honest and open," as Freud had once described his protégé to Jung (quoted in Lieberman 1985:98), Rank, during their many conversations in 1925, sought to persuade Freud to include a primary role for the pre-Oedipal mother in psychoanalytic theory—in addition, naturally, to keeping the role of the Oedipal father intact, but in a secondary position.

At no time did Rank ever minimize the place of fathers in our psyche. It would be sheer "nonsense" to do so, as he told Freud. Rank was a father himself. But he insisted that mother's will comes first in our psyche, then father's will. What's so hard to understand about that?

In every letter Rank sent Freud in 1925 he was warm and conciliatory, not wanting to cut ties with his beloved Professor to whom he remained deeply grateful for hiring him as his personal secretary, the first paid member of the psychoanalytic movement, funding his PhD studies at the University of Vienna, and elevating him to the No. 2 position in the psychoanalytic hierarchy.

Rank repeatedly insisted that, as a matter of being "true to oneself," he was only seeking to improve psychoanalytic theory and therapy, merely adding to what Freud had already discovered. "And so we would like to regard our arguments," Rank (1924) had concluded at the end of *The Trauma of Birth*, "only as a contribution to the Freudian structure of normal psychology, at best as one of its pillars" (210).

As Freud's closest colleague in Vienna since 1906, author of many publications on psychoanalysis, including a mammoth book on the *Incest Theme*, Rank felt that he was contributing a second pillar to "the Freudian structure of normal psychology"—what Rank was now calling the "pre-Oedipal" pillar.

Seeking to extend the frontiers of psychoanalysis, as he'd been doing with unflagging energy for almost two decades, Rank declared to Freud that he was proposing "something I certainly consider very important, and which others, too, already consider indispensable for an understanding of the cases and for a therapeutic influence on them" (Lieberman & Kramer 2012:210).

Like many highly creative people, Rank often suffered from mood swings, whose existence was well known to Freud. In 1918, while stationed in Krakow, Rank had written Freud: "The more frequent exchange of our emotional states, which you encouraged recently, would doubtless affect me favorably if I didn't fear affecting you the opposite way with my almost constant reports of bad mood" (79).

Because Freud had allowed Rank to interpret his dreams, their relationship was on a more equal footing than that between Freud and Ferenczi. At times, as seen in the letters Rank and Freud exchanged over the "David and Goliath" dream, the Freud-Rank relationship might even be said to have verged on "mutual analysis," although obviously Rank deferred to Freud as his revered teacher and the creator of psychoanalysis—but never at the condition of sacrificing his own integrity.

Even in the face of Freud's growing anger at Rank for publishing *The Trauma of Birth*, Rank's respect and admiration—indeed, love—for Freud remained unequivocal. On August 31, 1925, Rank wrote Freud after visiting him at his vacation home in the Austrian mountains:

> Due to my hasty departure from Semmering, I couldn't convey to you the deep sense not only of appreciation, but also of unfading closeness to you and your life's work, that I am only now truly beginning to feel. But I probably wouldn't have been able to tell you this even had I stayed longer, for such a thing can hardly be said without becoming banal. Yet I know that this time you also understand, as in old times—yet newly—and that means everything to me. (Lieberman & Kramer 2012:241)

But by then Freud was fed up with Rank's harping on the role of mothers in our earliest psychic life, both loving and punitive, caring and powerful, generous and threatening. Freud considered these views a sign of Rank's "creative discovery" mania.

Three weeks earlier, on August 7, 1925, Freud had told Eitingon: "He's in no hurry to retract his [pre-Oedipal] theories; there, too, much has solidified" (240). A week later, on August 14, in a letter to Ferenczi that must have terrified Rank's best friend, who was already slipping away from him, Freud now likened his attitude toward Rank to "an absolutism moderated by treacherous assassination" (Freud & Ferenczi 2000:222).

In the same August 14 letter to Ferenczi, Freud revealed that he had begun to draft a new manuscript, *Inhibitions, Symptoms and Anxiety*, to undermine Rank, who had no idea that Freud was girding his loins for a "treacherous assassination," this time to be witnessed by the whole psychoanalytic world.

Still assuming that he had been "forgiven" by Freud, Rank wrote Freud in October 1925 about "my great desire to return to my old relationship to analysis and its champions, and I'd be grateful for your further help with this, as I need it for my psychological healing, and it may be useful for analysis, too" (Lieberman & Kramer 2012:243).

In late 1925, Rank—having been abandoned by his only friend, Ferenczi—felt emotionally vulnerable and depressed in the face of the continuing withering attacks on him by Jones and Abraham, but was still holding on with integrity to his pre-Oedipal innovations in theory and therapy, which he never renounced. During their talks in 1925, Freud had left him with the distinct impression that the master would form a new, reorganized Secret Committee out of the shattered fragments of the old one.

From America, where he was delivering new lectures on *The Trauma of Birth*, Rank wrote to Freud in November 1925 that his pre-Oedipal ideas were being well received, adding "nor do I renounce anything here" (Lieberman & Kramer 2012:247). In the same letter, he explained how he was expanding the reach of psychoanalysis to the "huge territory" of social work, a profession that he foresaw as playing a leading role in the future of psychotherapy:

> What I've accomplished so far: a whole group of serious people working, a real force, is becoming supportive of psychoanalysis. If all goes as I predict . . . this will be the key to the development of psychoanalysis in America, perhaps in the world, for this center comprises not only psychiatrists, but also the huge territory of the 'social workers' and the entire problem of education and instruction, social concerns, and character.
>
> . . . But I hope, dear professor, you won't misunderstand me; I think I see things quite objectively. Personally, I'd be glad to work with all who wish to work and not fight. . . . While I am rather alienated from the idea of the former Committee and have outgrown it, I'm happy with the reorganization you suggest. I glimpse a good omen, too, because the group you prefer doesn't have the pettiness of the other group (Abraham, Jones), and provides in Ferenczi scientific tolerance, in Eitingon social sensitivity, and in your daughter the non-medical-pedagogical. I think I'd work well with this group, personally and objectively, if the members are willing, and confidently hope I can win back your daughter's trust. (247–249)

But Freud had deceived Rank, and was now intent on removing him permanently from all his leadership positions in psychoanalysis.

◆§

On April 12, 1926, Rank visited *Berggasse 19* to contest the arguments made against him, personally, in Freud's newest book, *Inhibitions, Symptoms and Anxiety*—the first work by Freud not read in advance by Rank, managing director of Freud's publishing house, the *Verlag*, since 1919. Before 1926, Rank had edited and proofread every book written by Freud prior to publication.

Deeply wounded by Freud's "treacherous assassination," Rank went to confront Freud face-to-face. *Inhibitions* was Freud's first full-throated attack on *The Trauma of Birth*, which he'd never before criticized in public, only in private letters exchanged with members of his inner circle.[1]

In *Inhibitions*, Freud (1926a) writes: "Rank's contention—which was originally my own—that the affect of anxiety is a consequence of the event of birth and a repetition of the situation then experienced, obliged me to review the problem of anxiety once more" (161).

Reiterating the castration theory at the core of the Oedipus complex, Freud rejects Rank's emphasis on the emotional pain and anxiety of separation from mother. Birth "is not experienced subjectively as a separation from the mother, since the foetus, being a completely narcissistic creature is totally unaware of her existence as an object" (130).

The *first* internalized object in the infant's psyche is the father, insists Freud. Father's power over the child is symbolized by the super-ego, heir to the Oedipus complex.

For Freud, the emotional experience of separation anxiety derives from fear of castration, not from the child's fear of its powerful mother. Moreover Freud claims: "At birth no object existed, and so no object could be missed" (170).

On the one hand, he recognizes the merit of Rank's "discovery of [the] extensive concatenation" between birth and physiological anxiety (151). On the other hand, he denies the traumatic emotional consequences of separation from the *Urmutter*.

Plunging a dagger into Rank's heart, Freud had fulfilled his promise to Ferenczi to "assassinate" Rank. In *Inhibitions*, Freud (1926a) concludes: "[I]t becomes impossible to shut one's eyes any longer to the far-fetched character of [Rank's] explanations" (136). Burying Rank for good, he adds, in a devastating coda: "Rank's theory ... floats in the air instead of being based upon ascertained observations" (152).

During the emotionally charged encounter between the two on April 12, 1926, the last time they would ever meet, Rank evidently accused Freud, to his face, of not having "any more insight than a small boy" (Jones 1957:172).

"Rank seems to be retracting nothing," Freud complained to Eitingon the day after Rank's visit. "Our conversation about my last book on anxiety revealed irreconcilable differences. Practically, he seems to be holding on to his technique. Moroever, he indicated that he has come much further in his insights although he correctly assesses his own state as manic" (Freud & Eitingon 2004:452).

There can be no doubt that Rank experienced extreme mood swings during his "David-and-Goliath" battle with Freud. "Rank increasingly feared what would happened to him after Freud's death," according to historian of psychoanalysis Paul Roazen (1974). "For Freud, Rank now became the favorite come to slay the father" (404). Intent on destroying Rank's reputation permanently, Ernest Jones (1957) distorted Rank's emotional state in his Freud biography, diagnosing it as insanity, a "psychosis" (45).

Jessie Taft (1958), who knew of Rank's "extreme swings of mood" (98), asserts that Rank "managed to live for twelve years with a 'psychosis' that seemed not to interrupt the creative drive, the therapeutic practice, or the teaching engagements, maintained to the time of his death in 1939" (113n.51).

After April 1926, Freud and Rank never spoke again, although they continued their debate in print. From then on, Freud called Rank a *Hochstaplernatur* (Gay 1988:471), which means an "imposter by nature" or a "confidence trickster."

In response to Freud's "treacherous assassination" of him in *Inhibitions, Symptoms and Anxiety*, Rank moved to Paris with his wife, Tola, and their daughter, Helene, to become a psychotherapist for blocked artists, mostly women who sought to reclaim the creativity of their wills—the vital power of their life force—from patriarchal domination.

In a lecture he delivered at the University of Pennsylvania School of Social Work, Rank (1996) responded to Freud's rejection of his argument that mother is internalized in our mental life beginning with birth:

> Freud rightly emphasizes the fact that we know too little about the newborn and its sensations to be able to draw compelling conclusions about it. But the same would be true—in spite of isolated observations of children and even child analyses—to a great extent for the child itself, in whom hitherto much too much "adultism," especially adult sexuality, was projected.
>
> Freud's caution in relation to sensations of the suckling remains but is also valid for his assumption that the mother does not represent an object for the newborn. I mean we do not know this absolutely, or rather it amounts to the same thing as a quibble over words. For it is certain that the newborn loses something as soon as it is born, indeed even as soon as birth begins, something that we can express in our language in no other way than loss of an object, or

if one wants to be more precise, as loss of milieu. It is just the characteristic quality of the birth act, that it is a transitional phenomenon par excellence, and perhaps just this determines its traumatic character. In parturition, one might say, the ego finds its first object only to lose it again immediately—and this may possibly explain many peculiarities of our psychical life. (118–119)

On May 6, 1926, from Paris, Rank sent a 70th birthday gift to Freud: the standard edition of the complete works of Nietzsche. Today, this set of 23 volumes, bound in white leather, sits on a bookshelf in Freud's London home at 20 Maresfield Gardens, now converted into a museum.

With this gift, Rank was pointing to the intellectual debt Freud owed Nietzsche, the great precursor of psychoanalysis, whose influence Freud had always refused to acknowledge, just as Freud was now refusing to acknowledge Rank's attempt to introduce pre-Oedipal theory and therapy into psychoanalysis. Harold Bloom (1973) calls the poet's refusal of precursors "the anxiety of influence."

In his "Literary Autobiography," a record of all his writings up to 1930, Rank (1981) observes that psychoanalyst Charles Odier had credited him in 1926 as the first to see "the primal source of the super-ego in the pre-Oedipal (maternal) inhibitions. The pre-Oedipal superego has since been overemphasized by Melanie Klein without any reference to me" (37).

The neurosis, Freud once told Ferenczi, "is the motherland where we first have to secure our mastery against everything and everyone" (Freud & Ferenczi 1993:247). "I do everything only for the cause, which again, is basically my own," Freud confided to Ferenczi. "I proceed thoroughly egoistically" (33).

At age 90, however, Amalia Freud—the *Urmutter* herself—would not allow claims of "self-causation" by her son. "I am the mother," she declared to at least one guest in 1926 at her son's 70th birthday party, bringing a wicker basket of fresh eggs as a gift (Roazen 1974:46).

In *The Denial of Death*, Ernest Becker (1973) observes that Rank "understood that the psychoanalytic movement as a whole was Freud's distinctive *causa-sui* project: it was his personal vehicle for heroism, for transcendence of his vulnerability and human limitations" (109).[2]

According to Esther Menaker (1982), Rank attributed Freud's *causa-sui* project to his "attempt to blot out his mother-origin in order to deny his mortal nature. For to be born of woman is to share one's fate with all other living creatures whose birth inaugurates the inevitability of death" (89).

Without identifying Freud by name, but almost certainly having his former mentor in mind, Rank (1941a) writes in *Beyond Psychology* that man's "fear of woman as a threat to his immortality, betrayed itself in innumerable tabus imposed on his sex life and that of the woman" (223).

Yet Freud never underestimated the trauma of birth, an idea he expressed as early as 1908, after a talk by Rank himself at the Vienna Psychoanalytic Society on the myth of the birth of the hero. Summarizing Freud's view in the minutes of this meeting, Rank (1996), who was then secretary of the Society, noted: "[A]ct of birth as a source of anxiety" (28).

In a footnote added to *The Interpretation of Dreams* in 1909, Freud repeated that the "*act of birth is the first experience of anxiety, and thus the source and prototype of the affect of anxiety*" (ibid.; italics in the original). It was this footnote, "an incidental reference of Freud's," as Rank (1996) later explained in his American lectures, that had inspired him to write *The Trauma of Birth* (116).

What, then, was the "David and Goliath" battle between Freud and Rank about? It clearly wasn't about the trauma of birth, which both men accepted. It was, at bottom, about the absence of the will of mothers in psychoanalytic theory.

8

The will of the mother

According to Freudians like Ernest Jones and Peter Gay—and maintained to this day by legions of academics in the humanities—Freud's self-analysis in the 1890s was a brilliant success and established the Oedipus complex as the nodal point for the attainment of emotional maturity.

In his correspondence with Wilhelm Fliess, Freud struggled against almost insuperable odds to reach the neurotic harbor of his own Oedipus complex, writes Gay (1988), by "subjecting himself to a most thorough-going self scrutiny, an elaborate, penetrating, and unceasing census of his fragmentary memories, his concealed wishes and emotions" (97).

But this census overlooked one person—the *Urmutter* of psychoanalysis, Freud's mother, Amalia: "[T]here is no evidence," reports Gay (1988), "that Freud's systematic self-scrutiny touched on this weightiest of attachments, or that he ever explored, and tried to exorcise, his mother's power over him" (505).

While all other relationships in life were ambivalent, Freud (1933) repeatedly declared the relationship between mother and son as "altogether the most perfect, the most free of ambivalence of all human relationships" (133). Freud never idealized the mother-daughter relationship, which, he insisted, was fraught with conflict and ambivalence from the start.

Intellectuals in the humanities sympathetic to Freud have difficulty grasping that Freud's failure to see "the will of the mother" explains virtually everything wrong with the development of psychoanalytic theory about women—and about the practice of psychoanalytic therapy—during much of the 20th century.

In a recent book lauding Freud's genius in discovering the Oedipus complex, psychoanalyst Harold Blum (2022) refers, but only glancingly, to "Freud's unconscious ambivalent relation to his mother" (62). However, he does not follow up, as if this lapse mattered not at all for the rule of the father's will at the core of the Oedipus complex.

Who was Amalia Freud? Even today, after an avalanche of books and articles on every aspect of Freud's work and life, almost nothing is known about his mother except for a few scattered reminiscences.

"She was charming and smiling when strangers were about," writes Judith Bernays Heller (1973), the maternal granddaughter of Amalia, "but I at least

Otto Rank and the Creation of Modern Psychotherapy. Robert Kramer, Oxford University Press.
© Robert Kramer (2025). DOI: 10.1093/9780197698303.003.0008

always felt that with familiars she was a tyrant, and a selfish one. Quite definitely, she had a strong personality and knew what she wanted" (338).

"I really feared" her, adds Heller. A "fine-looking" but exceptionally vain woman, Amalia "had a volatile temperament" and was somewhat shrill and domineering—the emotional opposite of Sigmund's father, Jakob, who "remained quiet and imperturbable, not indifferent, but not disturbed, never out of temper and never raising his voice." Even in his seventies, "Professor Freud would always find time [on] a Sunday morning to pay his mother a visit and give her the pleasure of petting and making a fuss over him" (335–336; 339).

Martin Freud (1958) writes of Eastern European women like his grandmother, Amalia: "They had little grace and no manners . . . certainly not what we should call 'ladies.' They were highly emotional and easily carried away by their feelings. . . . These people are not easy to live with, and grandmother . . . was no exception. She had great vitality and much impatience" (11).

Oliver Freud, also a grandson of Amalia's, observed that she was "very self-willed" (Roazen 1993:189). Another relative, a female, "said she had found it hard to take what she called their grandmother's 'authoritarian character'" (ibid.).

According to psychoanalysis, human beings are unable to keep secrets from anyone who has eyes to see. The unconscious is written on the body and the face.

Examined closely, the expression on Freud's face in Figure 8.1, an August 1925 photo—the same month in which Freud wrote *Inhibitions, Symptoms and Anxiety*, his polemic against Rank—can only be described as ghastly. In the photo, taken on the occasion of his mother's 90th birthday, Freud's mouth is ajar. His lips are parted, his eyes two pools of pain. His right arm hangs limply, as if it does not want to be there, at his mother's side. The hollow wreckage of his cancerous jaw is clearly visible on the right side of his face.

Until he died in 1939, Freud suffered through 33 operations and was forced to wear a series of painful prosthetic devices, severely limiting his hearing and speech—the very means, ironically, by which psychoanalysis, the "talking cure," was supposed to relieve neurosis. None ever fit properly.

"I am constantly tortured by something," Freud complained to Max Eitingon (Romm 1983:71). For the rest of his life, Freud would call the prosthesis a "monster" (Jones 1957:99), "an uninvited, unwelcome intruder whom one should not mind more than necessary" (Romm 1983:33), "my dear neoplasm" (Clark 1980:439), a "permanent, never-to-be ended misery" (Hyman 1962:298).

No other photograph of Freud, not even those taken during his youth, reveals so much of his infantile pain. This is a man who is suffering greatly, and not just from oral cancer. It is not an exaggeration, I suggest, to describe Freud's countenance as the tortured look of a small boy chained in fear, love, and hate

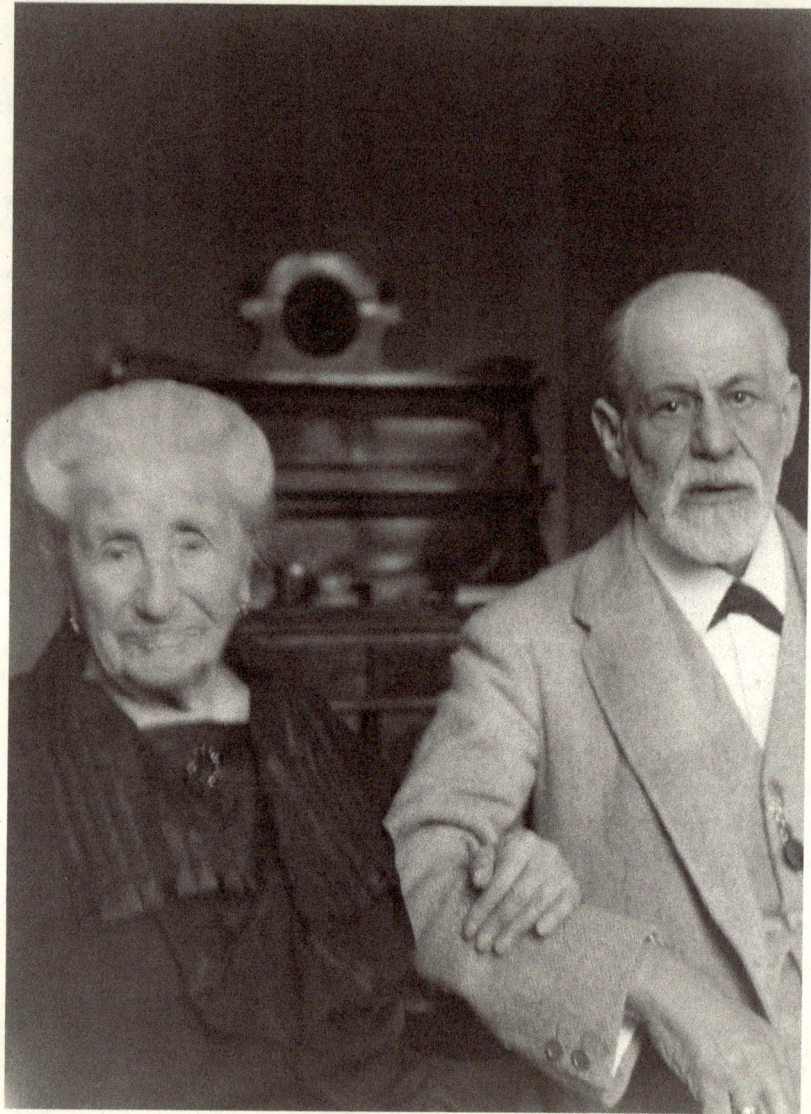

Figure 8.1 Freud and his mother, 1925
Credit: Everett Collection/Bridgeman Images

to his mother. According to Rank's pre-Oedipal thesis in *The Trauma of Birth*, there is no lack of ambivalence in the mother-child relationship, even for the small boy.

What made Freud, at age 70, regress to small boyhood in the presence of his 90-year-old mother?

The expression on Amalia's face, although somewhat blurred, is one of enormous narcissistic pride. Undoubtedly, this is a picture of a commanding mother, a woman with an iron will, a woman who does not intend ever to be separated from him. But to what extent, one wonders, does the "small-boy-in-Freud" *want* to break his mother's arm lock?

While we can—and should—be empathic toward Freud's pain, written all over his body and face, his refusal ever to explore and try to exorcise "his mother's power over him" (Gay 1988:505) raises considerable doubts about the extent of his emotional maturity *as an adult*, and the dire consequences its absence may have had for psychoanalytic theory and Freud's rules on how to practice therapy.

For two decades a favorite son of Freud's, Otto Rank knew everyone in Freud's family intimately. Like Ferenczi and other members of the inner circle, he had made courtesy calls on Amalia. Since Freud did not like to entertain, Rank and his wife, Tola, sometimes threw Christmas parties for Freud and his family, including Amalia.

When Freud's cancer was discovered in April 1923, Dr. Felix Deutsch could not bear to tell Freud of its malignancy, fearing that Freud would commit suicide rather than undergo the agony of major surgery. "If the disease is malignant," Freud had told Deutsch, "then I will have to see how one can disappear from this world with decorum" (Freud & Ferenczi 2000:103n). Instead, Deutsch recommended minor surgery to remove "leukoplakia"—a precancerous white patch or plaque—from Freud's mouth.

Informed by Dr. Deutsch that the cancer was, in fact, malignant, the Secret Committee met in August 1923 to debate how to tell Freud that he needed another, major surgery to remove parts of his jaw and palate. Who would tell him? Hanns Sachs suggested Freud's daughter, Anna.

But "Rank, striking to a deeper level, suggested Freud's old mother," writes Ernest Jones (1957:98), who was present at the meeting. Keenly attuned to the nature of the power that Amalia wielded over her son, Rank felt that only "Freud's old mother" could be enlisted to persuade him to undergo major surgery.

In *Inhibitions, Symptoms and Anxieties*, Freud (1926a) declared that "Rank's theory floats in the air instead of being based on ascertained observations" (152). But Rank had had plenty of opportunities in social settings to observe the relationship between Freud and his mother.

Might Rank's long-standing awareness of Amalia's powerful will explain why he told Freud, at their last meeting in April 1926, as Jones (1957) recounts, that "he couldn't credit Freud with any more insight than a small boy" (172)? Jones probably heard this directly from Freud himself, and it also appears in a letter Freud sent to Ferenczi (Freud & Ferenczi 2000:444). With this unvarnished remark, which no doubt infuriated Freud, Rank could only have been referring to Freud's unwillingness ever to analyze his mother's power over him.

Rank was not the only one to notice this gaping hole in Freud's life-long self-analysis. A few days before his own, final meeting with Freud in August 1932, Ferenczi confided to A.A. Brill that he agreed with Rank's critique: Freud, said Ferenczi, had no more insight than that of a small boy; "[T]his," writes Jones (1957), "happened to be the very phrase that Rank had used in his time—a memory that could but heighten Freud's forebodings" (172).

For years Ferenczi and Rank had talked endlessly with each other about Freud's personality, ideas, character, and feelings. As the two closest associates of Freud, and brilliant psychoanalysts in their own right, Freud dominated their lives, intellectually and emotionally.

What else can these assessments by Rank and Ferenczi be than a devastating indictment of Freud's "systematic" self-scrutiny? Psychoanalytic treatment, Freud had insisted from the beginning of his self-analysis, was founded entirely on truthfulness. Insight is all.

In their identical critique of Freud, Rank and Ferenczi were saying that the father of psychoanalysis, tragically, was stuck for a lifetime in the pre-Oedipal phase, like a bone lodged in his throat, refusing—self-destructively—to reach the neurotic harbor of his own Oedipus complex.

Defending the arguments he made about the role of powerful mothers in *The Trauma of Birth*, Rank had written Freud forthrightly in August 1924: "[W]hat remains is a portion of truth and reality that one cannot banish from the world by closing one's eyes. I have the definite impression that you don't wish to see certain things or that you can't see them, for sometimes your objections sound as though you hadn't read or heard what I actually said" (Lieberman & Kramer 2012:209).

A month later, Rank repeated: "I have the impression that you don't want to be convinced, and from your standpoint, I can understand that very well" (218). He was pointing, diplomatically but firmly, to Freud's refusal to examine his tortured relationship with the powerful mother to whom the father of psychoanalysis paid a reluctant call every Sunday morning. "It was a family joke that Freud's stomach would be out of sorts on these visits," writes historian of psychoanalysis Paul Roazen (1974:46). Freud always came late to his mother's apartment on Sunday mornings.

Echoing Rank's critique of Freud's blindness, Ferenczi (1932) wondered in his *Clinical Diary* about "the ease with which Fr[eud] sacrifices the interests of women in favor of male patients" (187).

Freud, concluded Ferenczi, "may have a personal aversion to the spontaneous female-oriented sexuality in women: idealization of the mother. He recoils from the task of having a sexually demanding mother, and having to satisfy her.

At some point his mother's passionate nature may have presented him with such a task. (The primal scene may have rendered him relatively impotent)" (188).

In making the father's powerful will the core of Oedipal theory, suggests Ferenczi, Freud was denying his shame, humiliation, and infantile rage at being the helpless object of Amalia's will, sexual or otherwise. Thus, he projected the fear of his powerful mother onto Jakob, by all accounts a mild-mannered father, never out of temper.

Ferenczi had spent decades immersed in Freud's thoughts and emotions, poring over each word in his letters and publications, scrutinizing every nonverbal gesture of the master, trying to understand what motivated him to create psychoanalysis. They exchanged over 1,240 letters. As regular visitors to Freud's home at *Berggasse 19*, both Rank and Ferenczi were well aware of Amalia's character.

In the third week of February 1926, Freud published *Inhibitions, Symptoms and Anxieties*, without allowing Rank, managing director of the psychoanalytic publishing house, to see the manuscript first, as he had always done before.

On February 24, Freud dispatched a printed copy of his anti-Rank tract to Ferenczi in Budapest, who read it immediately, as he always did with Freud's books. In the early 1920s, mail delivery between Budapest and Vienna took only one day.

Ferenczi interpreted the new book's "treacherous assassination" of Rank as a disguised attempt by Freud to bury his tortured relationship with his mother, Amalia. Unless Ferenczi did something to help Freud in his time of need, he knew that he would be the next victim of the Professor's "boiling rage" (personal communication, André Haynal).

On February 26 Ferenczi sent a remarkable letter to Freud, inviting him to go into therapy with him: "I will come to you for a few months and place myself at your disposal as an analyst—naturally: if you don't throw me out" (Freud & Ferenczi 2000:250)—as Freud had just "thrown out" Rank. For years, Ferenczi had been dissatisfied with Freud's own analysis of him, spread out over three short periods in 1914 and 1916 (Falzeder 2015: 246).

Unlike those who infantilize Ferenczi by refusing to take him at face value, I believe that by offering to analyze Freud, in addition to wanting to complete his own analysis, Ferenczi was unselfishly and sincerely offering an extraordinary gift to the Professor, his friend and mentor: an opportunity to experience emotionally—*perhaps for the first time*—the genuine possibility of healing in the therapeutic relationship.

"I am also [not] that psa. Superman whom we have constructed," Freud once admitted to Ferenczi (Freud & Ferenczi 1993:221). In a slip of the pen, Freud had forgotten to write the word "not" in this confession of humility. But surely Ferenczi saw at once that Freud's slip was an all-too-human cry for help.

And who better than Ferenczi, the only one trusted by Freud now that Rank had been thrown out, to help Freud in a time of such great need?

"My own analysis [with Freud]," Ferenczi (1932) confided to his *Clinical Diary*, "could not be pursued deeply enough because my analyst . . . could not follow me down into those depths" (62)—the same pre-Oedipal depths plumbed so fearlessly by Rank in *The Trauma of Birth*.

Although Ferenczi loved Freud, he was taken aback that Freud would not follow his own advice: "[S]urely infantilism is destined to be surmounted," Freud (1927) insisted. "Men cannot remain children forever; they must in the end go out into 'hostile life'" (49).

With respect to how Freud's unwillingness to exorcise the power of his mother, Amalia, might have harmed his own unfinished analysis with Freud, Ferenczi (1932) asked poignantly in his *Clinical Diary*: "Is it not possible, or even probable, that a doctor who has not been well analyzed . . . will not cure me, but, instead, will *act out* his own neurosis or psychosis at my expense?" (92–93; italics added).

Ferenczi always considered himself the analyst for the most difficult cases. Freud was now desperately ill. Not only was he suffering from cancer, he also had serious heart problems.

By fully experiencing the deeply empathic understanding of Ferenczi, the proud but anguished creator of psychoanalysis might, at long last, become more open to his own buried feelings, more open to experiencing feelings that seemed to him so terrible that he had never been willing to acknowledge their existence in himself—*acting them out, instead, with patients in the analytic setting*.

Like Rank, Ferenczi maintained that therapeutic healing occurs only in the here-and-now, in the person-to-person relationship between patient and analyst. No interpretation of past traumas, not even the sexual or other traumas Freud, as a child, might have experienced at the hands of Amalia, would be able to heal his emotional suffering. Change occurs in the present. Only an authentic, person-to-person relationship between Ferenczi and Freud in the here-and-now could heal the pain.

What would the emotional experience of analysis with Ferenczi have been like for Freud in the role of patient? How might Ferenczi have conducted himself in the role of analyst?

No one can know for sure. But it seems safe to conclude that Ferenczi, no matter how awed he was by Freud's genius, would have treated Freud along the lines of the tender encounters he describes so movingly in his *Clinical Diary*: "Should it even occur, as it does occasionally to me, that experiencing another's and my own suffering brings a tear to my eye (and one should not conceal this emotion from the patient), then the tears of doctor and of patient mingle in a sublimated communion, which perhaps finds its analogy only in the mother-child relationship" (Ferenczi 1932:65).

With Ferenczi's loving help, Freud might become more open to working through the pain of his archaic childhood, more open to loosening the chains that tied him to his tormented past, more open to letting go of defenses against threatening feelings—more open, in short, to warming the frozen sea inside his soul.

Then 70, Freud, claiming he was too old for analysis, declined Ferenczi's invitation to go into therapy because, as he explained in a curious aside, it would be "harmful for my loved ones!" (Freud & Ferenczi 2000:252)—in other words, analysis with Ferenczi evidently would open up for scrutiny his hostile feelings about "my loved ones" —including Amalia? —which he was unwilling to do.

In April 1923, Freud, on first learning of his cancer, had told Dr. Deutsch, "It will be difficult to do that to the old woman" (103n.1). Now that Rank had been "assassinated," it was not too difficult for Ferenczi to surmise that Freud had projected his ambivalent, even murderous, feelings toward his mother onto Rank (personal communication, André Haynal). Freud himself seemed to know, at some level of awareness, about the "psychic root" of his condition, yet, simultaneously, he did not want to know.

"There may indeed be a psychic root," Freud wrote to Ferenczi in February 1926, thanking him for his offer of analysis, "but let's not forget, dying also has its psychic root, and it remains quite doubtful whether it can be mastered through analysis, and finally, whether at seventy years of age one doesn't have a good right to rest of any kind" (252).

In response to Freud, Ferenczi suggested, with astonishing candor, that overcoming resistance to emotional insight was possible even for the creator of psychoanalysis: "[P]lease keep in mind that, as soon as your disinclination (should I say resistance?) has been halfway overcome, I can come to Vienna immediately" (253). There can be little doubt to what "resistance" Ferenczi was referring.

No one in psychoanalysis believed in the transforming power of insight more than Freud. "Being totally honest with oneself is a good exercise," he once told Wilhelm Fliess (Masson 1985:272). Psychoanalytic treatment, Freud had insisted from the beginning of his self-analysis, is founded on truthfulness, ripping away all veils, facing the darkest truths of the soul, fearlessly filling in all the gaps of memory.

Yet on this single point Freud did not want to know. "I have to blind myself artificially in order to focus all the light on one dark spot," Freud once told Lou Andreas-Salomé. "[F]or my eyes, adapted as they are to the dark, probably can't stand strong light or an extensive range of vision" (Freud, E. 1960:312).

If the two men closest emotionally to Freud—Rank and Ferenczi—agree, then one must take their conclusion about Freud's inhibited, symptomatic, and anxious psyche quite seriously. As Judith Dupont, the editor of Ferenczi's *Clinical Diary*, observes: "Freud could not renounce defending himself. . . . [I]t was to take more than half a century before Ferenczi's ideas and insights would be more or less assimilated by the psychoanalytic community" (Ferenczi 1932:xii).

In his American lectures, Rank leveled a veiled accusation that Freud had buried his feelings about his powerful mother. Always discreet, Rank refused to name names, but, nevertheless, he argued that the small boy "must, so to speak, make his father bad, in order to keep his picture of the good mother clear" (Rank 1996:142–143).

According to E. James Lieberman (1985), "Rank knew more about Freud than anyone else but did not retaliate with gossip or backbiting even though the Freudian establishment labeled him mentally ill" (xvii).

The powerful mother, said Rank (1996) in his American lectures, without naming Amalia, "*he has never seen, but only the later displacement of her to the father, who therefore plays such an omnipotent part in his theory.* The image of the bad mother" pointed out Rank, in the most penetrating critique of Freud's repudiation of femininity ever made, "is present in Freud's estimation of woman, who is merely a passive and inferior object for him: in other words, 'castrated'" (101; italics in the original).[1]

"What is more, if Freud," writes psychoanalyst Patrick J. Mahony (1987), "consequently neglected the psychic reality of the mother's castration of her son, he likewise underplayed the son's matricidal wishes" (149).

The Interpretation of Dreams, Freud's most revealing work, is at once a maternal return and an open refusal of the whole. Pregnant with metaphors such as "dark woods, narrow defiles, high grounds and deep penetrations," the *Dreambook* reveals unmistakably in its sexual imagery that "we are exploring a woman's body," according to literary critic Stanley Edgar Hyman (1962), "that of Freud's mother" (333).

The overdetermined nature of Freud's writing, especially the metaphors he uses, corresponds perfectly to his theory of the unconscious, which is a hermeneutics of suspicion (Ricoeur 1970). Freud's language often reveals his unconscious in plain sight, like Poe's purloined letter, at the same time that the master remains in the dark.

Derivatives of Freud's unconscious are manifest throughout the *Standard Edition* of his writings and emerge periodically in his letters, while in his conscious awareness Freud appears to be oblivious. This is perhaps the deepest meaning of psychoanalyst Jacques Lacan's much misunderstood claim that Freud's unconscious is structured like a language.

According to Didier Anzieu (2021), Freud, during his self-analysis in the 1890s, always used "the metaphor of female fertility" (469) in his letters to Fliess, while, at the same time, he was congratulating Fliess for finding "the way to stem the power of the female sex" (478).

Tragically, during his life-long self-analysis, Freud could never differentiate himself—never separate—from the powerful *Urmutter* of psychoanalysis, as Ferenczi and Rank were the first to note.

"The crucial conflict between his desire to lose himself in his mother, and to separate from her in order to achieve individuality," writes art historian Jack Spector (1973), "gave rise to Freud's Faustian restlessness and his never quite satisfied attempt to find a father figure with whom to identify" (64).

In addition to Ferenczi and Rank, many others saw uncanny signs of infantilism in Freud's adult behavior. The poet Hilda Doolittle (1956), known as "H.D.," recounts a startling experience in therapy with Freud, then 78 years old:

[Freud] is beating with his hand, with his fist on the head-piece of the old-fashioned horsehair sofa. . . . I was not aware of having said anything that might account for the Professor's outburst. . . . The Professor said, "The trouble is—I am an old man—*you do not think it worth your while to love me.*"

The impact of his words was too dreadful—I simply felt nothing at all. . . .

Anyhow, he was a terribly frightening old man, too old and too detached, too wise and too famous altogether, to beat that way with his fist, like a child hammering a porridge-spoon on the table. (21–23; italics in the original)

Martha Bernays noticed this trait long before Ferenczi, Rank, and H.D. did. As Jones (1953:148; italics in the original) reports in his Freud biography, Martha wrote to her 37-year-old fiancé in 1886, shortly before they were married, signing her letter "Mother":

Dear Sigi:

. . . First regain some calmness and peace of mind which at present is so entirely wrecked. You have no reason whatever for your ill-humor and despondency, which borders on the pathological. Dismiss all these calculations, and first of all become once more a sensible man. At the moment you are like a spoilt *child* who can't get his own way and cries, in the belief that in that way he can get everything.

Don't mind this last sentence, but it is really true. Take to heart these truly well-meant words and don't think badly of

Your faithful
Mother

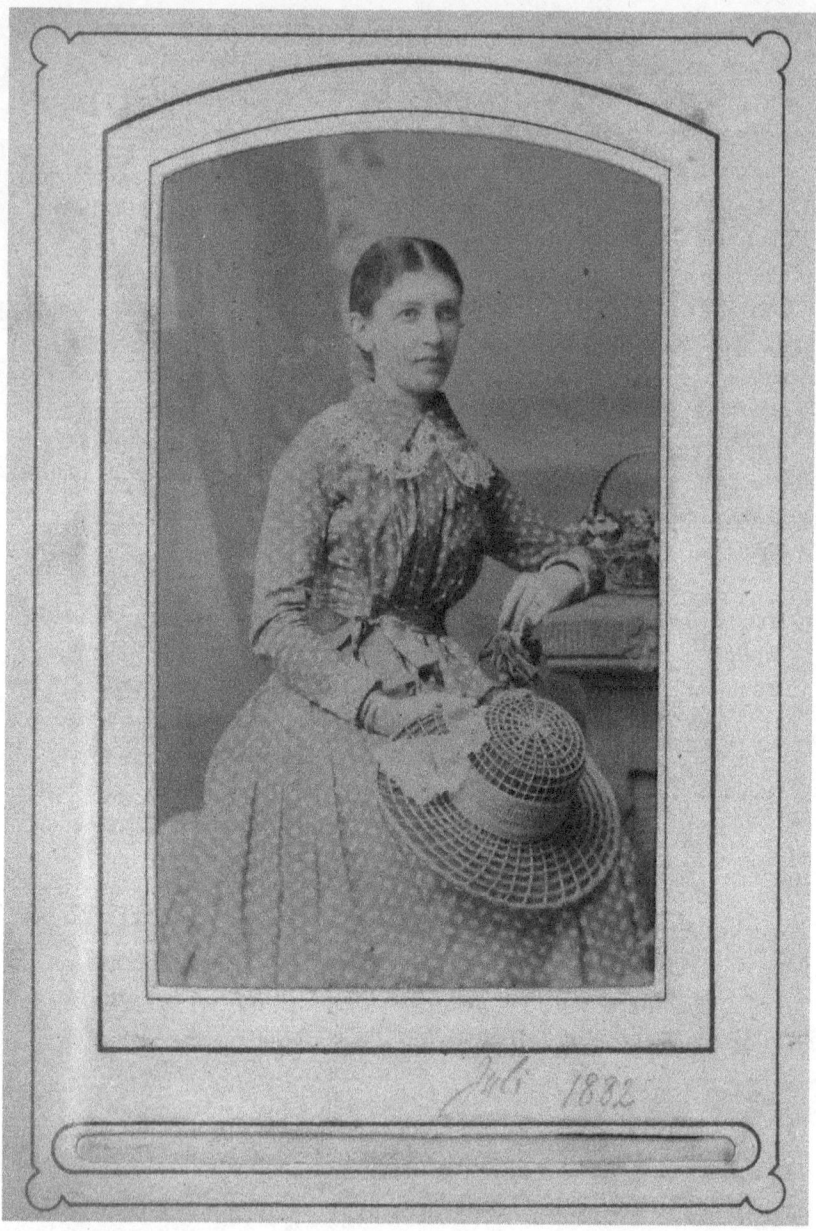

Figure 8.2 Martha Freud, 1882
Credit: Library of Congress Prints and Photographs Division

According to historian Paul Roazen (personal communication), Martha "laid out Freud's morning clothes each night before going to bed, and put the toothpaste on his toothbrush."[2] A regular visitor to the Freud household for 20 years, Rank would have had many opportunities to observe signs of Freud's infantilisms.

"Still stranger with such a supreme psychologist was the fact, on which we were all agreed," writes Jones (1955) of how the Secret Committee saw Freud's character, "that he was also a poor *Menschenkenner*" (412)—literally, not a "good judge of human nature." In other words, he lacked what today is called emotional intelligence—the sign of mature adulthood.

After Rank told Freud to his face, in private, that he had "no more insight than a small boy," Freud lashed back angrily, calling Rank a confidence trickster, a *Hochstaplernatur*.

In *The Secret Artist: A Close Reading of Sigmund Freud*, Lesley Chamberlain (2000) observes:

> When Freud fell into hostile relations with others, he looked away from what he should have seen, namely his own acts of self-repetition and vengeance. He called Rank a confidence trickster, but who exactly was the confidence trickster? To avoid confrontation with the truth, Freud split this fallible part of himself off and called it Rank. (55)

Freud's refusal to analyze Amalia's power over him, according to psychoanalyst Christopher Bollas, accounts in large measure for classical psychoanalytic technique: "What Freud could not analyze in himself—his relations to his own mother," says Bollas, "was *acted out* in his choice of the ecology of psychoanalytic technique" (quoted in Zaretsky 2004:275; italics added)—i.e., transference.

9

Transference versus relationship

Transference does not emerge automatically from within patients like spontaneous combustion. Although each of us carries images in our minds of significant people in our early lives, and we often see others through these templates, transference is something else. In psychoanalytic therapy, transference is *provoked* by the impersonal—emotionally distant—behavior of the analyst.

"The analytic technique creates transference," Ferenczi (1932) avers in his *Clinical Diary*, "but then withdraws, wounding the patient without giving him a chance to protest or go away; hence interminable fixation on the analysis while the conflict remains unconscious" (210).[1]

What was the connection, in Freud's formulation of therapy, between transference and cure? "Essentially," Freud had told Jung in 1906, the "cure is effected by love." By "love," Freud meant the *patient's* love of the analyst. Absent this love, "the patient does not make the effort or does not listen when we submit our translation [of the Oedipal unconscious] to him" (McGuire 1974:12–13).

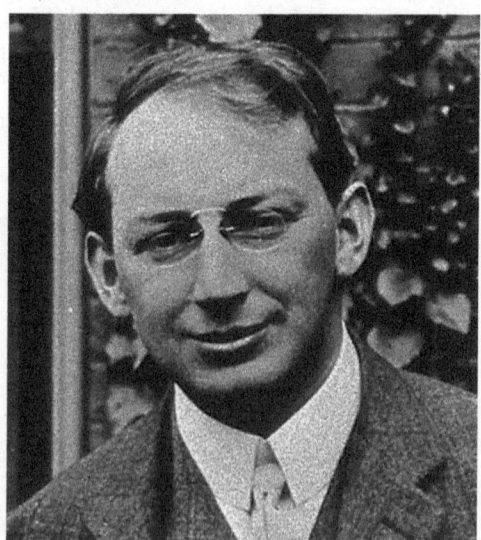

Figure 9.1 Sándor Ferenczi, 1909
Credit: Wellcome Collection

Otto Rank and the Creation of Modern Psychotherapy. Robert Kramer, Oxford University Press.
© Robert Kramer (2025). DOI: 10.1093/9780197698303.003.0009

According to Ferenczi, Freud cared about helping patients in the early stages of his career as a psychotherapist, but was frustrated by his continuing lack of success. By the early 1920s, Freud had become cynical about therapy and, instead, exploited his patients, luring "transference love" in the same way a small boy demands unconditional love from his mother. "Psychoanalysis," writes Ferenczi (1932) in his *Clinical Diary*, referring to Freud, "lures patients into 'transference'" (199).

Ferenczi observes that Freud, dismissive about the healing possible in psychoanalysis, had become "more and more impersonal (levitating like some kind of divinity above the poor patient, reduced to the status of a mere child, unsuspecting that a large share of what is described as transference is artificially provoked by this kind of behavior), [Freud] postulates that transference is created by the patient.... [This gives] him the opportunity to enjoy his superiority, and *to be loved without any reciprocity* (a situation of almost *infantile grandeur*), and moreover he even gets paid for it by the patient" (93–94; italics added).

Ferenczi explains how interminable analysis leads to unresolvable transference, observing in his *Cinical Diary* that "one finds far too much [transference] arising in analysis, which analysts in their ignorance are not equipped to resolve (he would have to know himself and his behavior much better to be able to do this)." Scathingly honest, Ferenczi continues:

> The analysis provides a good opportunity to carry out unconscious, purely self-seeking, ruthless, immoral, indeed so to speak criminal actions and similar behavior guiltlessly (without a sense of guilt), such as a sense of *power over* a succession of helplessly devoted patients who admire him without reservation. Sadistic pleasure in their suffering and their helplessness. (199; italics added)

Disillusioned with Freud's manipulative practice of psychoanalysis, Ferenczi's critique that transference does not emerge spontaneously from within patients but is largely created by the impersonal, unfeeling behavior of analysts—a critique that Rank shared—is the most devastating ever made of the core technique of psychoanalytic treatment. For fear of enraging Freud, however, Ferenczi never expressed it publicly, reserving his views for the privacy of his diary, which was not published until 1988, over half a century after his death.

For Rank, provoking transference prevents experiencing feelings in the present moment, by both therapist and patient. "To Rank's way of thinking," according to Will Wadlington (2012), recently retired after having practiced Rankian therapy for four decades, "patients find the analyst's [transference] interpretations comforting, and a way to avoid feeling in the moment" (388).

To the extent that analysts deliberately create conditions for transference to arise they are manipulating patients to *live in the past*. Under the sway of transference, neither is fully present, engaged with the other, in the relationship. In fact, there is no relationship taking place. What is therapeutic, Rank (1996) said in his American lectures, "is just that which is new, that which lies beyond the 'transference'" (230).

"[T]he transference," insisted Freud (1923b), at a time when Ferenczi and Rank were beginning a campaign to persuade other analysts to build an authentic relationship with patients in the here-and-now, "plays a part scarcely to be over-estimated in the dynamics of the process of cure" (247). Yet, by then, both Ferenczi and Rank knew that Freud did not believe that psychoanalysis cured patients. Was Freud referring, perhaps unconsciously, to his *own*—always out-of-reach—cure?

Ferenczi and Rank had realized that under the "infantilizing" spell of transference—created purposefully by a Sphinx-like analyst who is not permitted to show feelings during therapy—almost any "interpretations" would do to convince patients of the correctness of the analyst's "insights" into their unconscious—at least until the inevitable "resistances," grounded in the *Todestrieb*, Freud's death drive, flared up.

All the platitudes of psychoanalysts about the need for "neutrality," "abstinence" or—as Anna Freud (1966) always insisted—staying "equidistant from the id, the ego and the super-ego" (28) covered up this basic fact, clearly visible to Ferenczi and Rank in how Sigmund Freud constructed the ecological setting of therapy. "There was a kind of manipulation, exploitation involved," explains psychiatrist Thomas Szasz (Sullum 2000).

Although celebrating Freud's incomparable gifts as a writer, literary critic Harold Bloom criticizes psychoanalysis for promoting transference. In "Reading Freud: Transference, Taboo, and Truth," Bloom (1983) asks bluntly:

> Why should it be genuinely therapeutic to generate an illusive relationship [i.e., transference] merely in order to dissipate it? Is there any analogue available to us that might illuminate so odd a transaction? How has psychoanalysis won social acceptance of so knowing an illusion, of so imaginary and consciously deceptive a false connection? (309)

Bloom is saying that an illusory, manipulative, false connection could not possibly be a means to heal psychological suffering.

By the mid-1920s, Ferenczi and Rank "had proposed that the curative component of psychoanalytic therapy was not the interpretation of the transference" (Merkur 2010:67). They had reframed the meaning of "transference," even while continuing to use the term, to mean an authentic relationship in the here-and-now. Ferenczi and Rank were arguing, against Freud, that the analyst needed to show a *genuine caring* and *empathy* for the patient's suffering. Transference, in the Freudian meaning, was a manipulation by analysts for the covert purpose of retaining *power over* patients, not sharing *power with* them.

In an untranslated work published in German in 1926, Rank writes of the beginning phase of relationship therapy: "We give the patient the mother love [*Mutterliebe*] sought for since his earliest childhood" (Rank 1926:39). In the same work, Rank was the first psychoanalyst to use the term "here-and-now" (9). Moreover, since the "here-and-now" of the present moment moves more swiftly than the blink of an eye, he was also the first to use the term "then-and-there" (24n.).[2] Every relationship, he insisted, and therefore also the one with the therapist, "always results freshly from the I" (206), and is completely new and unprecedented. Later, Rank (1936a) would argue in *Will Therapy*:

> The undischarged, unreleased, or traumatic experiences are not repressed into the unconscious and there preserved, but rather are continued permanently in actual living. . . . Here in actual experience, as in the therapeutic process, is contained not only the whole present but also the whole past, and only here in the present are psychological understanding and therapeutic effect to be attained. (40)

Along with Ferenczi, Rank regarded the demonstration of "mother love" by analysts as an essential first element in the healing process of psychotherapy.

Since feeling evokes feeling, patients return gratitude, said Rank, even love, toward their analyst, who, they feel, has demonstrated true caring for their anguish, suffering, and loneliness. Someone was finally listening to their feelings. For Rank, the expression of empathy—or love—had to be mutual for relationship therapy to be an experience of healing.

But there are limits to love. In an untranslated book, Rank (1927) insists that, once demonstrated, the analyst's genuine "mother love" for the patient, if taken to excess, is likely to become an "opiate" (23) that would lead patients to cling to their analyst like a child clings to its mother.

As a result, Rank was the first to focus on the dynamics of the *separation* phase of therapy. From the dreams of his patients, he intuited that the prospect of separating from the therapist was reviving vague, fleeting memories of the painful separation anxiety first felt at birth, and recorded pre-verbally, unconsciously, in the body's implicit memory.

While necessary for healing, learning how to love others on the patient's part (as Freud had told Jung) is not sufficient, insisted Rank. Discovering, and expressing, the power of their own "creative will," is essential, said Rank, to help patients learn how to affirm their creative life force, their difference. Instead of *power over*, Rank advocated *power with*.

For self-leadership or self-empowerment to emerge during the end phase, he argued, the patient needs to learn how to will, not only how to love, although experiencing both love and will over the course of therapy is necessary for healing.

But if a patient's creative will is not affirmed and actualized, the "mother love" offered by the therapist might become an opiate, leading patients to feel guilty for hurting the feelings of therapists by abandoning them at the end phase of therapy. The therapist must be wise enough to help the patient gain independence even from therapy itself.

"The last and decisive step of therapy," writes Rank (1927), "is the weaning of the patient from this opiate, which can take place only by active intervention in setting a time limit, a process that, after a designated time period, withdraws the 'drug' from him" (23).

After experimenting for a while with end setting, and watching how his patients reacted, Rank finally decided that it would be best to set this date in collaboration with them, not arbitrarily. He was always open to shortening or lengthening the time period if patients expressed a need to do so. Decades before researchers studied the subject, Rank employed what today would be termed "evidence-based best practices" for ending therapy (Wollan 2020:17).

Virginia Robinson said that "as far as she knew in the late twenties and early thirties Rank was not using a *fixed time limit* for beginning and ending, 'but made use of ending with each patient differently'" (quoted in Menaker 1982:106; italics in the original).

Social worker Ethel Seidenman (1978), who was in therapy with Rank from 1936 to 1938, recalls how Rank, in a most natural and humane way, initiated their conversations regarding the end phase:

"Let me ask you whether you feel like terminating our interviews." I said that I had not come to this decision, but actually, I feel the problems that brought me to him in the first place are figments of the past. Perhaps we could think about this. Rank suggested that it might be a good idea if we schedule a few appointments, perhaps two or three, to review our experience and see whether there are some loose ends that we might clear up.

Although I was entirely in agreement, I began to feel sad because my experience with Rank was a great experience. We agreed that our next sessions would be in New York. When I got up to leave he shook my hands warmly and said we will meet again next week. (62)

At the next session, writes Seidenman, "we settled into our chairs and when he asked me what was on my mind, I reminded him that we had decided on concluding our interviews and I gather that I have some feeling about this."

> "This is usually the case," he said. "Let us talk about it." I was surprised how quickly my anxiety subsided. "Where would you like to start?" I started with my beginning experience that brought me to him. The problem of "not wanting to be uprooted; fearful, and with anxiety."
>
> As I finished saying this, I added, "I am no longer plagued with these problems that interfered with my work and social life. I was afraid to make close relationships with people even with my colleagues. It is a great relief that I don't feel this way any more."
>
> ... [Rank's] personal quality is unique. He is an artist who touches the core of me. Even when we were discussing my problematic situations, I frequently felt like singing. (63)

Having learned in the beginning and middle phases of the relationship to love themselves and the therapist, patients learn during the end phase how to bear the anxiety and guilt of separating as the painful, but necessary, price for self-actualization, for creative expression of their unique selves—for "singing," as it were.

In a charming footnote in *The Trauma of Birth*, Rank (1924) mentions a "little girl of three years"—who probably was his own daughter, Helene: "[W]hen directly asked by her mother as to the cause of her fear of bees, she explained with many contradictions that she wanted to go into the bee's body and yet again not to go in" (14n.1).

In other words, Helene wanted—and, at the same time, didn't want—to return to the safety and security of her mother's womb. Observing Helene's ambivalent behavior may have planted the seeds for what Rank later came to call the expression of willing and counter-willing in the therapeutic setting, when patients learn how to navigate the narrow channel between regress and progress, the will to merge, staying embedded in the womb of therapy, and the even more urgent will to separate, and realize themselves as independent.

"Relationship therapy," observes Susan Lanzoni (2018) in *Empathy: A History*, "required what Rank called 'conscious empathic identification'—a studied attunement to the client's spontaneous living and feeling, conveyed with an awareness of radical acceptance" (140).

When did Rank invent the principles of relationship therapy? No one can be certain, but in 1919, deeply moved by the pregnancy of his wife, Tola, Rank

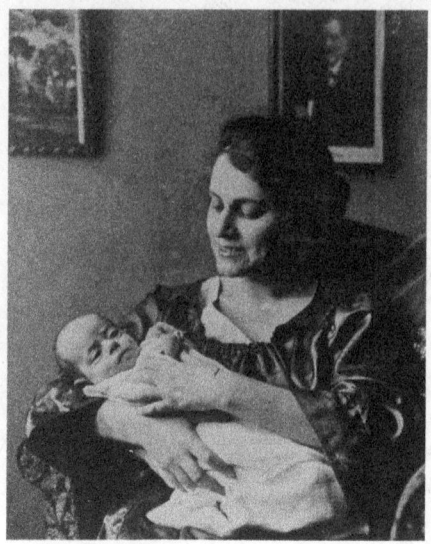

Figure 9.2 Tola Rank holding her newborn, Helene—named after Helen of Troy—with photo of Freud behind her, 1919

Credit: Ruhama Veltfort for the Estate of Otto Rank

shared with Ernest Jones (1957) his growing appreciation that "the essence of life was the relation between mother and child" (58).

In 1921, at the Vienna Psychoanalytic Society, Otto Rank gave a lecture "on the relation between married partners; they, he maintained, always repeated in essence those between mother and child (on both sides alternately)" (ibid.), an idea that was unheard of in psychoanalysis before Rank conceived it. Each partner projects the experiences of his or her own mother-child relation on the other and simultaneously identifies with the other's projections, generating a continual circuit of feelings.

Jones and Abraham, rivals of Rank and Ferenczi on the Secret Committee, were opposed to this idea, now widely accepted in couples and family systems therapy, as well as to Rank's earlier remark that "the essence of life was the relationship between mother and child."

From 1921 through 1924, Ferenczi and Rank collaborated to overcome Freud's pessimistic conclusion, as he told Ferenczi (1932), that "psychoanalysis as a therapy may be worthless" (186).

Freud often deprecated therapy in private conversations with members of the Secret Committee, but would dangle its benefits before an unsuspecting public, who, he knew, would not pay for psychoanalytic treatment if they learned that Freud secretly believed it to be worthless, merely an opportunity for scientific research into the unconscious and to obtain an income from the fees of patients.

In 1924, simultaneously with the publication of *The Trauma of Birth*, Ferenczi and Rank had argued in *The Development of Psychoanalysis* that the process of healing occurs only in a genuine relationship between therapist and patient. An authentic relationship in the here-and-now is the locus of healing, with empathy at its core.

The arid requirement for emotional distance during "scientific" investigation of the patient's Oedipal unconscious, had led to "an unnatural elimination of all human factors in the analysis," wrote Ferenczi and Rank (1924:40–41), marking the beginnings of what would later be termed *humanistic psychology*.

The simultaneous publication of *The Trauma of Birth* and *The Development of Psychoanalysis* was part of a political campaign by Ferenczi and Rank to shake up the Secret Committee—and make the analytic community worldwide realize that acting coldly, unfeelingly, was not a helpful way to practice therapy.

The German title of Ferenczi and Rank's book was *Entwicklungsziele der Psychoanalyse*, rendered as *The Development of Psychoanalysis* in the English translation by Caroline Newton, an American social worker who'd been in relationship therapy with Rank in Vienna.

But a more accurate translation would have been: *The Developmental Aims of Psychoanalysis*. "Why are we doing therapy in the first place?," Ferenczi and Rank were asking in their joint book. What kinds of feelings will patients be experiencing, in their relationship with us, during therapy? What, exactly, are the *developmental* rather than the *research* aims of psychoanalysis?

The purpose of their work was to contest the idea, held by Freud, that the aim of psychoanalysis was research into the Oedipal unconscious rather than healing, which, Freud informed Ferenczi and Rank and others in the inner circle was impossible anyway. "What we criticized in our joint work," Rank told Freud, "was just that any analytical therapist could, as researcher, over-extend his analyses, causing them to fail therapeutically" (Lieberman & Kramer 2012:189).

Neither Ferenczi nor Rank was ready to accept Freud's "therapeutic nihilism," as Ferenczi (1932:93), in his *Clinical Diary*, termed Freud's disparaging attitude toward therapy.

However, because Ferenczi was extremely reluctant to challenge Freud, Rank took the lead in conceptualizing new approaches to the practice of psychoanalysis. As a prolific author, Rank was the senior partner in their collaboration.[3]

At the center of their campaign to save psychoanalysis from Freud's "therapeutic nihilism" was Rank's revolutionary new work, *The Trauma of Birth*, which focused on the powerful role of mothers in our emotional life, a role Freud had ignored in his Oedipal theorizing.[4]

Without Ferenczi's support, Rank knew that Jones and Abraham would defeat him in what was turning out to be a fierce battle inside the Secret Committee over the future of psychoanalysis. Transference versus relationship? An unfeeling analyst versus an empathic one?

All relationship therapy is "active," Rank (1924) had argued in *The Trauma of Birth*, and "purposes an effect through volitional [*willkürliche*] influence and a change resulting from it" (203)—the seeds of what Rank would later call *will therapy*.

The Trauma of Birth was also Rank's first, sketchy exposition of *Lebensangst* and *Todesangst*—life fear and death fear, which later became the core principle of his *existential therapy*.

At the moment of birth, proposed Rank, each new arrival on the planet emerges to find its first object, mother, only promptly to lose her again: the primal anxiety.

The word anxiety (*Angst*) derives from the Latin *angere*, which means "to squeeze or strangle"—suggesting the fear of strangulation that the newborn inevitably feels as its tiny, fragile body is squeezed out into the air, experiencing a peristaltic crush, gasping for a flow of oxygen that it has never had to breathe in before. Both mother and fetus face the prospect of death during the birthing process.

The newborn, maintains Rank, suffers *separation anxiety* the moment it is thrust out of the womb, whether through natural birth or Caesarean section, facing the possibility of strangulation by its umbilical cord and of not getting enough oxygen into its raw lungs to survive.

This is the physiological trauma of birth. The term "separation anxiety" did not exist at that time in the vocabulary of psychoanalysis, focused as it was solely on "castration anxiety."

Because of "the change from a highly pleasurable situation to an extremely painful one," adds Rank (1924) in *The Trauma of Birth*, "[the newborn] immediately acquires a 'psychical' quality of feeling" (187). The trauma of separation at birth is more than physiological; it is a psychological trauma as well.

The anxiety of experiencing *difference* for the first time is felt acutely during the process of being born. It is "*the first psychical content* of which the human being is conscious" (50; italics in the original)—heralding what Rank later termed his *psychology of difference*.

The tiny creature has been thrown into life. Suddenly, it feels alone, helpless, fragile, vulnerable—and experiences in its body, pre-verbally, what Kierkegaard memorably called "fear and trembling."

Separation brings suffering. The trauma of birth—from Greek, *trauma*, "wound"—is an original wound and the birth of existential loneliness.

To be born is forever to be fragile, vulnerable, and lonely. Only love can heal the feeling of loneliness that difference evokes in the tiny, trembling creature forced out of its warm, protective home into a cold alien world.

In psychotherapy, argues Rank, the mother-child relationship ought to be the template for the encounter between patient and analyst, who unite in deep sharing in order for the patient, during the end phase, to learn how to bear the anxiety of separating with less suffering than before.

The therapist is a Socratic practioner of "midwifery," says Rank (1924) in *The Trauma of Birth* (181). By overcoming his own birth trauma, Socrates "establishes his claim to be the forerunner of Psychoanalysis" (182).

$$\clubsuit$$

The trauma of birth is transmuted by culture into the myth of "the Fall," the story of Adam and Eve's expulsion from the Garden of Eden, where loneliness, self-consciousness, anxiety, guilt, and death do not exist.

With birth the feeling of Oneness, of wholeness, that was experienced by the fetus in the womb is lost. We seek for a lifetime to regain, no matter how circuitously, the lost feeling of Oneness we felt in Eden.

"[T]he whole process of culture," maintains Rank (1924) in *The Trauma of Birth*, "as reflected in myths, is only a human creation of the world on the pattern of one's own individual creation" (85–86).

A ceaseless yearning for Oneness, he adds, is a major impetus for the creation of art, music, myth, poetry, religion, and philosophy—in other words, for all of culture. Culture is everything that does not exist in nature. Culture serves as a shield against the existential anxiety of loneliness, according to Rank, and creates a humanly significant world.

"Not only is the patient always conscious that the cure must one day be finished," says Rank, "but every single hour demands from him the repetition in miniature of the fixation and severance, till he is in the position finally to carry it through" (215) at the end phase—which is a triumph of spiritual rebirth, hard-won, but nevertheless an expression of self-determination.

The trauma of birth, writes Rank, ends only with the trauma of death, which is the final separation and the final union. "Everyone born sinks back again into the womb from which he or she once came into the realm of light" (114).

Since the first home of every human being is the womb, the relationship the fetus has with its mother, argues Rank, serves as an unconscious model for all our other relationships during the rest of our lives—within therapy, the family, friendship, love, marriage, the group, the village, the city, the organization, and the nation-state.

All these relationships, according to Peter Sloterdijk (1998), the most important philosopher in Germany today after Jürgen Habermas, are external recreations of the spherical womb—what Sloterdijk coined the term "spherology" to characterize.

Many philosophers, most notably Martin Heidegger, have focused on death as the foundational problem of human existence. However, because human life begins at birth, "*natality*," proposes Hannah Arendt (1998) in *The Human Condition*, "not *mortality* may be the central category of political, as distinguished from metaphysical, thought" (9; italics added).

Each person "is unique," adds Arendt, "so that with each birth something uniquely new comes into the world. With respect to this somebody who is unique it can be said that nobody was there before" (178). About the mystery of birth, a new being arriving on the planet from Nowhere and Nothing, she observes: "the new, therefore, always appears in the guise of a miracle" (ibid.).

In *The Life of the Mind*, Arendt (1978) attacks psychoanalysis, which, she argues, "discovers no more than the ever-changing moods, the ups and downs of psychic life" and whose "results and discoveries are neither particularly appealing nor very meaningful in themselves" (35).

Indeed, for Arendt, "the *monotonous sameness* and *pervasive ugliness* so highly characteristic of the findings" of Freud (who is not named in her text, but is clearly meant) contrast "so obviously" with the "enormous variety and richness" of each individual (ibid., italics added). Psychoanalysis is, as Rank emphasized, a psychology of likeness rather than a psychology of difference.

Freud, suggests Arendt, had neither a theory of natality nor a theory of creativity, the two being correlates of each other. For Arendt, the greatest political theorist of the 20th century, the nation-state is an extension, a grand symbolic disguise in non-bodily form, of the womb. The word "nation" comes from the Latin, *nasci*: "to give birth," which is why so many nation-states refer to themselves as the "motherland."

Willing, argues Arendt (1998) in *The Human Condition*, is ontologically rooted in natality and the "web of human relationships" (184) in which we are embedded, beginning with our time inside the womb.

One of the reasons Arendt wrote *The Human Condition* was to criticize her former lover, Martin Heidegger, who, in his single-minded obsession with death, had ignored the awe-inspiring miracle of birth, a mystery beyond the capacity of science or philosophy to understand.

According to Arendt, Heidegger—whose name, like Freud's, she does not mention in *The Human Condition*—was as patriarchal as Freud was. Arendt's *The Life of the Mind* contains two volumes, *Thinking* and *Willing*. There's no evidence that Arendt read Rank, but her vocabulary—"natality," "web of human relationships," "willing"—echoes that of Rank.

Psychoanalyst Julia Kristeva (2001) observes that Arendt rejected Freud "to save the freedom of the 'who' at the heart of an optimal political plurality, and to not hand it over to some uncontrollable unconscious" (67), a position diametrically opposed to Freudians like literary critic Jacqueline Rose.

As we saw in Chapter 3, Rose remains willing to hand over the freedom of the "who"—as expressed in the exercise of self-leadership, and, indeed, in all of political life—to the *Todestrieb,* the death drive, which "could be said to sabotage once and for all the vision of man in control of his mind" (quoted in Sehgal 2023:18).

In *Better Never to Have Been: The Harm of Coming Into Existence,* the anti-natalist philosopher David Benatar (2006) argues that, due to the pain and suffering of human existence, we would've been better off never having been born, an argument first made by the ancient Greek philosophers.

However, like these male philosophers, all of whom minimized or dismissed the mutual love obtainable within a genuine relationship, Benatar elides the obvious fact that the lives we *share with others* make our existence meaningful, even in the face of death.

In *Being Born: Birth and Philosophy,* Alison Stone (2019), a female philosopher at Lancaster University in the U.K., provides a systematic account of how philosophers have ignored mothers and birth throughout the history of Western thought.

Stone resonates strongly with the relational theme at the core of Rank's *The Trauma of Birth,* taking from him "an insight into the lasting power in our lives of a kind of separation anxiety" (19). She asserts:

> [O]ur condition is one of *relational mortality.* Because our selves and personalities are relational through and through—because we are born—our deaths, too, are relational and shade into one another continuously. A more individualistic view is that my own death and the deaths of others are radically different; one version of that view is found in Heidegger's *Being and Time.* (6; italics in the original)

Disputing Heidegger's proposition that we die alone, Alison Stone writes of "relational mortality" in terms that Otto Rank and Hannah Arendt would have endorsed:

> I argue instead that each individual's death is bound up with the deaths of the others with whom that individual has had close relationships—so that if one of these others dies, then a part of me dies, while when I die, part of those others dies too: death is always shared. Consequently, my death and those of others are to be feared because these deaths spell the end of our relationships, the point when we will be separated forever. (ibid.)

In a 1938 lecture at the University of Minnesota, Rank (1996) explains how a succession of separations marks all of human life, starting with separation at birth and ending with separation at death. An inability to bear the anxiety of separation plays a significant role in human suffering. Only through an authentic relationship, he argues, can the suffering that commences at birth be relieved, even if only temporarily:

[T]he capacity to separate is one of life's major functions. Life in itself is a mere succession of separations, beginning with birth, going on through several weaning periods and the development of the individual personality, and finally culminating in death—which represents the final separation.

... In the process of adaptation, man persistently separates from his old self, or at least from those segments of his old self that are now outlived. Like a child who has outgrown a toy, he discards the old parts of himself for which he has no further use. . . . The ego continually breaks away from its worn-out parts, which were of value in the past but have no value in the present.

The neurotic, however, is unable to accomplish this normal detachment process. He cannot live through and emancipate himself from the various fundamental separation stages in life.

Owing to fear or guilt generated in the assertion of his own autonomy, he is unable to free himself. . . . He stays fixated, so to speak, upon a particular worn-out part of his past that he cannot sever himself, and his whole present behavior is directed and symbolized in terms of this *unaccomplished* separation. (270; italics in the original)

Summing up his philosophy of healing, Rank says that a mutual relationship is essential to allow vulnerable human beings to feel more whole, more connected to others and to themselves. "Simply speaking, this is the definition of relationship: one individual is helping the other to develop and grow, without infringing too much on the other's personality" (271).

10

Feelings

Otto Rank was among the first psychoanalysts to use their own feelings as an instrument to register—and empathize with—the suffering of their patients. "He was a very tender person, an extremely devoted one," said his wife Tola Rank, an eminent psychoanalyst in her own right. "And he was always wrapped up in his deep feelings" (quoted in Lieberman 1985:201).

In 1924, at the time of publication of *The Development of Psychoanalysis* and *The Trauma of Birth*, analysts around the world held to Freud's view that the feelings experienced by patients during the therapeutic hour were transferred from their past: they were not real.

"Rank," said psychoanalyst Clara Thompson, "was the first to point out that in doing this the patient was led away from the living present, the area of real feeling" (quoted in Lieberman 1985:237). Of all the members on the Secret Committee, only Ferenczi accepted Rank's view.

"I like Rank's sadness," said Anaïs Nin (1966), "his tenacity, his caring about people. He cares. He cares tremendously about everything" (336). In his consulting room, Rank responded authentically, not as a blank screen. He did not "hide relevant feelings from the patient" (Lieberman 1985:xxxvii). He held his ground and stayed connected.

In a book never translated into English, Rank (1928) explores at length the varieties and gradations of feeling. As the epigraph to a chapter entitled "Feeling and Denial," Rank quotes Goethe: "*Gefühl ist alles*"—"feeling is all" (75).

"Psychoanalysis has contributed relatively little to understanding the emotional life," observes Rank; "in the psychoanalytic literature [the word 'feeling'] is scarcely used, although in essence our whole emotional life rests on feelings and is directed by feelings" (ibid.). Typically, Rank used the words "emotion" and "feeling" interchangeably.

By attuning himself to the feelings that flowed, in a circuit of projection and identification, between a client and himself, Rank was transgressing the norms of psychoanalytic practice. In the Vienna of the 1920s, remembers psychoanalyst Margaret Mahler, "it was anathema even to speak of analysis with emotion, much less infuse one's therapeutic work with emotion. A good analyst, an 'insider analyst,' could not show *any* emotion under *any* circumstances" (quoted in Stepansky 1988:81–82; italics in the original).

Otto Rank and the Creation of Modern Psychotherapy. Robert Kramer, Oxford University Press.
© Robert Kramer (2025). DOI: 10.1093/9780197698303.003.0010

"The characteristic of that time," recalls Sándor Radó, who was in analysis with Karl Abraham from 1922 to 1925, "was a *neglect of a human being's emotional life*. Everybody was looking for oral, pregenital, and genital components in motivation. But that some people are happy, others unhappy, some afraid, or full of anger, and some loving and affectionate—read the case histories to find out how such *differences* between people were then absent from the literature" (quoted in Roazen & Swerdloff 1995:82–83; italics added). The analyst's "listening to the patient as well as the patient's production of thoughts were oriented by theories" (78), rather than the feelings of either one in the here-and-now.

Rank and Ferenczi maintained that the feelings of patients were being discounted by analysts who were rigidly following Freud's recommendations to behave coldly like a "surgeon." Empathy, according to Rank, is based on identification with the other. No other emotion is more capable of helping us feel, at a deep level, what another person is feeling. "[F]eeling reacts most of all to feeling and is influenced by it," Rank (1932b) wrote in *Modern Education* (71).

As Ferenczi (1932) confided to his *Clinical Diary*, patients had reproached him: "You don't believe me! You don't take seriously what I tell you! I cannot accept your sitting there unfeeling and indifferent while I am straining to call up some tragic event from my childhood" (1). The major obstacle to healing, according to Ferenczi, was *"Insensitivity* [Fühllosigkeit] *of the analyst"* (ibid., italics in the original).

In *Truth and Reality*, Rank (1936b) noted that Freud "scarcely approached the problem of the emotional life" (16–17). Going one step further than Ferenczi, in *Will Therapy* Rank (1936a) criticized Freud for reducing *all* feelings to a derivative, however disguised, of sexuality: "[T]he emotional life develops from the sexual sphere; therefore [Freud's] sexualization in reality means emotionalization" (233).

"Libido," Freud (1921) had written, "is an expression taken from the theory of the emotions" (90). Emotion or libido is the cause of neurotic disorder. Increases in emotion, according to Freud, are unpleasurable. Analysis, said Freud, means "working through" and eventually uprooting, to the extent possible, the unruly feelings of the patient. Feelings are irrational. The analyst makes the unconscious conscious by providing cognitive insight (i.e., "transference interpretations") to the patient, thereby subduing the pressing drive for the irrational to emerge from the patient's unconscious.

The confusion between sexuality and emotions extended throughout the 20th century, and continues, even today, among many psychoanalysts. "Emotions have long been seen as less than fully real, as mere epiphenomena, as derivative from those essential motivators, the instinctual drives," explains psychoanalyst Donna Orange (1995). "Since emotion signified trouble, a psychoanalytic cure meant *reducing* or *eliminating emotion*. Making the unconscious conscious, full of cognitive insight, should render emotional signals from the unconscious almost unnecessary" (89; italics added).

Since 1939, the year of Freud's death, scores of articles in the official psychoanalytic journals have lamented the absence of a psychoanalytic theory of feelings or emotions (Weinstein 2001:15–51), but no progress was ever made. The chorus included such distinguished analysts as Marjorie Brierly, David Rapaport, Bertram Lewin, Ernst Kris, Charles Brenner, Jacob Arlow, John Gedo, Leo Rangell, Edith Jacobson, Arnold Modell, Frank Lachmann, Robert Stolorow, Michael Franz Basch, Ethel Spector Person, John Munder Ross, and Adrian Applegarth.

"Fifty years after Brierly's statement [in 1937], William Meissner noted that the psychoanalytic psychology of affective experience remains to be written" (40). Such critiques persist.

In 2023, a leading psychoanalyst in the U.K. wrote: "One of my children around the end of her second year came walking through the kitchen at breakfast time with a breezy air and announced, 'I feel happy.' I was struck by a child so young having words for feelings" (Hinshelwood 2023:xiii). Yet, in the same breath, seemingly without realizing that he was indicting his field for its continuing failure to understand feelings, this same writer adds: "Despite psychoanalysts lacking a theory of affects, here is a two-year-old who had herself a rudimentary theory" (xv). A two-year-old has a theory of feelings but— psychoanalysis now over 125 years old—does not? How, one wonders, could this be possible?

The answer goes back to Freud's own extreme distrust of feelings. Writing in his *Clinical Diary*, Ferenczi (1932) points to the "[p]ersonal causes for the erroneous development of psychoanalysis" (184):

> One learned from [Freud] and from his kind of technique various things that made one's life and work more comfortable: the *calm, unemotional reserve*; the unruffled assurance that one knew better; and the theories, the seeking and finding of the causes of failure in the patient instead of partly in ourselves … and finally the pessimistic view, shared with only a trusted few, that neurotics are a rabble, good only to support us financially and to allow us to learn from their cases: psychoanalysis as a therapy may be worthless. (185–186; italics added)

Although patients provided the means to support him and his family financially, Freud disparaged the practice of psychoanalysis. At various times, in addition to calling patients "negroes," Freud called them *Narren* (nuts), *Gesindel* (rabble) and *Quälgeister* (pests). "To Binswanger's question about his position towards his patients, Freud answered: 'I could wring their necks, all of them'" (quoted in Falzeder 2016:94). To Karl Abraham, Freud explained: "[T]hose cases in which

I took an excessive personal interest failed, perhaps just because of the intensity of feeling" (quoted in Freud & Ferenczi 1993:xxxv).

In *Freud's Patients: A Book of Lives*, Mikkel Borch-Jacobsen (2021) presents the most detailed documentation of Freud's clinical practice ever published: "[W]ith a few ambiguous exceptions, such as the treatments of Ernst Lanzer, Bruno Walter and Albert Hirst," concludes Borch-Jacobsen, "Freud's cures were largely ineffectual, when they were not downright destructive" (9).

Ideologically committed to positivism, Freud's lifetime mission was to conquer feelings—which he saw as irrational—for science. According to Rank (1941a), writing in *Beyond Psychology*, "From the point of view of [Freud's] rational psychology, 'feminine' traits of emotionalism appear 'irrational,' whereas in reality they represent human qualities of a positive nature" (241).

As Anna Freud told Max Eitingon, describing her own nearly four years of analysis with her father—which focused on his attempts to eradicate her lesbian desires—"Papa always makes it clear that he would like to know me as much more rational and lucid than the girls and women he gets to know during his analytic hours, with all their moods, dissatisfactions and passionate idiosyncrasies" (quoted in Young-Bruehl 1988:156).

Never mentioning the I–Thou relationship anywhere, Freud speaks in the terminology of I–It: *wo Es war, soll Ich werden*: where It was, there I shall become. "It is a work of culture—not unlike the draining of the Zuider Zee" (Freud 1933:80), which was completed in 1930 for the purpose of building an enormous dike to keep out North Sea flooding in the Netherlands.

What did Freud mean by analogizing the aim of therapy to the draining of the Zuider Zee? In *Beyond Psychology*, Rank (1941a) explains that Freud, "by comparing his achievement to the drainage of the Zuider Zee as a piece of progressive engineering, prided himself on having made it 'psychological,' that is, of having brought it, so to speak, under the individual's control" (39).

Baffled by the appeal of psychoanalysis as a therapy, Harold Bloom (1991) observes, "I take it that a successful [psychoanalysis] is an oxymoron. I do not know anyone who has ever benefited from Freudian or any other mode of analysis, except for being, to use the popular trope for it, so badly shrunk, that they became quite dried out. That is to say, all passion spent" (200)—like the draining of the Zuider Zee.

Although Freud (1937) conceded in "Analysis Terminable and Interminable" that even a "thorough analysis" could never drain *all* feelings, he retained a deep-seated "hostility" (Gay 1988:537) to feelings, which, since they derived, no matter how disguised, from "the It," *das Es*, he insisted were irrational— just as his women patients, like his own daughter, Anna, with "all their moods, dissatisfactions and passionate idiosyncrasies," were, at bottom, irrational.

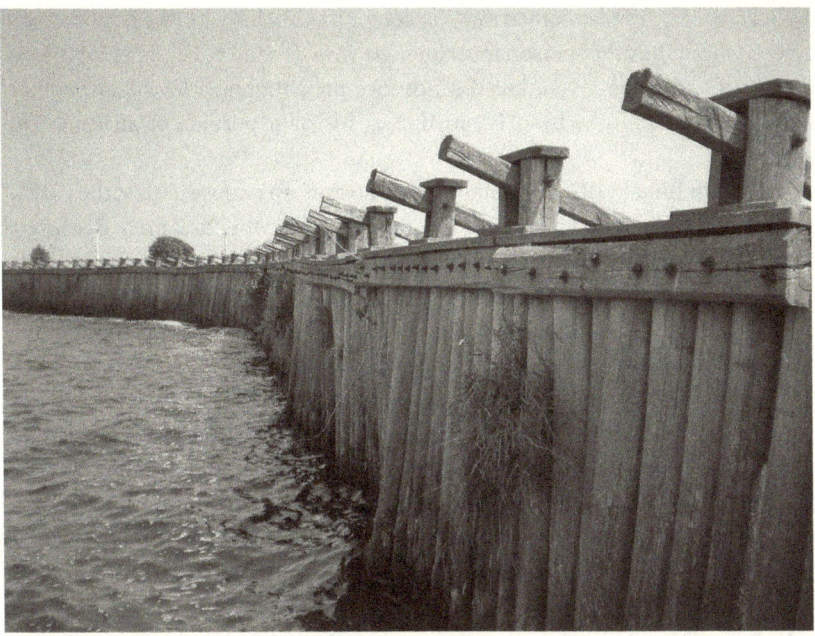

Figure 10.1 The Zuider Zee dam

Credit: Photograph by Atsje via Wikimedia Commons. Reproduced under a CC BY-SA 3.0 license

"In place of a reciprocal, 'personal' communication within an I-Thou relationship," said psychiatrist Ludwig Binswanger (1942), "we find a one-sided—irreversible—relationship between doctor and patient, and an even more impersonal relationship between researcher and the object of research" (62).

In *The Question of Lay Analysis*, Freud (1926b) insisted on an "inseparable bond between cure and research" (256). By equating the two, countered Rank, Freud justified his failures as a therapist since he could always claim he'd found something new about the Oedipal unconscious in his research, even if the patient never got better.

Psychoanalytic technique requires *Indifferenz*, Freud said—the analyst's "indifference" to the suffering of the patient. "We must see to it," added Freud, "cruel as it may sound, that the sufferings of the patient . . . do not come to an end prematurely" (quoted in Gay 1988:304).

The word *Indifferenz*, although translated as "neutrality" in the three places it appears in the *Standard Edition* of Freud's writings, has a more callous connotation than "neutrality." According to Freud scholar Ernst Falzeder (personal communication), "if Freud had meant 'neutrality' in the benevolent or non-intrusive sense, he would have used the perfectly adequate German word *Neutralität*."

To Ferenczi, Freud enjoined that the doctor must behave as "the perfectly cool object, whom the other person must lovingly woo" (Freud & Ferenczi 1993:468). Freud wanted to be loved, but did not love his patients, a love that Ferenczi sought, unsuccessfully, from Freud during his own periods of analysis with him.

As Martin Buber (1923) maintained, the doctor can choose to treat the patient as an *It* or a *Thou*. Freud mandated that doctors treat patients as an *It*. Because of the necessity of a power imbalance, the analyst and patient were to be physically together but otherwise engaged in an *I–It*, not *I–Thou*, relationship.

The premise was that analysts, as objective researchers into the Oedipal unconscious, know more about the psyches of patients than the patients do themselves. Transference is *power over*—not *power with*—patients.

Freud (1912) urged "emotional coldness" (115) in analysts, who needed, he said, to model themselves on the surgeon. Pointing to this admonition, a lodestar for generations of analysts, Rank observes in a 1927 lecture at the University of Pennsylvania School of Social Work that Freud's "[s]urgical therapy is uprooting and isolates the individual emotionally, as it tries to *deny* the emotional life" (Rank 1996:169; italics in the original).

In *Beyond Psychology*, Rank (1941a) adds: "In respecting emotional expression as a positive will manifestation without condemning it as 'resistance,' I shifted the emphasis from the individual's past to his present self, thereby allowing it a much more active role than that of merely being an object upon which the therapist operates [like a surgeon]" (49–50).

Although Freud argued for "emotional coldness," Rank knew that he routinely violated his own prescriptions and, at times, even invited patients to dinner, gave them gifts, engaged in spirited exchanges, joked, and gossiped during the analytic hour. Freud "did not himself live up to the proclaimed ideals that he held aloft for others" (Roazen 1995:xxii). According to Freud scholar Ulrike May (2018), Freud followed no technical rules, showing a cold side to patients he didn't like and a warm side to patients he did, even those who thought psychoanalysis to be worthless. Freud regularly showed both sides to the same patient.

In the only detailed account of how Freud worked before he was diagnosed with cancer in 1923, Freud is seen as "suggestive and seductive, and partly also very active, but at the same time he kept his distance in the analysis, as he did in most cases" (Koellruter 2016:66).

No matter how inconsistently Freud practiced psychotherapy, for decades the feelings experienced by patients in the here-and-now were dismissed by analysts as irrelevant to the treatment. The patient's feelings were not real; they were "transferred" from the past and needed to be interpreted as such. Moreover, the analyst's feelings were also not real, dubbed "counter-transference," and needed to be expunged through a "training analysis" that was to be continued for the rest of life.

In the mid-1950s, Anna Freud cautiously offered what she called "technically subversive thoughts" about the "real relationship" between patient and analyst:

> With due respect for the necessary strictest handling and interpretation of the transference, I still feel that somewhere we should leave room for the realization that analyst and patient are also two people, of equal adult status, in a real personal relationship to each other. I wonder whether our—*at times complete*—neglect of this side of the matter is not responsible for some of the hostile reactions which we get from our patients and which we are apt to ascribe to "true transference" only. But these are technically subversive thoughts and ought to be "handled with care." (Freud A. 1954:373; italics added)

In 1974 Anna Freud criticized relationship therapy for contradicting her father's approach to psychoanalysis, which was based solely on "conflict within the individual person . . . aims, ideas, and ideals battling with the drives to keep the individual within a civilized community." Psychoanalysis, she added, should not "water this down to every individual's longing for perfect unity with his mother, i.e., to be loved only as an infant can be loved. There is an enormous amount that gets lost this way" (quoted in Young-Bruehl 1988:457).

Almost 40 years later, social worker Steven Kuchuck (2021), president of the International Association for Relational Psychoanalysis and Psychotherapy, said: "I had early teachers and supervisors stress the importance of making sure that emotions never registered on my face. . . . Although less and less emphasized by many, it is still an essential goal for some analysts" (25–26).

At a time when Freudians were deriding the feeling-oriented curriculum of the University of Pennsylvania School of Social Work for being "anti-Oedipal," Rank, Jessie Taft, and Virginia Robinson were teaching their students the principles of relationship therapy. They were also teaching them how to become self-empowered, drawing on their own feelings, while simultaneously helping clients—most of whom were minority or female or both—find the creative will within themselves to break the chains of what Rank (1941a) in *Beyond Psychology* called the "masculine ideology" (235–270) of psychoanalysis.

In *The Free World: Art and Thought in the Cold War*, Louis Menand (2021) wonders about the sway of masculine ideology in America during the better part of the 20th century. "Why that ideology was so powerful and its effects so widespread, why men of every political view and in every walk of life seem to have subscribed to it, is one of the enigmas of postwar American history"

(543). Menand identifies three culprits for enforcing "the regime of subordi-nation" (548): patriarchy, sexism, and misogyny, but manages to overlook an obvious one—Sigmund Freud.

During the period Menand is writing about, many of the most influential academics and opinion leaders were mesmerized by the writings of Freud, whose ideas about women held sway among vast swathes of American intel-lectuals. Some analysts, writes historian of psychoanalysis Eli Zaretsky (2015), "wielded terms like *femininity, the mother,* and *vaginal orgasm* as weapons against assertive women" (31; italics in the original).

For example, psychoanalyst Benjamin Spock's *The Common Sense Book of Baby and Child Care* advocated that mothers stay at home to take care of their kids instead of working outside the home. Dr. Spock's book, Menand (2021) reports, "sold 18.5 million copies between 1946 and 1964" (545), during a period when male Freudian psychoanalysts occupied the chairs of virtually every psychiatry department in American medical schools.

By the 1930s, adds Zaretsky (2004), Dr. Spock "had stopped practicing anal-ysis because of his disquiet over an 'intensely feministic' female patient who 'argued fiercely against every interpretation for over two years'" (327).

Spock refused to affirm or even acknowledge a woman's will emerging inside the analytic setting in the form of counter-will, treating it, instead, as "resis-tance" to be overcome or as an expression of "penis envy." Spock believed that women, by resisting his interpretations, didn't *want* to get better—an unconscious expression of the *Todestrieb*, the death drive.

"[T]he professional conflicts between a male-dominated [Freudian] psychi-atry and female social workers," notes historian of humanistic psychology Roy deCarvalho (1999), "were crucial in the dissemination of Rank's psychological thought and the early popularity of [Carl] Rogers" (132).

Society has never held Freud accountable for turning his back on women patients who pleaded with him to take their cries of sexual trauma seriously. Freud refused to listen to their feelings. Instead, he constructed an *entirely* male-focused developmental theory that ignored the three most important stages of every woman's life: menstruation, pregnancy, and menopause.[1]

Following Freud's neglect of these issues, psychoanalysts remain virtually oblivious to them—up to the present. According to psychoanalyst Michael Moskowitz (2014), in Freud's theory "the generic human being happens to be a white male."

A century ago, Otto Rank criticized the gaping hole in Freud's understand-ing of women. The psychoanalytic theory of sexuality, Rank (1924) said in *The Trauma of Birth*, "has given predominance to the man's point of view and has almost entirely neglected the woman's. . . . [A]s a rule, we tacitly represent the sexual relations only from the man's point of view . . . from an insufficient understanding of the woman's sexual life" (36–37).

Drawing on Rank's teachings about the patriarchal bias of psychoanalysis, Jessie Taft and Virginia Robinson learned from him that, in Freud's Oedipal narrative, women had no will, power, or identity of their own. Silhouetted against an omnipotent father-figure, the mothers of Anna O., Little Hans, Dora, the Rat Man, and the Wolf Man—the most famous cases of Freud—were not persons with wills of their own.

"There is a pre-Rank vision," notes Anaïs Nin (1966), who understood that Rank's introduction of the creative will had offered women a psychology of self-empowerment and strength, "and there is an after-Rank perspective" (290).

In an essay entitled "Sons and Daughters," penned in the late 1920s, Rank (1989) writes of "the daughter who stands up for her own right by opposing her father's will after a conventional marriage"—not an attitude that Freud would have countenanced with his own lesbian daughter, Anna. Rank adds:

> We can find antecedents of a daughter's revolt against the father, for instance, in Samuel Richardson's *Clarissa* (1748), and in Jean-Jacques Rousseau's *Nouvelle Héloïse* [1761]. Most recently the subject was treated in Rudolph Besier's popular play, *The Barretts of Wimpole Street* (1931), which centers upon the love of Elizabeth Barrett for Robert Browning, who eventually rescues her from the house, or one might say from the clutches, of an inhuman, tyrannical father. (61)

"*Was will das Weib?*," Freud had asked Princess Marie Bonaparte in 1925, at the height of his battle with Rank over *The Trauma of Birth*: "What does a woman want?" (Jones 1955:421).

Rank (1936b) answered in *Truth and Reality*: "The emotional tone is an index of the '*what*' of the will" (48; italics added). Returning to Freud's question in his last book, *Beyond Psychology*, Rank (1941a) added: "She has always wanted, and still wants first and foremost to be a woman, because this and this alone is her fundamental self and expresses her personality, no matter what else she may do or achieve" (254).

It's not surprising, therefore, that female social workers felt so strongly empowered by Rank's will therapy. Moreover, these women greatly appreciated that, in *The Trauma of Birth*, Rank was the first psychoanalyst to focus a spotlight on pregnancy and childbirth. The pregnant body had received no attention by analysts before Rank.

In *Women's Bodies in Psychoanalysis*, Rosemary Balsam (2012), Yale clinical professor of psychiatry, shows how the "vanished pregnant body" (31–54) has barely begun to be seen in psychoanalytic theorizing. "Rank's ability to draw attention to childbirth as a central bodily female experience and a vital trope in our own minds is surely a highly valuable vision" (Balsam 2013:713).

Along with Karen Horney (1924) and a few others, Rank tried to prevent "the war against women" (Lament et al. 2016) in Freud's making of psychoanalytic theory. "Psychoanalysis has both waged 'hot' war on women overtly and 'cold' war covertly over the years," writes Balsam (2016), "by colluding with cultural stereotypes offered as 'theory,' starting with Freud and his Viennese circle" (83). The war waged over the years against Rank by Freudians was the same war they waged against women.

In *Three Essays on The Theory of Sexuality*, Freud (1905) went so far as to claim that "libido is invariably and necessarily of a masculine nature, whether it occurs in men or women" (218), a claim he maintained throughout his life.

In the midst of his "David and Goliath" conflict with Rank, Freud (1925) published an essay entitled "Some Psychic Consequences of the Anatomical Difference Between the Sexes," in which he asserted that "the elimination of clitoridal sexuality is a necessary precondition for the development of femininity" (255).

Freud added: "I cannot evade the notion (though I hesitate to give it expression) that for women the level of what is ethically normal is different from what it is in men. Their super-ego is never so inexorable, so impersonal, so independent of its emotional origins as we require it to be in men" (257).

These and similar remarks led Rank—along with Ferenczi—to conclude that Freud showed no "more insight than a little boy" (Freud & Ferenczi 2000:444) when it came to understanding mothers and women in general. In other respects, of course, Rank considered Freud an intellectual giant, a superb rhetorician, whose greatness as a master of the German language he could only envy.

In none of Freud's writings, however, was the master able to visualize erotic feelings from a woman's point of view, just as he never saw any sign of their powerful will or moral development. "The repudiation of femininity," said Freud (1937), "can be nothing else than a biological fact, a part of the great riddle of sex" (252). When Freud wrote this, Rank could only have read it as Freud's final repudiation of his own mother, Amalia, writ large.

As psychoanalyst Jill Gentile (2018) notes: "For Sigmund Freud, the repudiation of femininity was the mother of all repudiations. In one of his last and most influential essays, 'Analysis Terminable and Interminable,' written in the dark year of 1937, he identifies this repudiation as 'psychological bedrock' (for both sexes) based on the 'biological fact' of sexual difference. Men reflexively shrink from the feminine, defined for Freud by passivity and subjugation, as an expression of castration anxiety. Women, on the other hand, perversely reject

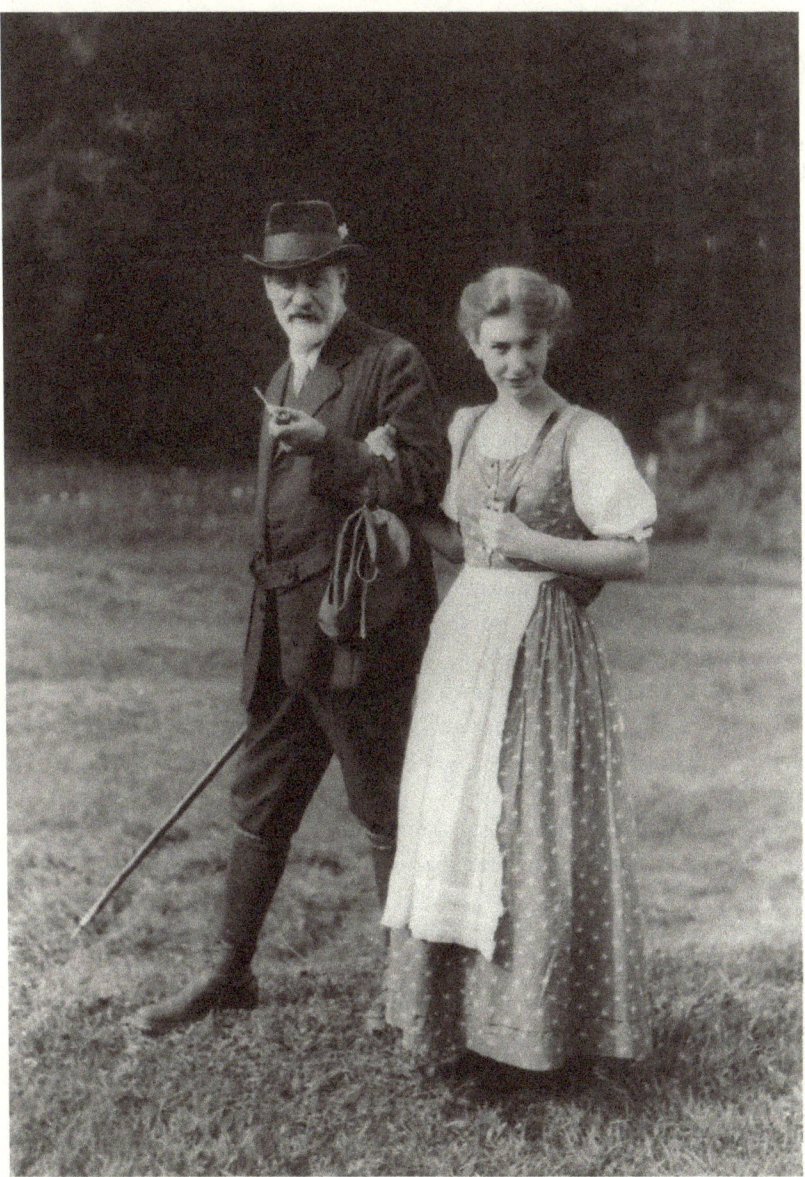

Figure 10.2 Freud and Anna, 1913

Credit: Collection Bourgeron/Bridgeman Images

femininity because it is a mark of their shame—the shame of lacking a penis" (n.p.).

Psychoanalysts Bertram Cohler and Robert Galatzer-Levy (2008) observe that "female sexuality had to forever remain unknown to Freud and his daughter" (23). They explain:

> [T]o assert female desire would have meant to disrupt the bond between Anna and Freud. Father and daughter colluded to maintain a mystery so that they might repeat the drama of Oedipus and Antigone. Both pairs of fathers and daughters could not have maintained their bond in the face of a fully avowed female genital sexuality. . . . In the case of Anna and Freud, this required a denial of the reality and intensity of ordinary female sexuality, a denial that distorted the psychoanalytic vision of women's sexuality for decades. (ibid.)

In *The Question of Lay Analysis*, which, not coincidentally, was written in the year that Rank left Vienna for Paris, Freud (1926b) admitted that "We know less about the sexual life of little girls than of boys. But we need not feel ashamed of this distinction; after all, the sexual life of women is a '*dark continent*' for psychology" (212; italics added).

But was the sexual life of women really a "dark continent" for psychology? This now famous and infamous term, which Freud wrote in English, is a trope for Africa, a trope that corresponds to Freud's denigration of his patients, most of whom were female, as "negroes."

A glance at any artwork by Gustav Klimt, Oscar Kokoschka, or Egon Schiele—which could be found in exhibition halls, galleries, or museums a short distance from *Berggasse 19*—makes it evident that Freud was unwilling to see the powerful sexuality of the females these artists were portraying so vividly in *fin-de-siècle* Vienna.

These artists depicted a range of women, oscillating between maternal and sexually provocative, sometimes blending the two in one painting. They all celebrated the sexual freedom of women. Freud never showed the slightest interest in the work of these artists, who would have been amused by Freud's puzzlement, which they certainly did not share, about the "dark continent" of female sexuality.

In 1931, a few months after the death of Freud's mother, Amalia, whose funeral in September 1930 he declined to attend, sending Anna in his place, Freud published an essay entitled "Female Sexuality."

In a letter, Rank informed Jessie Taft (1958) about an English translation of Freud's essay that was about to appear in an American psychoanalytic journal. Freud, Rank wrote drolly to Taft, has "discovered [female sexuality] only now to exist" (175). With Amalia gone, Freud could now finally find the courage to write on the subject, which the master had never approached directly before. Perhaps female sexuality was a "dark continent" only for Freud and not for psychoanalysts like Karen Horney and Otto Rank?[2]

🐦

In *Revolution in Mind: The Creation of Psychoanalysis*, George Makari (2008) claims that Freud made "an objective science of subjectivity" (4). Makari elides the fact that Freud created psychoanalysis subjectively, from his own self-analysis.

Freud taught the impossibility of self-knowledge—and he was quite right because he was speaking autobiographically. Throughout his lifelong self-analysis, Freud tragically never understood himself, or his own feelings, projecting his bewilderment onto the whole world: thus justifying the need for interminable analysis.

That Freud had no appreciation of female sexuality, even though he accepted women as psychoanalysts, renders Makari's claim of "objectivity" absurd. In what way can the misrepresentation in Freud's theory of half the human species be considered "objective science"?

Yale's Rosemary Balsam (2012), a training and supervising analyst, argues that the female's capacity to become pregnant and give birth remains breathtakingly occluded in psychoanalytic theorizing.

Echoing Balsam's critique, Michaela Chamberlain (2022) remarks in *Misogyny in Psychoanalysis* on what she sees as the misogyny still rampant in psychoanalysis. Even today, in psychoanalytic training institutes worldwide, argues Chamberlain, former CEO of the London Bowlby Center and a training and supervising analyst herself, "the fundamental experiences of pregnancy, birth, and menopause continue to be overlooked. Ironically for a field whose main currency is reflection, the different treatment of women is bypassed because misogyny is institutionalized in psychoanalysis" (x).

"Decades of psychoanalytic literature," adds Joan Raphael-Leff (2016), a psychoanalyst and social psychologist, "labelled the mother merely as the baby's 'object' rather than a subject in her own right and [John] Bowlby notoriously stipulated that a 'safe base' means twenty-four-hour maternal devotion, seven days a week, 365 days a year, which negates the mother as a person" (173).

The first psychoanalyst to make mother "a subject in her own right" was Otto Rank. Two of Rank's greatest advocates in America, Esther and Bill Menaker, played a major role in the introduction of second-wave feminism.

Published in 1963, *The Feminine Mystique* emerged from Betty Friedan's will therapy in the 1950s with Bill Menaker, husband of Esther Menaker, a pre-eminent exponent of Rank's thought.

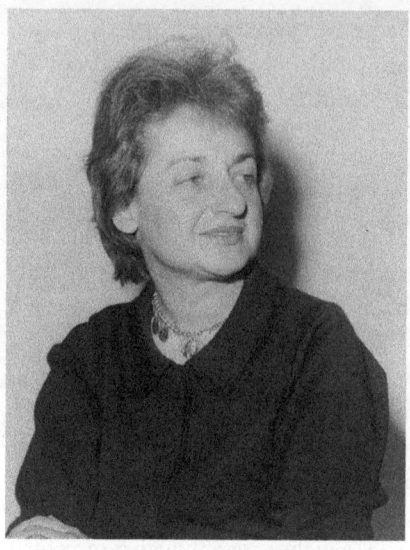

Figure 10.3 Betty Friedan

Credit: Photo by Fred Palumbo, World Telegram staff photographer. Restored by Adam Cuerden via Wikimedia Commons.

Coined by Friedan, the term "feminine mystique" was intended to criticize the widely held assumption in American society that women can find fulfillment only in marriage, housework, and child rearing, as Dr. Spock and other Freudians had argued.

In Friedan's last chapter, entitled "A New Life Plan for Women," *The Feminine Mystique* echoes Rank's views on life fear, *Lebensangst*, and its relation to the difficulties inherent in developing one's capacity for self-leadership, views that Bill Menaker shared with Friedan during their therapy. "It is easier to live through someone else than to become complete yourself," writes Friedan (1963) about her own life fear. *"The freedom to lead and plan your own life is frightening if you have never faced it before"* (326; italics added).

> [Bill] Menaker asked her why she confined herself to "'playing the role' of suburban housewife." . . . Her experience with Menaker proved so positive, in fact, that she approached him several years later, after receiving the contract for what would become *The Feminine Mystique*. Believing that his expertise would lend her work "more authority," Friedan proposed that they collaborate. Had her editor not nixed the idea, the name of an authorizing "eminent male psychoanalyst" might therefore have graced the cover of *The Feminine Mystique*—a mindboggling notion, given the book's ultimate trajectory. (Plant 2016:74)

Although later criticized for not paying attention to the needs of women of color, lesbians, or the poor, Friedan identified a prevailing belief, rooted in the Freudianism of the 1950s, that middle-class White women did not want to work, become educated, participate in political discourse, or lead movements for social change. By the time Friedan died in 2006, *The Feminine Mystique* had sold over 3 million copies and been translated into many languages (Friedan 2013).

In her autobiography, *Misplaced Loyalties*, Esther Menaker (1995b) reveals what it was like for her and her husband, Bill, to be analyzed in Vienna in the early 1930s—Esther by Anna Freud and Bill by Helene Deutsch. Both analyses were harmful, not helpful, writes Esther Menaker, since they were conducted under "classical" conditions with Anna Freud and Helene Deutsch showing only emotional coldness to Esther and Bill.

"Bill was interested in Rank when we were in Vienna," Menaker told Todd Dufresne (2007). "Once when he was looking through a Rank book, Helene Deutsch made a point of saying that it was a very bad book. Well, since Bill had a very bad time of his analysis with Deutsch, he probably went right out and bought the book! We brought back to America an interest in Rank, which was heresy. Anna Freud knew I was interested, but said nothing—which is the analyst's privilege" (31).

Reviewing Menaker's autobiography, Paul Roazen (2002) writes: "Esther Menaker's *Misplaced Loyalties* should be a classic for those who cannot accept the organizational legends about the field" (109).

11

How did Rank practice therapy?

In 1924, immediately after publishing *The Trauma of Birth*, Otto Rank went on a lecture tour to America to explain his new "pre-Oedipal" theory and practice of short-term therapy. Recognized as Freud's right-hand man, he brought "a method to cut down neurosis at the main trunk instead of picking at leaves and twigs," recalls psychiatrist Abram Kardiner. "We all flocked to him" (quoted in Lieberman 1985:234).

At that time, everyone in Rank's audiences knew that Freud's therapeutic method included a process of *attachment*, called "transference," but were puzzled by why there was no provision for *detachment*. Psychoanalytic treatment was getting longer and longer. Patients were being soldered into the couch, virtually for life, by the withering heat of transference. *Would analysis ever end?* No one knew.

Freud had written virtually nothing about how to end analysis—only how to begin it. Analysis was becoming interminable, which was certainly good for the financial health of analysts but not necessarily good for the mental health of patients.

By the early 1920s, writes Ferenczi (1932) in his *Clinical Diary*, psychoanalysts had developed an "[u]nconcern regarding the length of the analysis, indeed the tendency to prolong it for purely financial reasons: if one wants to, one turns the patients into taxpayers for life" (199). Even today a typical analysis lasts three to seven years, with many lasting a decade or longer, under the assumption that *more* analysis is *better* (Werbart & Lagerlöf 2022).

A century ago, Rank surprised his American audiences by focusing on the *end phase* and the patient's *separation anxiety* at the prospect of leaving the therapist, now seen as a mother surrogate.

More is not better, argued Rank; *better is better*. After a lecture at Yale University, Rank was asked by an audience member if he would elaborate on how he conducted short-term therapy—which Rank had begun to experiment with almost as soon as he started practicing therapy to support his family.

He smiled and answered, "I analyzed first according to Freud's technique and then gradually developed a shorter one, a technique that is getting shorter and shorter, so I am almost afraid that soon I won't have to see the patient at all" (Rank 1996:250n.10). The audience laughed, but behind Rank's witty response was a profound point he made in *Will Therapy* about the end phase of therapy:

Otto Rank and the Creation of Modern Psychotherapy. Robert Kramer, Oxford University Press.
© Robert Kramer (2025). DOI: 10.1093/9780197698303.003.0011

For no matter whether symptoms appear again or not, the patient always finds himself in doubt in the end phase as to whether or not he is healed, a doubt which in truth the Freudian analyst as a rule shares with him and tends to solve by prolonging the treatment. . . .

One of my patients solved this problem with a chance visit sometime after the ending of the treatment, when he remarked that he assumed that he had not been analyzed at all, for otherwise he would always have had to ask whether or nor he had been cured. (Rank 1936a:267)[1]

Like all therapists, Rank sometimes failed. For example, he was unsuccessful in relieving the emotional suffering of Elizabeth Severn, a 45-year-old woman who saw him in New York City for three months in 1924.

Severn, then practicing as a psychoanalyst, went by the title "Dr." although she had no academic degree or training in the field of therapy. According to Clara Thompson, who knew Severn well, she was "one of the most destructive people I know" (quoted in Fortune 1993:115). After being referred to Ferenczi by Rank, who was unable to help her, Severn was in analysis with Ferenczi from summer 1924 until his death in 1933. The chief protagonist of Ferenczi's 1932 *Clinical Diary*, Severn was treated by Ferenczi for four or five hours a day.

In a book published in 1933, and recently reprinted, Severn asserts, "The greatest objection to be made against Psychoanalysis [as practiced during the 1920s and 1930s] . . . is, in my opinion, its rigidity. Being devised as a systematic and observational method, it lacks in *flexibility* and humanness in its personal application to sick people" (Severn 2017:51; italics in the original).

Psychoanalyst Arnold Rachman (2018) reports that Severn described her therapy in 1924 with Rank as a "'three-month course' with an education focus on Rankian theory. . . . She described the experience with Rank as follows: '[I]f you could recall the feelings of being born, every subsequent difficulty in your life would be eliminated. An extraordinary theory don't you think?. . . . Rank was one of those analysts . . . Freud's pupils, who decided they knew as much as Papa did, if not a little more . . . I found him completely wrapped up in the one idea of the birth trauma, and incapable of thinking of anything else'. . . . Severn said that the therapy with Rank '. . . didn't help me any'. . . . Severn's observations about Rank," writes Rachman (2018), "closely paralleled Freud's and Ferenczi's evaluations [of Rank]" (110). Concludes Rachman: "Rank, for all his shortcomings, helped her change her life by referring her to Ferenczi" (113).

Rank, while usually confident about his capacity to help patients, especially those blocked in expressing their creativity, at times confessed his bafflement about the mysteries of the human psyche. It would have been out of character for Rank to "lecture" Severn on his birth trauma theory. He never did so with any other patient. It's more likely that he *encouraged* Severn's "resistance" to him as a sign of latent strength or "counter-willing," the first inkling of the emergence of the creative will—an aggressiveness that she demonstrated with both Rank and Ferenczi.

Never posing as an expert, Rank valued the condition of "not-knowing" as an opportunity to learn more about his craft as a therapist. He was always willing to "access his ignorance," the fundamental skill in helping others, according to Edgar Schein (2009:91). An artist who visited Rank to relieve a creative block in 1927, Myron Chester Nutting recalls:

> . . . Rank said, "Well, I will tell you something that you may find rather comforting. I don't understand what happens." He said, "You don't understand, and neither do I." He just simply knew that from experience he could expect that certain things could happen if they were handled rightly and if the person's psyche and personality could be influenced for the better along certain lines. But he wouldn't pretend at all to try to give me a lecture on why it was happening because he said, "I don't know." (quoted in Lieberman 1985:272)

In contrast to his failure with Severn, Rank had many successes as a clinician. "Rank is like a tender watching mother," wrote Wilda Peck in a journal she kept

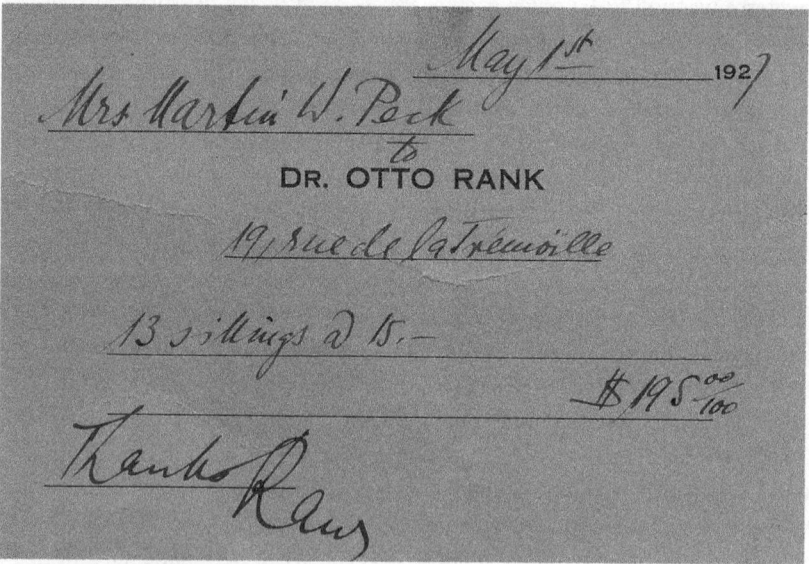

Figure 11.1 Rank's invoice, 1927. In Paris, Rank charged five dollars less than Freud, but triple what New York analysts were then charging. He offered a reduced fee to social workers.

Credit: Ruhama Veltfort for the Estate of Otto Rank

of 31 sessions with Rank in Paris in 1927 (quoted in Lieberman 1985:270). She was unhappily married to Dr. Martin Peck, a psychiatrist who'd undergone a training analysis with Rank, and recommended that she visit him.

Guilty about not loving her husband, Peck felt all alone. She wanted to change, and, at the same time, didn't want to change. There's no right way to love, Rank counseled Peck, only your own way. Everyone is different. "The thing I am to accept is love," she discovered. "All I haven't had, all I've wanted, flows through Rank, the medium, to me. I accept" (ibid.).

When Peck asked whether patients fell into groups, he answered, "No. Each one works out his problem in his own individual fashion. . . . It isn't possible to generalize or find types; it would be dangerous to do so" (ibid.).

"I had orginally accepted P's [Martin Peck's] estimate of you as the rigid sci-entist that he was looking for and wanting," Wilda Peck told Rank, "not the great flexible, all-embracing mind. Every idea I have has been not only agreed with, but backed up and reinforced by your knowledge and authority. Really an emotional experience" (ibid.).

She was learning not to be afraid to love or be loved, even when there was risk involved. Relationship therapy was an emotional, not an intellectual, experience. "To accept love," wrote Peck in her journal, "one must accept risk of pain. . . . Not free love, but loving freely" (ibid.).

Rank said, "[T]he problem of human relationship is the most important in the world today" (ibid.:269); he summed up the aim of his relationship therapy as "freedom from the mother, adjustment to the environment, and discovering of abilities" (ibid.).

After her therapy, Wilda Peck, who had studied to be a professional librarian, went on to become a noted painter and print artist.

Social worker Phoebe Crosby's experience of being in therapy with Rank occurred in June and July of 1927. On the first day, Crosby told Rank, "I had never been able to really love. My emotional life was poor and thin" (Crosby & Janus 2017:448). "No, of course I hadn't loved," recalled Crosby, "because I was constantly blaming my failures on other people, and trying to make them over to suit my ideas" (449).

> During these early sessions, Rank taught me two words, "projection" and "iden-tification." I began to see that I had always projected myself onto other people, trying to change them, trying to put myself across, to impose my ways on them, instead of identifying with them, getting myself enough inside them to understand them, to see them with empathy. (ibid.)

As Crosby struggled to come to terms with her alienation from others, and her inability to love herself, she was surprised to discover that she was *learning to feel her own emotions* more deeply than she had ever felt them before. Very soon after her therapy began, Phoebe Crosby began to experience a visceral welling inside her, the stirrings of love—empathy—for herself and for Rank.

> Slowly and painfully there emerged from the talks two things I must do. I must love him, the analyst, and I must love myself. (ibid.)
> "Emotion is the only reality," were his words at one time. (450)
> I remember very clearly another question and answer. I said, "Is this process of identification that you are trying to teach me one kind of love?" "The only kind worth having." (451)
> I don't know how Rank did it, but he managed to end each session on a constructive, even cheerful note. It did not seem a contrived thing. It was as if at that moment, he let his natural buoyancy, his joy in life, come through. (ibid.)

Crosby recalls beginning to experience a "rush of feeling" for herself and for Rank, a feeling that continued to expand, allowing her to identify with "my childhood on the farm," with a river that flowed into an ocean, and, finally, with everything in the universe. "The ocean is the universe," exclaimed Rank with joy. Always striving, whenever the moment was right, to connect the microcosm of his patient's psyche to the macrocosm of the universe, the All, he said, "You are not satisfied now unless you love the universe!" (452).

> One more lesson was to be learned. I would say that it was the hardest, except by this time I was so aware of Rank's goodness and wisdom and capacity for helping that with such a guide nothing seemed impossible.
> *Separation.* The next step in loving. Loving and leaving. You do not really love unless you are able to "leave" the beloved. And leaving can be terribly destructive unless at the same time, you are able to love the thing you leave.
> It was nearly time for the analysis to end. The two months allotted to it were almost over. I had learned at great cost to love myself and Rank and now I had to leave him.
> One thing that helped was that I realized that this was no strange thing that was being suddenly thrust upon me. He had been preparing for it almost from the beginning, with as I now saw it, incredible skill. He had known all the time that it would be like this. I had not known, now I did. We were doing it together. (ibid.; italics in the original)

Social worker Jessie Taft, then 44, describes her first interview with Rank in 1926. Two years younger than Taft, Rank was

. . . quiet, brief. . . . No doubts were expressed by him, no fear of my age. . . . He did not promise anything. He merely agreed to try, on the basis of time at my disposal. I can only recall one remark from that interview in response to something I had presented about myself. "Perhaps the problem lies there." And that was all, but in that one sentence I began to make myself over before anyone else should have the chance. (Taft 1958:x)

Unlike others who had frowned on her lesbian desires, Rank valued Taft's sexuality as essential to her way of being and encouraged her, even in the face of societal disapproval, to accept her "difference" wholeheartedly, without ambivalence, guilt, or anxiety. In a 1927 lecture given at the University of Pennsylvania School of Social Work, Rank (1996) said that same-sex relationships "are sometimes much more satisfactory from an emotional as well as from an ethical viewpoint than are the heterosexual ones" (187).

While training to become a psychoanalyst during the last decades of the 20th century, Stephen Kuchuck (2021), a gay social worker, writes that "the entire analytic community and literature confirmed that I was damaged. . . . Not once did I hear a teacher, supervisor or student question this—an experience that was dispiriting and embarrassing when not dissociated" (24). Much has changed since then, and gay and lesbian therapists are now welcomed by the analytic community, but this was not the case for the better part of the last century.

Relationship therapy, concluded Jessie Taft (1933), perhaps autobiographically, is "an opportunity to feel in the present and gradually begin to take responsibility for one's own feelings and impulses in all their ambivalence, with as little denial, rationalization and justification as possible" (94).

Taft summed up her learnings from Rank in one beautifully-crafted sentence: "Therapy is a process in which a person who has been unable to go on with living without more fear and guilt than he is willing to bear, somehow gains the courage to live again, to face life positively instead of negatively" (283).

In the fall of 1927, at the urging of Taft, Virginia Robinson (1968) went to see Rank for one hour a day over the course of six weeks.

I began in the first hour with a description of my family where no problem existed for me and continued with family history until my interest flagged— as did Rank's. Dreams interested him and served me well to take me into the fundamental problems of relationship, the problems he was working on in his lecture series [at the University of Pennsylvania School of Social Work]. These were problems of denial, identification and projection to show how the self builds itself up through *likeness* and *difference* in a search for its own identity. Figures in my current professional and living situations appeared in dreams for this purpose rather than figures from the past.

I realize today more vividly than at the time how brilliantly and considerately Rank made use of these to show me my "patterns" in relationship. I remember today the sense of illumination when he said *"perhaps what the self really seeks is identity; does it ever accept difference?"* (21–22; italics added)

To accept one's own difference and that of the other is the biggest challenge in any human relationship, said Rank, and usually comes to a peak of emotional tension during the end phase of therapy, when separating from the therapist is essential for discovering the power of one's creative will, one's difference. "[T]he emotional life," wrote Rank (1932b) in *Modern Education*, "is extensively an expression of individual will" (69).

"To take over into [oneself] the responsibility for separation without denial of the value of the other is a development so rare that it may easily not happen once in a lifetime," said Robinson (1930:123) in her PhD dissertation, published as *A Changing Psychology in Social Case Work*. Robinson drew extensively on Rank's writings on difference and likeness in her chapter on "The Problem of Relationship" (115–127).

After their experiences of therapy with Rank, Jessie Taft and Virginia Robinson lived happily together for the rest of their lives, creatively balancing their desire for difference and their need for likeness. These two pioneer feminists, both long-time professors at the University of Pennsylvania School of Social Work, were among the first same-sex couples in the United States to adopt children (Frederiksen-Goldsen et al. 2009).

"If one were to pick out the particular attitude which finally led Rank to a new comprehension of the therapeutic task ...," wrote Taft in her introduction to *Will Therapy*, "one might well select his complete respect for the personality of the neurotic patient" (Rank 1936a:xi). Deeply grateful to Rank for valuing her sexual orientation, Taft became his friend, translator, and greatest advocate in social work.

Over half a century before the term "diversity" became popular, Rank's psychology of difference, as taught by Jessie Taft and Virginia Robinson, included unconditional respect for the overlapping identities of gender, race, ethnicity, and sexual orientation, a respect that Black writer Nella Larsen, who included a lesbian subplot in her 1929 novel *Passing*, had also sensed in Rank (Blackmore 1992).

Far ahead of her time, Jessie Taft "developed a large corpus of feminist therapy" (Deegan 1991:387). She "was surrounded by women; their ideas, issues, friendships, life-styles, and institutions" (384). Her 1916 University of Chicago PhD dissertation, *The Women's Movement from the Point of View of Social Consciousness*, "reads as a deeply felt examination of the predicament of American

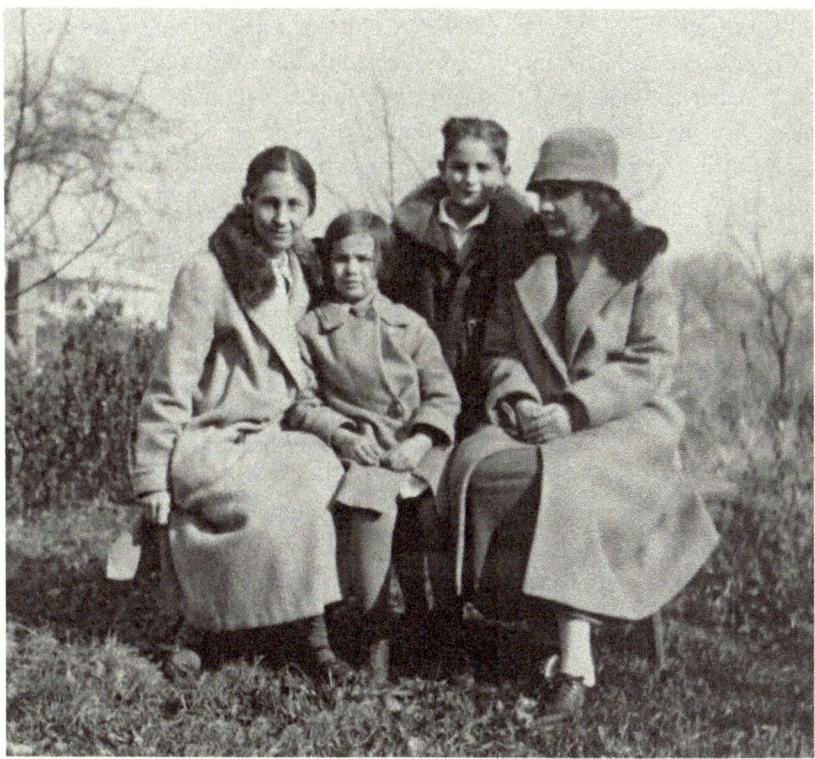

Figure 11.2 Jessie Taft and Virginia Robinson with adopted children, Martha and Everett, 1923. From left to right: Jessie, Martha, Everett, Virginia.
Credit: Everett Taft via Wikimedia Commons

women at the dawn of the 20th century" (Mertens 2012:60). Feminist scholars call it "the best testament of feminist pragmatism that's ever been written" (ibid.).

Scorned by male psychiatrists who promoted Freud's psychology of likeness, Rank's psychology of difference inspired legions of students at the University of Pennsylvania School of Social Work to become agents of social change in order to develop the capacity for self-leadership of those who embody "difference" in society—unwed mothers, the poor, the disabled, the elderly, racial and sexual minorities.

The most vivid account of how Rank practiced his art of healing was written by Anaïs Nin, whose therapy with Rank for inability to finish a novel resulted in an explosive release of her creative will.

In Paris, over the course of ten months, from November 1933 to August 1934, Nin and Rank "began a profound mental exchange, which did not end for Nin until her death in 1977" (Spencer 1997:97). Nin kept a diary of her conversations with Rank. When she began, she had expected that he would rush to classify or diagnose her, as did her previous analyst, a Freudian. But she found Rank intent on discovering a woman neither of them knew. She sensed immediately that Rank was drawing on his own feelings and intuition to understand her, as an artist would.

"Impression of keenness, alertness, curiosity," recalls Nin (1966) of her first encounter with Rank in November 1933:

> His joyousness and activity immediately relieve one's pain, the neurotic knot which ties up one's faculties in a vicious circle of conflict, paralysis, more conflict, guilt, atonement, punishment, and more guilt. Immediately I felt air and space, movement, vitality, joy of detecting, divining. The spaciousness of his mind. The fine dexterity and muscular power. The swift-changing colors of his own moods. The swiftness of his rhythm, because intuitive and subtle.
>
> I trust him.
>
> We are far from the banalities and clichés of orthodox psychoanalysis.
>
> I sense an intelligence rendered clairvoyant by feeling. I sense an artist. (286)

In her account of how Rank helped her to unlearn subjugation to the traditional roles of women, Nin (1976) writes, "[Rank] focused on the strongest element in my divided and chaotic self. No matter what disintegrating influences I was experiencing, the writing was an act of wholeness. . . . He was challenging my creative will" (59–60). In his first act of challenging her creative will, Rank had asked Nin to leave her diary with him—to *separate* from it—instantly spurring her to react with strong counter-will. No!

"When Rank cut off Nin's diary supply," writes Ruth Charnock (2011), "it was an attempt to wean her off the diarization or narrativization of experience, to encourage her to exist in the present and to channel her creative energies into producing fiction rather than the diary" (149). She needed to wean off it, at least temporarily, in order to be "reborn" spiritually as a mature artist, willing to risk more of herself in the writing of fiction.

As Rank listened empathically to Nin as she shared her most intimate hopes, dreams, and fears, he recast his work *The Myth of the Birth of the Hero*—transforming it, one might say, into *The Myth of the Birth of the Heroine*.

"You tried to live your life like a myth," he told Nin (1966), after reading and returning her diary to her. "Everything you dreamed or fantasized, you carried out. You are a myth maker" (272). Nin reflects: "As he talked, I thought of my difficulties with writing, my struggles to articulate feelings not easily expressed. Of my struggles to find a language for intuition, feelings, instincts which are in themselves elusive, subtle, and wordless" (276). She concludes:

Rank. I have a blurred memory of vigorousness, of muscular talks. Of sharpness. . . . Rank waits free ready to leap, but not holding a little trap door in readiness which will click at the cliché place. He waits free. You are a new human being. Unique. He detours the obvious, and begins a vast expansion into the greater, the vaster, the beyond. Art and imagination. With joyousness and alertness. (289)

When the therapy ended, Rank and Nin began a sexual relationship (Bair 1995). His marriage to Tola had begun to deteriorate after 1926. She'd never wanted to leave Vienna due to her closeness to Freud, who treated her as a daughter-in-law, and supported her membership in the Vienna Psychoanalytic Society. The Ranks' daughter, Helene, was considered by Freud as if she were his own grand-daughter.

From Paris, where her husband had established a successful therapy practice, Tola returned regularly to Vienna to visit Freud and his family, but never accompanied by Otto. By September 1934, having for a long time been ready to separate from Tola, Rank offered to marry Nin and gave her the signet ring he'd received from Freud at the creation of the Secret Committee. On October 13, 1934, while traveling on a ship from Paris to New York, Rank gushed in a letter to Nin:

I not only want you but I also want you to take care of me and I want to take care of you, too: you know! You must come [to New York] soon. All my "magic" is with you and I can't give anything to anybody—not even to myself. . . . I am like the sea: As deep and as changeable. But with you I am not changing—just

deepening

deepening

deepening

Rank wrote the words "deepening" in the form of a visual poem to show Nin that he was diving into the depths of his soul. One day later, he penned another letter to Nin, this time about the "cosmic" meaning of the feelings and love they shared for each other:

I don't know whether I expressed what I feel, but you know anyway how I feel, and that's most important. This cosmic love enables us to create otherwise from the surplus, the overflow of our love![2]

After considerable inner turmoil, Nin declined his marriage proposal, unwilling to abandon her other lovers, of whom there were many, including Henry Miller and his wife, June. With her lovers and in her fiction, Nin enjoyed trying on different, overlapping identities. For Nin, as for Nella Larsen, one identity was never enough.

When she learned in 1939 of Rank's death, Nin wrote, "In the face of death, one asks oneself invariably: Did I see enough, hear enough, observe enough, love enough, did I listen attentively, did I appreciate, did I sustain the life? Did Rank die not knowing perhaps how much or how deep was his gift, how vivid his human presence?" (quoted in Spencer 1982:127).

Rank's "metaphysics of creativity," concludes Helen Tookey (2003) in a profound study of Nin's fiction, "both inspired her personal project of self-creation and, she later came to believe, could inspire other women to fulfil the potential that the feminist movement was beginning to awaken" (72).

As a therapist, Rank always affirmed the will of his patients to *connect deeply with him*, while simultaneously supporting their equally strong will, during the end phase, to *differentiate from him*, thus giving them an opportunity, perhaps for the first time in their lives, to integrate love and will.

From the very first sessions, Rank looked for signs that might reveal when his patient, feeling a mixture of dread and hope, wanted, at once, to hold on and let go, to stay connected and leave. When these signs of ambivalence, at first faint, became increasingly visible, a critical moment was on the verge of arriving, a moment that pointed toward a need for jointly setting the ending.

It was a *phase*, insisted Rank, not a single event, that was needed to end therapy. During the end setting phase, said Rank (1936a) in *Will Therapy*, he would "prize" the patient's will to separate as an expression of creativity, "the act of will as such, instead of condemning it" (270) as resistance to continuing the analysis as Freud had done.

Rank's approach was nimble, never formulaic, shifting from person to person, hour to hour, according to the needs of the situation and each person, but had an end in sight from the beginning—the spiritual "rebirth" of the person, now self-empowered with a vibrant, creative will.

"Having an end in sight right from the beginning focuses the mind," argue Burns & Burns-Lundgren (2015), "and avoids coasting along with no sense of urgency" (30), as in the case of interminable psychoanalysis, which continues to be promoted by many analysts today.

In the second paragraph of "Analysis Terminable and Interminable," his final word on the subject of psychotherapy, Freud (1937) scorns Rank's time-limited relationship therapy.

Rank, writes Freud (1937), had pointed to "the possibility of a child's 'primal fixation' to his mother not being surmounted but persisting as a 'primal repression'" (216). Sadly, as we have seen, the father of psychoanalysis was himself primally fixated on his powerful mother, Amalia, and refused help from Ferenczi, when offered in 1926, to heal his suffering. Insisting on the need for interminable analysis, Freud continues:

> Rank hoped that if this primal trauma were dealt with by a subsequent analysis the whole neurosis would be got rid of. Thus this one small piece of analytic work would save the necessity for all the rest. . . . [It] was a child of its time . . . designed to adapt the tempo of analytic therapy to the haste of American life. . . . The theory and practice of Rank's experiment are now things of the past—no less than American "prosperity" itself. (216–217)

But Freud was wrong. Neither Rank's experiment nor American prosperity were things of the past.

It is not widely known that Freud loathed America. "America," Freud once joked, "is a mistake; a gigantic mistake, it is true, but none the less a mistake" (Jones 1955:60). Historian of psychoanalysis Ernst Falzeder (2015) quotes many other sayings by Freud denigrating America, almost all which mention women in the same breath. For example:

> American women "make fools" of their men, they "are an anti-cultural phenomenon. . . . In Europe, things are different: men take the lead and that is as it should be. . . ." "[I]n America the father ideal appears to be downgraded, so that the American girl cannot muster the illusion that is necessary for marriage. . . ." To Blumgart he wrote: "None of you [Americans] has ever found the right attitude toward your women." (314)

According to psychoanalyst Patrick Mahony, Freud displaced the rage he felt toward his powerful mother Amalia onto his anti-Americanism. "Freud's biographers err in writing he rarely spoke of the pre-oedipal mother," says Mahony (quoted in Falzeder 2015:325). "The over-determined fact is that he felt always compelled to speak about her, disguised as America. Her demonic power made him regress into an infantile, paranoid state of aggrievement and petulancy that lasted all his life. He tried to control the oedipal but especially pre-oedipal mother by spatially constricting her in his symbolic geography" (ibid.).

What was the price Freud paid in emotional and physical suffering for refusing help from Ferenczi to exorcise the power of his mother over him? According to Thornton Wilder, Freud (1992) once told him "that it might some day be shown that cancer is allied to 'the presence of hate in the subconscious'" (297–298). No wonder that Jacques Lacan (1977) would later call for a return to "the truth in Freud's mouth" (121)—referring to his oral cancer. Like Rank and Ferenczi, Lacan recognized that the truth speaks where there is pain.

While Freud was dismissing Rank's ideas about the centrality of an authentic relationship to the healing process of therapy, these ideas spread across America, through thousands of female social workers taught by Jessie Taft, Virginia Robinson, and their heirs at the Penn School and the even larger numbers of social workers, counselors, and therapists influenced by the enormously popular writings of Carl Rogers.

Rank's ultimate goal was to allow the genuineness, acceptance, and empathy he demonstrated during the therapeutic relationship to spark the emergence of his client's creative will during the end phase, which today "is often experienced as its most productive period" (Burns & Burns-Lundgren 2015:30). At the end phase, according to the latest outcome studies, there is even evidence that interpretations have the potential to be harmful (Zilcha-Mano et al. 2023).

Rank was intent on helping transform his patient's *negative* will, which had turned inward toward creation of a neurosis, into the outward expression of the creative energy—the passion, power, and life force—of their *positive* will. A student of the arts and humanities, Rank considered psychotherapy to be a performing art—an improvisation. "The therapist may do whatever he believes is pertinent to the process and *moment of therapy* with a particular individual," said Rank, "as long as he takes responsibility for, and deals helpfully with, what he precipitates in the patient" (quoted in Lieberman 1985:xxxvii; italics in the original).[3]

Mary Plowden, a social worker who experienced therapy with Rank in the late 1930s, told E. James Lieberman (1985):

> With Rank there was no dogma. Everything was open from minute to minute. Nothing was imposed on you. Rank was not looking for disease, he was not trying to eradicate anything. He wanted you to open up and be as you might want to be but didn't dare to. He had an overwhelming force but it did not take away from anything else—it gave you a force of your own. (xxxviii)

Yet another account of Rank as a therapist, and a vivid example of what Rollo May (1969) in *Love and Will* called the creative power of the "daimonic," which Rank termed "counter-willing," can be found in a letter Henry Miller sent in 1933 to Anaïs Nin—a letter that convinced her to go to Rank for therapy. Two years earlier, Nin had begun a stormy sexual relationship with Miller and also simultaneously with his wife, June. Miller, having been overwhelmed by the vast Old World scholarship in Rank's *Art and Artist*, published in English a year earlier, made an appointment to see Rank in his Paris consulting room at 5:30 p.m. on March 6, 1933.

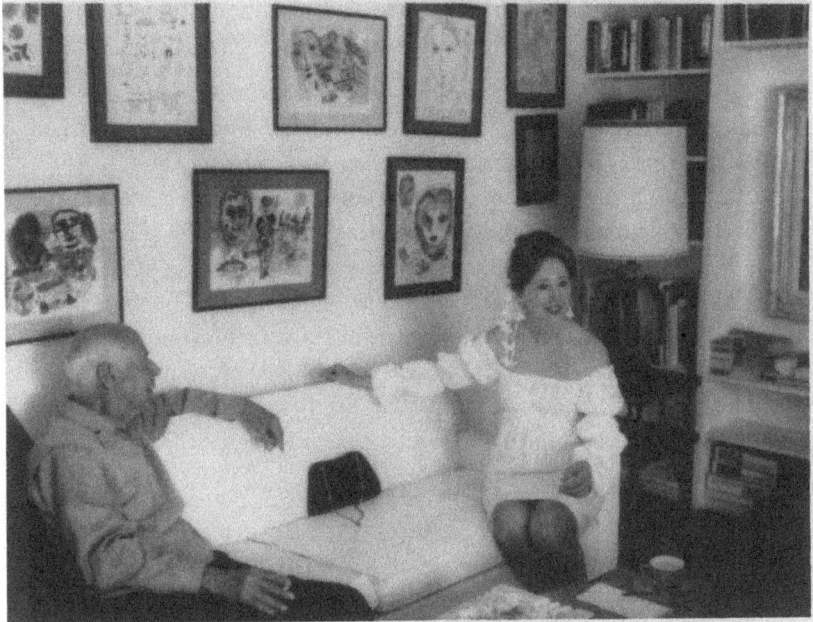

Figure 11.3 Henry Miller and Anaïs Nin

Before doing so, Miller, shared with Nin his feelings of timidity in visiting Rank, who was then famous in Paris, having lectured to acclaim at the Sorbonne and elsewhere. "I am going to Rank in full panoply," he told her, "but closing in on the problem more and more, getting supersaturated so that when the discharge comes it will be a cloudburst. I want it to rain blood" (Stuhlmann 1979:107).

And rain blood it did—for all of one hour. Miller left Rank's office a different man, never to return. Even for Rank, who pioneered limited-term therapy, it may have been the shortest analysis on record.

As soon as Miller arrived, Rank immediately intuited that he did not need "a tender watching mother" or "mother love." Instead, as an indomitable force, Miller needed a high challenge, a vibrant confrontation between two powerful creative wills, those of Rank and Miller, connecting with and challenging each other. In this case, the therapy would consist of a spirited duel of wills, not a sharing of tender feelings.

Every patient is different, according to Rank, who used his artistic temperament to create a new therapy each time. In a breathless fourteen-page letter to

Nin, Miller, no longer intimidated by Rank, exulted at the outcome. In the space of one hour,

> [W]hat had been achieved was no less than a brilliant, an artistic cure ... cured as one could possibly be. . . . Cured I was of certain terrible timidities. . . . What I needed was the high challenge, the acid test, and I got it. . . . I felt my wrist stronger, firmer, my aim more accurate, a deadly aim. Yes, this is a dramatization. . . . Perhaps I exaggerated when I said over the phone that he employed the word "amazing." Perhaps that is my representation of it; but it was there, whether he used the word or not; it shone in his eyes, it revealed itself even more by his temporary bewilderments. Read into this all you want of ego, make the necessary subtractions—it remains a fact that I conquered, and not the least important fact that I consider the conquest a victory over myself, my Romantic self, if you will. (108)

Rank would have been delighted by Miller's letter, which Nin likely showed him, for after all, Miller's response was Rank's aim in the first place. In *Art and Artist*, Rank (1932a), had written that, in therapy, just as in artistic creation, the process of unlearning is "a separation which is so hard, not only because it involves persons and ideas that one reveres, but because the victory is always, at bottom and in some form, won over a part of one's own ego" (375).

No one has written more subtly about the vital need for sparking a patient's creative will within the therapeutic relationship than Rank. In his most radical innovation, Rank was the first therapist to locate the *center of change* in the creative will of his patients. In contrast, Freud, and almost all psychoanalysts even today, insist that the analyst's *interpretations* are at the center of change, and that "resistance" to interpretations must be overcome through the long process of working through.

Pointing to Freud's own self-centeredness, which was evident to anyone who knew him well, Rank (1936a) dryly remarked in *Will Therapy*: "Apparently the narcissism of the analyst has compensated for his passivity, so that he has related all reactions of the patient, as far as they do not permit of being put back on an infantile pattern, to his own person" (10). By "infantile pattern," Rank was referring, of course, to transference.

Instead of promoting transference, said Rank, he was choosing to place the client "as chief actor, in the center of the situation" (ibid.). According to Esther Menaker (1982), for Rank "transference reactions are not cultivated as they are in a classical analysis, but are in effect *pulled out by the roots*" (117; italics added).

In a Copernican turn, Rank had shifted the source of therapeutic results from the helper to the person being helped, an idea many psychoanalysts today would find inconceivable or bewildering. The emergence of the patient's will during therapy, usually in the form of defiance or counter-will, was seen by Freud as "resistance" to his Oedipal interpretations, and needed to be overcome.

"Rank moved out of the classical tradition," observed Jessie Taft (1958), "into a completely reversed conception of the role of the therapist as secondary, leaving to the patient the *active role of the creator* in the therapeutic process" (124; italics added).

Clients want their feelings to be understood and accepted, not analyzed. We yearn, at once, to experience closeness and autonomy, connection and authenticity, union and separation, love and will. Both yearnings need to be experienced if the therapeutic relationship is to be healing. According to Rank, "authenticity"—becoming and being one's self and constantly evolving one's "I" throughout each of the developmental stages of life—is the definition, the *sine qua non*, of mental health.

Creative solutions to human problems, said Rank in *Will Therapy*, emerge while therapist and client grapple with the reality of each other's existence—each party expressing the creative energy of their own will—and with the tension each experiences between the desire for likeness and the need for difference.

The main work of the therapist, Rank said, is to help clients find the courage to unlearn out-of-date values, assumptions, beliefs, emotions, and expectations they've been taking for granted all their lives, and give birth and contin-ual rebirth to a new, healthier, more creative self—a forever growing and evolving "I."

The process of giving birth and rebirth to a new self extends throughout life, since the human being is dynamic not static. Rank originally entitled his book on relationship therapy *Dynamic Therapy*, changing it only later, during Jessie Taft's translation process, to *Will Therapy*.

Joining together in feeling, said Rank, therapist and patient, rather than per-manently losing their separate identities, may experience sublime moments of connection in which they find and then re-create themselves. In the simultaneous dissolution of their difference in a greater whole, the two sur-render their separate identities for a moment, only to have individuality returned to them in the next, reenergized and enriched by the experience of "loss."

Relationship therapy, according to Rank, involves both parties learning how to give and take, surrender and assert, merge and individuate, unite and separate—without being trapped in a whipsaw of opposites. At rare moments, the two may unite so deeply that the patient may now find in this "enlarged self" the differentiation necessary for life.

The lifelong implications of yearning at each developmental stage to integrate our desire for union and separation, connection and individuation, likeness and difference—love and will—Rank would work out, systematically, in the years after he left Freud. Experiencing likeness and difference simultaneously, said Rank, reinforce rather than contradict each other. Today, Rank's dialectical thinking is commonplace among developmental psychologists:

> [Harvard's Robert Kegan] sees the central theme as two basic, but conflicted yearnings for humans, one for communion (the yearning to be included, to be part of, to be close to) and one for agency (the yearning to be autonomous, to be distinct, to choose one's own direction).... The conflict between communion and agency is a central construct in many developmental theories, including Piaget, Kohlberg, Loevinger, Maslow, Erikson and McClelland. (Dixon 1999:39)

The name of Carl Rogers could also have been included on this list of psychologists who saw the tension between communion and agency, likeness and difference, as central to therapy.

Considered to be "the most influential psychologist in American history" (Kirschenbaum & Henderson 1989b:xi), Rogers always acknowledged that a personal encounter with Rank in 1936 revolutionized the way he practiced therapy. "I became infected with Rankian ideas," said Rogers (quoted in Kirschenbaum 1979:95).

In *The Discovery of Being*, existential psychologist Rollo May (1983) observed that Rogers's "theory about human nature owes much to Otto Rank" (173n.11), whose ideas planted the seeds of client-centered therapy. As noted earlier, Rogers "has had such a major influence on social work practice, that his principles and tenets could be viewed as almost synonymous with our own professional standards" (Lewis 1991:166).

How did Rank inform Rogers's theory of human nature, and, in the process, lay the foundation for modern psychotherapy?

12

Carl Rogers meets Otto Rank

What was Rank's theory of human nature? "Rank is very diffuse, very hard to read," attests Ernest Becker (1973) in *The Denial of Death*, "so rich that he is almost inaccessible to the general reader" (xx). He adds, "Rank could have helped his own work enormously by putting conceptual order into his insights" (177). Readers, concludes Becker, need to put their "own order into the broadside of Rank's work" (ibid.).

In contrast to Freud, a past master of the German language, Rank's prose often wraps around itself, as if to protect its author from the existential anxieties it does so much to illuminate. "I crave simplicity," Rank once joked to Jessie Taft (1958) about his labyrinthine mind. "[T]he other"—complexity—"I have myself" (183). According to E. James Lieberman (1985):

> Ideas tumble over one another in Rank's writing like charms on a heavy bracelet. In some places they obscure the connecting chain. The linking argument is strong, but the material is dense and the connections may be lost to the untrained eye. By contrast to this jeweler-artisan writing, Freud's texts are those of a forester-scientist who guides the reader along a path so clearly marked that one cannot fail to see; one can refuse to follow, but there is little danger of getting lost. (93)

For Rank's patients, his dense prose didn't matter: "Rank's own writings," recalled Phoebe Crosby (1970), over 40 years after she was in therapy with him in 1927, "[are] still an unknown language. Never mind. *He* changed me, if his writings don't. And his change in me was from black to red. From ink to blood. From trying to work things out intellectually to giving myself more to feeling. So—*he* won't mind if I can't read him" (101–102; italics in the original).

Perhaps the best way to explore Rank's view of human nature may come from Carl Rogers, whose personal and moving writings are universally admired for their clarity and grace.

For this reason, I want now to relate an encounter in 1936 between a young American therapist and a famous Viennese psychologist excommunicated a decade earlier from Freud's inner circle for "anti-Oedipal" heresy.

Although, as I will show, Carl Rogers and Otto Rank differed on the meaning of Rollo May's "daimonic," the spiritual resonances between Rogers and Rank

Otto Rank and the Creation of Modern Psychotherapy. Robert Kramer, Oxford University Press.
© Robert Kramer (2025). DOI: 10.1093/9780197698303.003.0012

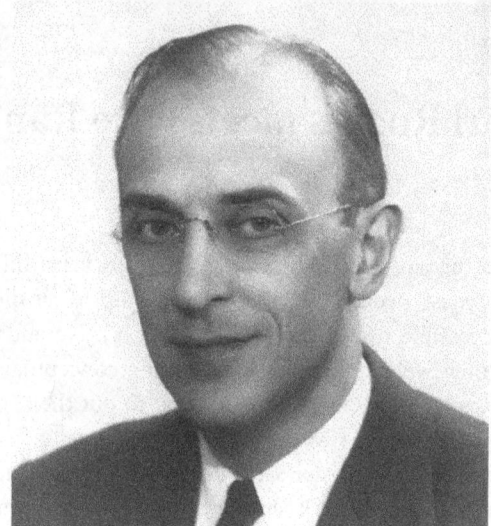

Figure 12.1 Carl Rogers, c. 1930
Credit: Carl Rogers Trust

are otherwise striking. I want to reveal, as fully as I can, the attunement between these two kindred souls, so different in culture and background, yet so similar in their grasp of human nature and the necessity of empathic understanding to affirm the creative will of human beings.

Then, by taking the experience of empathy to its deepest level, I want to lead us on a journey to the border of a realm beyond psychology, to the shores of the ineffable, the numinous, an "other-worldly" realm that Rogers (1986), just before he died, came to prize as "the transcendent, the indescribable, the spiritual" (199). A realm in which human beings may find themselves face-to-face with the Unknown and the Unknowable, "negotiating," said Rank (1932a) in his masterpiece *Art and Artist*, with "the Beyond" (49n).[1]

Here, if we are truly open to the awe and wonder that await us at the core of empathy, we may rediscover the spiritual meaning of love, and, perhaps just as importantly, be reminded of the sheer strangeness, the tragicomic absurdity, of existence itself.

What was the context for Carl Rogers's meeting with Otto Rank? In the 1920s and 1930s, as we saw earlier, psychoanalysts were unconcerned with a patient's feelings, paying virtually no attention to the "here-and-now" relationship taking place inside the consulting room.

Following Freud's medical model, the emphasis was on "treating" patients by coolly giving them interpretations of transference, not by listening with empathy to their feelings.

"In the medical model," writes Art Bohart (2006), a close colleague of Rogers's, "therapy is analogous to a medical operation. Interventions operate on clients to change dysfunctional behaviors, cognitions, affects. . . . The client is the 'dependent variable' on which the independent variable of the therapists' interventions operate" (220).

According to Freud, these interventions were interpretations, carefully dosed and timed, that were supposed to provide "insight" into the client's Oedipal unconscious. There *was* no other unconscious for Freud.

From 1928 through 1939, Carl Rogers served as director of the Child Guidance Clinic in Rochester, NY—his first professional position after studying for a PhD in clinical psychology at Columbia University's Teachers College, where he had been drawn to adopt "a rigorous scientific approach allied to a coldly objective statistical methodology" (Thorne 1992:7). At Columbia, Rogers was also impressed by the progressive education movement, which emphasized self-directed learning.

Not entirely satisfied with being trained just in research, Rogers was exposed during his Columbia years to clinicians practicing Freudian psychoanalysis. "If Rogers favored any one deep, therapeutic approach when he came to Rochester," writes his biographer, "it was *'interpretive therapy,'* the major goal of which is to help the child or parent achieve insight into his own behavior and motives, past and present" (Kirschenbaum 1979:86; italics added).

On his staff at the Rochester clinic were graduates of the University of Pennsylvania School of Social Work, where Otto Rank had been serving as a visiting professor since the mid-1920s at the invitation of Jessie Taft and Virginia Robinson.

In June 1936, intrigued by social workers who were telling him that *relationship therapy*—not *interpretive therapy*—was the emphasis of the Penn School, Carl Rogers invited Otto Rank to Rochester to conduct a three-day weekend introduction to his new practice of therapy (Evans 1975:28).

No longer calling himself a psychoanalyst, Rank was, by 1936, a "world-renowned psychologist whose major works could be read in English, French and German" (Lieberman 1985:355). In 1935, Rank had lectured at Harvard University at the invitation of Henry Murray, then the preeminent American student of "personology" (363).

Meanwhile, back in Vienna, Freud (1937) was preparing to launch his final attack on Rank in "Analysis Terminable and Interminable," a gloomy essay in which Freud reiterated the inexorable force of the self-destructive "death-instinct," the *Todestrieb* (243).

Resisting interpretations of their unconscious due to this *Todestrieb*, patients do not *want* to get better, said Freud. They behave toward the analyst "exactly like a child who does not like the stranger and does not believe anything he says" (239). Freud also made clear, in even stronger terms than ever before, his unwavering "repudiation of femininity" (252).

One month after visiting Rochester, in July 1936, Rank published two books: *Will Therapy* and its companion volume, *Truth and Reality*. Translated into English by Jessie Taft, *Will Therapy* was the first book ever published with the words "therapy" and "relationship" in the title.

Rank himself composed the title, which reads in full: *Will Therapy: An Analysis of the Therapeutic Process in Terms of Relationship*. Relationship therapy and will therapy were synonyms for Rank. Willing, argued Rank, is always relational.

"The whole psychoanalytic approach is centered around the therapist," Rank (1935) advised a group of social workers shortly before he met Rogers in 1936. "*Real therapy has to be centered around the client, his difficulties, his needs, his activities*" (262; italics in the original).

"Freud was very explicit," writes Jacob Arlow (2002), a former president of the American Psychoanalytic Association, "that everything had to be focused on the person of the physician" (1140), who, as the blank screen on which infantile sexual desires were to be transferred, was at the center of therapy.

By creating an authentic, respectful relationship based on empathic understanding, Rank had de-centered the therapist. The term "client-centered" would later be adopted by Rogers to describe his own work.

While no record exists of Rank's weekend with Rogers in 1936 at Rochester, I want to reconstruct what he might have said, drawing on Rank's *Will Therapy, Truth and Reality, Psychology and the Soul*, and *Art and Artist*, and the lectures Rank gave at Penn, Yale, and the University of Minnesota.

Over the course of the next two chapters, I will unpack Rank's theory of human nature based on passages from these books and lectures. In my reconstruction, I will also cite writings by philosophers, therapists, neuroscientists, biologists, and others that can help clarify what Rank meant.

The word "will," as we saw earlier, can hardly be found in modern psychology texts, having been replaced by such terms as "decision," "motivation," "agency" and "self-efficacy"—all euphemisms, in my view, for "will."

"Will may be defined as the life force," Rank once told a group of clinicians who asked what he meant by the word (quoted in Isono 2012:400). Both women and men experience the power of this life force. The "will," suggested Rank, is an emotional expression of the evolutionary energy coursing through the universe since the beginning of time, an energy derived, at bottom, from what today we'd call the explosive force of the Big Bang.

"Most patients don't ask for a definition," Rank said, "because each has an idea of his own and therefore does not feel it necessary to ask" (ibid.). How does one define "will" or "the life force" when no one has ever been able to define "life" itself? (Schrödinger 1944). Even biologists still lack consensus, says biochemist and molecular biologist Jamie Gómez-Márquez (2021) "to answer questions such as *What is life?* . . . some scientists and philosophers of science suggest that it is not possible to define life" (6223; italics added).

According to Rank, Freud had reduced all human nature, all thinking and feeling, all culture and art, all the creativity needed for scientific discoveries, to a disguised derivative of the sex drive. Although marveling at Freud's mastery of language, Harold Bloom (1981) asserts that "Freudian thought is necessarily antithetical to nearly any theory of the imagination" (215).

As the psychoanalyst most absorbed in studying inhibitions to creativity, Rank was the first to point out that because Freud had rejected feelings as "irrational," he could never account for art or even the discoveries of science—discoveries, like those of quantum physicists in the early 20th century, that require enormous creativity, and are just as full of feeling and intuition, as Einstein and other great scientists insist, as are the creations of artists.

Freud was unable to explain how from a sex drive common to all human beings there was produced not sexuality but artistic creation. "Sublimation" of the sex drive, writes Rank (1936b) in *Truth and Reality*, is an "insipid and impotent concept which prolongs a shadowy existence in psychoanalysis" (11).

Who or what was doing the "sublimation"? "An inexplicable 'remainder' had therefore to be admitted," observes Rank (1932a) in *Art and Artist*, "but this remainder embraced no more and no less than the whole problem of artistic creativity" (63). In the German sub-title of *Art and Artist*, Rank uses the term *Schaffensdranges*—"creative urge," an urge, maintains Rank, that great artists feel even more strongly than their sex urge.

The creative urge, insists Rank, is not a "sublimation" of the sex urge, although exceptionally creative people, like Anaïs Nin and Henry Miller, often have very strong sex drives (Jong 1993). As a biological process, sex can lead only to species *reproduction*, not cultural or artistic *production*, which requires a conscious feeling person to make something unprecedented, new, something that does not already exist in nature.

"[W]e fail to see," argues Rank (1932a) in *Art and Artist*, "how the sex urge, which is designed primarily to preserve the [species], should produce even the most primitive ornamentation, still less a higher art-form . . . unless we build the bridge of the individual will which converts the propagation of the species into a perpetuation of the [I]" (84–85)—the individual.

Art expresses the urge for immortality of the individual artist—a creative process above and beyond the sexuality of nature, according to Rank. Like all of culture, art is *super*natural, not natural. Art is unnatural. There is no art to be found in nature.

"The will," asserts Rank, is always "the expression of the individual, the indivisible *single* being, while sexuality represents something shared, something *generic* which is harmonious with the individually-willed only in the human love-experience and is otherwise in perpetual conflict with it" (85–86; italics added).

The species, Darwin had observed, is driven to maximize reproductive success, a battle against the finality of death. *Species* immortality is, therefore, the "purpose" of natural selection but does not allow for *individual* immortality.

For Freud, the primal force of sex was "a First Cause, to be believed in precisely because it is both fundamental to and inaccessible to experience" (Rieff 1959:35). Freud's lifelong "desire was always to find in emergence, sameness; in the dynamic, the static; in the present, latent pasts" (237). In contrast to Freud's psychology of likeness, as we have seen, Rank championed a psychology of difference in creative tension with likeness.

It is "only in the individual act of will," insists Rank (1936a) in *Will Therapy*, that "we have the unique phenomenon of spontaneity, the establishing of a new primary cause" (63)—and the potential for an *individual* will to immortality in contrast to a *species* will to immortality.

The laws of physics, maintains Rank, are unable to explain anything artistic. These laws, no matter how well scientists understand them, cannot account for Beethoven's Ninth Symphony, Martha Graham's dances, Emily Dickinson's poetry, or even the discoveries of the laws of physics themselves—discoveries that require conscious, willing, feeling human beings, like Einstein, Planck, and Heisenberg, collaborating and competing with each other to find them.

Schopenhauer, whose book *The World as Will and Representation* (1819) Rank had studied before meeting Freud, saw "the will as the most powerful driving force in all species. It constitutes the basis for the entire biological world and can be understood as the will for life.... [T]he will is expressed with undiminished force in every one of the billions of organisms that are produced" (Klein 1992:152).

Obviously, neither Schopenhauer, Freud, nor Rank knew of DNA, which was discovered much later by Rosalind Franklin, James Watson, and Francis Crick. There is, nevertheless, a parallel between Schopenhauer's "world as will," the urge that drives all human creatures, and the relentless force of DNA.

Now imagine you are Carl Rogers, an unknown 34-year-old who has yet to publish his first book, sitting in the audience, listening to the world-famous Otto

Rank. What might you have learned about how Freud and Rank differ in their understanding of human nature and their practice of therapy?

At Rochester in 1936, Rank may have begun by telling Rogers that Freud had borrowed Schopenhauer's "will" and renamed it *das Es*, the id or "the It," a term that Friedrich Nietzsche and Georg Groddeck, the father of psychosomatic medicine, had used before Freud.

According to Rank, willing is what it *feels like to be me*: the subjectivity of lived, embodied experience. The first-person experience of being embodied and of feeling alive, the "*I am*" experience, Rank calls an act of willing. The subjective experience of willing cannot be understood intellectually. It must be *felt viscerally in one's body*, according to Rank.

Over the eons of evolution, human beings discovered themselves to be conscious, to be alive. Consciousness in human beings, maintains Rank, means that the cosmos has become aware of itself. I am in the cosmos and the cosmos is in me. Human willing, observes Rank (1936b) in *Truth and Reality*, is "the cosmos manifested in [me] ... [so that] nature becomes ever more conscious of herself" (24).

To be conscious is to *feel emotions in my body* and, in so doing, eventually become aware of the prospect of my body's eventual decay, death, and disappearance. Only the human animal is self-consciously aware of the inevitabilty of its own death, which makes self-consciousness an often anguishing experience for the most sensitive souls.

In *Will Therapy*, Rank (1936a) argues that, at some point in the evolution of the universe, human beings became aware of themselves, manifesting their self-awareness through the "soul life of feeling and willing" (231). The feeling, willing mind created art with the aim of defying death and achieving *individual* immortality. Religion and the nation-state, on the other hand, were created, according to Rank, to promote *collective* or *group* immortality.

For Rank, the terms "soul life," "feeling" and "willing" are synonyms. An individual's feeling and willing constitute each other. The many varieties of feeling and willing are colors of the "soul."

Rank was the first to point out that Freud, due to his repudiation of femininity had also repudiated feelings, equating them with irrationality—with *das Es*, "the It." According to psychoanalyst Bruno Bettelheim (1990), "Freud believed that feelings and emotions were irrational and, therefore, suspect. . . . Freud could not see that if man's thinking is split off from his feelings, both become distorted" (50).

As a result, observes Rank (1936a) in *Will Therapy*, "the real I, or self with its own power, the will, is left out" (160) of psychoanalysis especially for women. Rank detected a striking contradiction in Freud's theory of human nature that no one had seen before. Even though Freud claimed to be a strict determinist, psychoanalysis had nevertheless managed to smuggle into its theory of human nature the power of willing—but *only* for men.

In Freud's Oedipal theory, men and fathers *have* powerful wills, since they are the sole source of the "above-I," the paternal super-ego internalized in everyone's unconscious at ages 4–6. But do women have powerful wills of their own? Not in Freud's Oedipal theory.

Influenced by his wife, Rank had been protesting against Freud's repudiation of women's will as early as 1924 with the publication of *The Trauma of Birth*, a book that had enraged Freud for revealing the will of the powerful "pre-Oedipal" mother, touching the third rail of Freud's own unconscious.

For both women and men, according to Rank, the life of feelings constitutes the "*I am*" experience, which is identical to what ancient peoples called the "soul." By celebrating the value of feeling and willing as an expression of the "soul life," Rank was returning to Nietzsche, who had criticized Schopenhauer's call for the abolition of all willing.

According to Schopenhauer, the more intense the willing, the more intense the suffering. Following the Buddha, Schopenhauer preached that Nirvana is the end of suffering, which means the end of willing.

Quoting from Schopenhauer's *The World as Will and Representation*, Rank (1924) writes in *The Trauma of Birth*: "[During] the *painless condition*, which Epicurus praised as the highest good and as the condition of the Gods, we are set free at that moment from contemptible will-pressure, we celebrate the sabbath of the penal-work of will" (141n.3; italics in the original).

Rank observes that Schopenhauer calls Nirvana "the deliverance from 'Will'" (ibid.). Opposing Schopenhauer and Freud, Rank favors, instead, Nietzsche's philosophy of willing. "But to eliminate the will altogether, to suspend each and every affect, supposing we were capable of this," Nietzsche (1887) had written, "what would that mean but to *castrate* the intellect?" (119; italics in the original).

Following Goethe, Nietzsche said that he had "fought against the separation of reason, sensation, feeling, and will" (quoted in Katsafanas 2018:133). These are all expressions of the soul, and cannot be separated, insisted Nietzsche. They are one. All together, they compose the whole of a human being's nature, male or female. By integrating reason, sensation, feeling, and will, Goethe had "disciplined himself to wholeness," added Nietzsche (ibid.).

Simply put, according to Rank, to know what "I want" means to know what "I will"—and answers Freud's infamous question, "*Was will das Weib?*" (What does a woman want?). *Wanting* and *feeling* overlap for Rank.

Intelligence, declare Nietzsche and Rank, is not the opposite of feeling. The rational life and the feeling life cannot be demarcated. Foreshadowing the findings of modern neuroscience, Nietzsche and Rank assert that rationality is impossible without the perspective and judgement provided by feelings. Certainly some emotions, if carried to excess, lead to harmful, destructive, irrational behavior. Not everything I want is good for me or for others.

But psychoanalysts like Freud and traditional cognitive models, according to neuroscientist Antonio Damasio (1994), don't understand that *"reduction in emotion may constitute an equally important source of irrational behavior"* (53; italics in the original).

Nietzsche infused intense feeling into all his writings, reflecting a conviction that feeling is nonrational but intelligent. Feelings are not the opposite of rationality. Without access to our feelings, which express purpose, meaning, and motivation, there can be no rational action. Rationality, argues Rank, depends on feelings, on the intelligence of the emotions.

For women and men, "the emotional tone," writes Rank (1936b) in *Truth and Reality*, "is an index of the *'what'* of the will" (48; italics added).

Without listening to our feelings and intuitions, we cannot know what we want. We use our feelings and emotions as bodily touchstones to tell us what we desire, what is important for us, what is meaningful.[2]

We use our feelings to make difficult decisions. Moreover, without listening to the feelings of others, we cannot know what *they* want. For Rank, in large measure, feelings constitute willing.

Neuroscientist Ernst Pöppel, when asked by an interviewer, "How do you make difficult decisions yourself? According to your intuition, or your understanding?," answered:

That is the wrong question, but that is not the fault of either of us. We use concepts like intelligence, consciousness, feeling, free will—that has been our tradition for 2,500 years—but these concepts conceal the fact that such functions do not exist independently of each other. There is no such thing as feeling in itself, perception in itself, no memory as such, they all derive from the anatomy of the brain; it is all unbelievably closely networked. Every feeling is also perception and memory, every rational process is embedded in emotional evaluation, every intuition is linked to behavioral intention. (quoted in Plamper 2015:245)

According to Rank, only when we express the power of our "creative will"— our life force—can we deploy our feelings to create art, culture, myth, philosophy, and religion in the heroic quest to transcend death, even while the species "demands," through its relentless, blind sexual will—*das Es*, "the It"—that we reproduce in order to maintain the immortality of the "germ plasm," the term used before the discovery of DNA.

All artists know that there can be no act of creativity without accessing their deepest feelings, which are embodied. Reason and feeling interact. But even today, writes neuroscientist Antonio Damasio (2018), "feelings have not been given the credit they deserve as motives, monitors, and negotiators of human cultural endeavors" (3).

The production of art, or any product of culture for that matter, can be accounted for only by the "emergence of conscious, feeling minds" (6), insists Damasio, by conscious human beings who use their imagination, empathy, and feelings to create something new. Only those capable of experiencing empathy and feeling can create or enjoy art, or appreciate what has been created. Feeling is a form of embodied cognition.

As philosopher Martha Nussbaum (2001) observes in *Upheavals of Thought: The Intelligence of Emotions*:

A lot is at stake in the decision to view emotions in this way, as intelligent responses to the perception of value. If emotions are suffused with intelligence and discernment, and if they contain in themselves an awareness of value or importance, they cannot, for example, easily be sidelined in accounts of ethical judgment, as so often they have been in the history of philosophy. Instead of viewing morality as a system of principles to be grasped by the detached intellect, and emotions as motivations that either support or subvert our choice to act according to principle, *we will have to consider emotions as part and parcel of the system of ethical reasoning*. We cannot plausibly omit them, once we acknowledge that emotions include in their content judgments that can be true or false, and good or bad guides to ethical choice. We will have to grapple with the messy material of grief and love, anger and fear, and the role these tumultuous experiences play in thought about the good and the just. (1–2; italics added)

Even more radically, argues Rank, if we allow feeling to infuse our bodies, its vital energy can, at times, connect our individual psyches to everything in the macrocosm, linking part to whole, the personal to the universal.

In *Truth and Reality*, Rank (1936b) proposes that human willing is a "temporal representative of the cosmic primal force" (10), an expression of the creative evolutionary process unfolding with immeasurable energy, force, and power in the universe—"the ALL," as Rank (1936a) terms the macrocosm in *Will Therapy*, capitalizing the word "ALL" for effect (219).

The "expansive self-feeling of the life force," maintains Ernest Becker (1973:151) in *The Denial of Death*, is what promotes the creation of culture, symbols, and art as a way to transcend death.

Expressed viscerally, through our emotions, "the strength of this force," says Rank (1936b) in *Truth and Reality*, "we call the will" (10). The universe lives in us. Each person is a whole composed of its parts, yet is also part of a larger whole. If the whole infuses the parts, the parts themselves will feel whole.

We are microcosmic parts of this ALL, according to Rank, seeking always, in disguised and varied forms, to return to the whole, a feeling of Oneness, union, with the macrocosm that we felt pre-verbally in the womb and then lost during separation at birth. An implicit memory of wholeness remains in the body.

"If there is a symbol for the condition of wholeness, of totality," writes Rank (1936a) in *Will Therapy*, "it is doubtless the embryonic state, in which the individual feels himself an indivisible whole and yet is bound inseparably with a greater whole" (190).

As a bodily experience, the trauma of birth is the *first* feeling of separation anxiety and simultaneously the *first* feeling of loss of wholeness. Empathizing deeply with the newborn's loss of wholeness, Rank observes:

> In the first developmental stages after birth, the child has lost not only the feeling of connection with the mother, but also the feeling of wholeness in himself. In relation to the outer world he becomes successively mouth, eye, ear, legs and so forth and, for a long time, in a certain sense all his life, remains related to the world partially, until he can establish again in his ego feeling [*Ichgefühl*] something similar to the original totality. (ibid.)

In the 20th century, Martha Graham, renowned as the mother of modern dance, expressed the primal force of her creative will by "channeling" the power of the macrocosm through every sinew, every part, of her body. In such moments, she felt most alive.

Determined to go beyond the rarefied techniques of classical ballet in order to create something new and raw, a reflection of her own vivid bodily experience of living fully, Graham was the very embodiment of what Rank calls willing. Her soulful dances pulsate with rage, loneliness, anxiety, tenderness, love, and the whole range of feelings that Freud strove to suppress in himself and in his female patients—including in his own daughter, Anna.

"[T]he influence of Rank," according to Martha Graham's biographer, Mark Franko (2012), "was fundamental" (11) to Graham's understanding of her own, fierce, unremitting creative will. A great admirer of Rank's *Art and Artist*, Martha Graham says of the creative will:

> There is a vitality, a life force, an energy, a quickening that is translated through you into action, and because there is only one of you in all of time, this expression is unique. And if you block it, it will never exist through any other medium

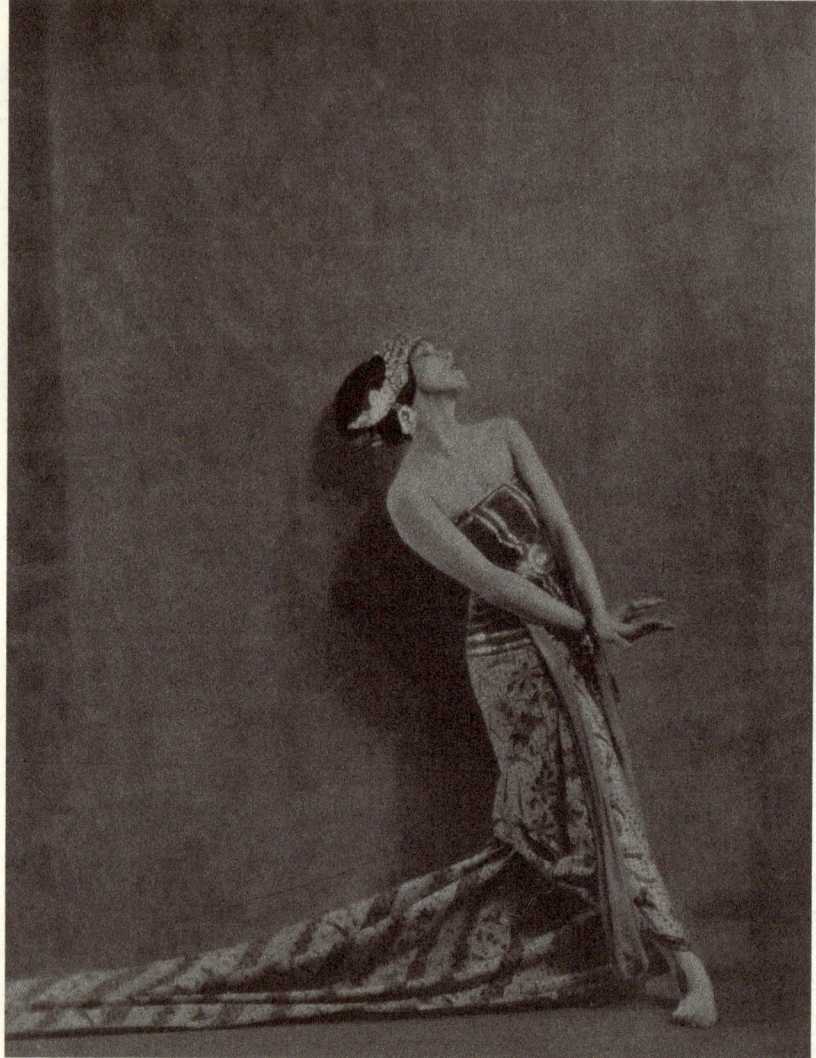

Figure 12.2 Martha Graham, 1922

Credit: Photograph by Nickolas Muray. Jerome Robbins Dance Division, The New York Public Library

and it will be lost. The world will not have it. It is not your business to determine how good it is nor how valuable nor how it compares with other expressions. It is your business to keep it yours clearly and directly, to keep the channel open. . . . You have to keep yourself open and aware to the urges that motivate you. Keep the channel open. (quoted in De Mille 1991:264)

For Martha Graham, willing is composed of the greatest joys, love, and ecstasies as well as the greatest sufferings, anguish, and dissatisfactions. The word "indifference" was not in Graham's vocabulary. "No artist is pleased," she said. "[There is] no satisfaction whatever at any time. There is only a queer divine dissatisfaction, a blessed unrest that keeps us marching and makes us more alive than the others" (ibid.). For Martha Graham, as for Rank, willing is always embodied.

As a therapist, Rank would strive to sense pre-verbally, intuitively, what he was feeling in his own body in the relationship with his patients, while registering, empathically, what they were feeling in their bodies.[3]

13

Willing = feeling alive = guilt-feeling

Willing is the experience of feeling the "cosmic primal force" that quickens us, that infuses our bodies, that makes us come alive, that propels our creativity. Human "*being*" is a verb, not a noun. To *be* alive is to *feel* alive, viscerally.

In *Will Therapy*, Rank (1936a) explains how he helped his clients "learn to will" (14)—learn to feel more powerful, more alive, more embodied, more whole in the present moment. Willing expresses itself uniquely for each of us. Willing = difference.

But accepting one's difference is painful. Although essential to self-empowerment, willing, according to Rank, inevitably leads to a feeling of existential guilt for being separate from the universe, "the ALL" (219).

Are we not forever in debt to another or an "Other"—someone or something outside ourselves—for the gift of our very existence? This is not guilt for wrong-doing. Existential indebtedness is a feeling of being grateful for the unasked-for gift of our life: a miracle.

To be sure, Rank acknowledges both Oedipal (paternal) and pre-Oedipal (maternal) guilt-feeling, but observes that they are surplus guilt; they come on top of an already present existential indebtedness, an indebtedness that is connected to our sense of awe, amazement, wonder, and gratitude for being alive, "the marvel of creation itself" (Rank 1941a:250).

"[W]e are not our own," argues Rank (1936a) in *Will Therapy*, "no matter whether we perceive the guilt religiously toward God, socially toward the father, or biologically toward the mother" (143).

For Rank, difference is the experience of separateness. It is only through some form of creative production or mutual love that the pain of living can be eased and the gift of life justified.

"I remember today the sense of illumination," writes Virginia Robinson (1968) of her therapy with Rank 40 years earlier, "when [Rank] said 'perhaps what the self really seeks is identity; does it ever accept difference?'" (22).

While focusing on willing in the here-and-now, Rank (1936a) does not ignore the past, which, he insists, lives in the present. "Thinking and feeling, consciousness and willing," argues Rank, "can always be only in the present" (54). *Gefühl ist alles.* "The feeling of experience [*Gefühlserlebnis*], purposefully and with

Otto Rank and the Creation of Modern Psychotherapy. Robert Kramer, Oxford University Press.
© Robert Kramer (2025). DOI: 10.1093/9780197698303.003.0013

intent, is made the central factor in the therapeutic task" (9), no matter how painful at times.

The therapeutic experience, says Rank, is "a learning to feel, a process in which the individual learns to develop emotions" (233)—the opposite of Freud's view, which claims that emotions are neurotic repetitions of infantile patterns, and need to be "drained" like the Zuider Zee.

For Rank, the experience of being in relationship therapy would mean learning how to *accept all our feelings*, both grateful and sorrowful, loving and angry, to become, as it were, a continual flow of our feelings—but keeping harmful, destructive emotions under control.

Early in their conversations, Rank told Anaïs Nin (1966): "The flow of life and the flow of writing must be simultaneous so that they may nourish each other" (283). Later, Nin (1967) said that "he had given me emotional freedom" (6) and that she was now able to live "by a flow, a trust in my feelings" (69). One cannot will unless one learns to trust one's feelings, but, at the same time, it is essential, insisted Rank, to value the fruits of intellect, insight, and rationality.

At a 1930 congress on mental health held in Washington DC, Rank (1996) delivered a keynote address criticizing Freud for stigmatizing feelings as "only a transference phenomenon" (221). In psychoanalysis, he added, there is a "complete lack of any satisfactory theory . . . of the emotional life" (222). Speaking as a discussant, Jessie Taft elaborated:

> A theory of the emotions that not only recognizes, but embraces, their inevitability, that is not trying to escape them or to reduce them to conditioned reflexes or infantile patterns that ought to be abandoned, gives us a new basis for self-respect, a new standard of values, and a very different concept of growth and maturity. As long as emotions are feared and condemned, as long we struggle to attain the lifeless ideal of a maturity that is not subject to the *negative separating affects*, so long are we bound to a standard that already spells defeat or success at the price of self-deception and a *deadening of all feeling*. . . .
> (quoted in Lieberman 1985:290; italics added)

By "*negative separating affects*," Taft is referring to Freud's failure to understand separation anxiety, and his insistence, related to this failure, that psychoanalysis be interminable, becoming, in the long run, a "*deadening of all feeling*"—"all passion spent," in the critique Harold Bloom (1991) leveled against psychoanalysis as therapy (200).

"The emotional impoverishment of psychoanalysis," adds Ernest Becker (1973) in *The Denial of Death*, "must extend also to many analysts themselves and to psychiatrists who come under its ideology. This fact helps explain the terrible deadness of emotion that one experiences in psychiatric settings, the heavy weight of the character armor erected against the world" (195n).

When we fully own the feelings that propel our acts of willing and creativity, according to Rank, our sense of selfhood and engagement with others changes.

Tenderness, empathy, and love are the feelings urging us to *unite* with others; assertion, anger, and hate are the feelings urging us to *separate* from others. Both uniting and separating—the two represent a continuum of feeling, not a binary opposition—are essential for living as a whole human being. Love is a softening of will; hate a hardening of will.

The objective of therapy, writes Jessie Taft (1933), is to "gradually begin to take responsibility for one's own feelings and impulses in all their ambivalence, with as little denial, rationalization and justification as possible" (94).

Much of the neurotic suffering in our life, says Rank, is due to a refusal to affirm ourselves as individuals, a refusal to become ourselves, a refusal to accept our difference—a fear or reluctance to *be fully alive*, to feel all our emotions, good or bad. When we are fully alive, we are in touch with all aspects of our embodied being.

Neurosis "is *self-willed*," argues Rank (1996) in his American lectures, "a sort of creation that can find expression only in this negative, destructive way" (252; italics in the original). Neurosis, one might say, is a creative achievement.

Both constructive and destructive, willing is expressed in creativity or lost in neurotic symptoms, that is, self-destruction. "This evaluation of illness as an expression of the individual creative force," adds Rank (1936a) in *Will Therapy*, "leads to a wholly different conception of the neurotic . . . [who] unites in himself potentially the possibilities of destructiveness as well as of creativeness" (226).

Rank is not referring to Freud's *Todestrieb*, a biologically-based "death drive," although his term "possibilities of destructiveness" may have a superficial resemblance. He's referring to the consequences of *Lebensangst* and *Todesangst*, fear of living and fear of dying—an ultimate existential anxiety: *Urangst*.

When we choose not to exercise our will, due to *Lebensangst*, we distort the primal life force into its own denial. The neurotic, insists Rank, is "a personality denying its own will, not accepting itself as an individual" (70), not accepting its own creative life force, its own feelings, its own capacity for self-leadership. Paradoxically, we seem to have been granted the freedom of will to "transform will to not-willing" (215).

Although a "creative achievement," says Rank (1936b) in *Truth and Reality*, neurotic suffering is a form of negative willing (10). When we refuse the existential burden of our freedom, we deny ourselves—our uniqueness, our difference.

"[T]he fundamental problem," adds Rank (1932a) in *Art and Artist*, "is *individual difference*, which the [I] is inclined to interpret as inferiority unless it can be proved by achievement to be superiority" (42; italics in the original).

My consciousness that *I am alive*, which cannot be explained by science, inevitably leads to self-consciousness—the awareness that I am a physical body that will age, shrivel, and die. Self-consciousness is the dawning realization that everything I call "myself"—my "*I am*," my bodily processes, my thinking, feeling, and willing—is fated to die.

Rank (1936a) practiced therapy by empathizing with the pain of his patients's "consciousness of living" (59). At bottom, argued Rank in his American lectures, "the real etiological factor of the neurosis consists in the fact that we have a psychical life"—a feeling of *Angst*, or dread, merely for existing, for being alive, unique, and separate from everyone else. "It is simply anxiety in the I and for the I" (Rank 1996:124). This is an existential condition, said Rank, not a psychiatric problem.

For any understanding of the universal suffering of human beings, isn't the strange *consciousness of living*—the dim awareness that we're embodied and alive, for a moment, on a speck of dust as it spins, meaninglessly, around the sun, itself only a slightly larger speck of dust in the vast, incomprehensible spaces of the cosmos—*the* single most significant fact of human existence?

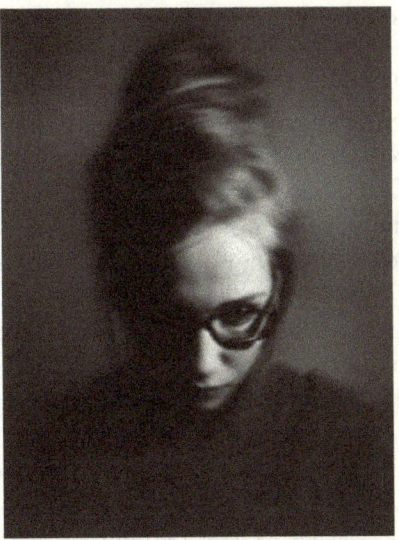

Figure 13.1 Anxiety
Credit: By Elīna Arāja via Pexels

Freud's unconscious is sexual, while Rank's is existential. Not a box in the mind whose contents can be uncovered, interpreted, and repackaged by analysis, Rank's unconscious is a mystery, shrouded in darkness.

"I would prefer that you listen," Rank had invited members of the American Psychoanalytic Association during a lecture he gave at their 1924 annual meeting, paraphrasing a famous line from *Hamlet*, "as if a traveler were relating to you his experiences in a yet undiscovered country" (Rank 1996:78).[1]

In *The Trauma of Birth*, to be sure, Rank declined to map any part of this "dark continent." Always just out of reach, the undiscovered country is an infinite past stretching backward into the impenetrable darkness of the universe "before" our arrival on the planet and stretching forward into an equally impenetrable darkness "after" our departure.

Emerging at conception from Nothingness, and returning at death to Nothingness, we are astounded by the eerie similarity of the two black holes called "before" and "after."

Enigmatically, our *conscious awareness of being alive* has suffered a much deeper repression than even the repression of our sexual desires, which can be revealed. Rank's unconscious, on the other hand, can never be revealed. At best, it can only be intuited—through a glass darkly—with the symbols of art, music, myth, poetry, religion, or philosophy.

In my collection of Rank's American lectures, I coined the term "existential unconscious" to encapsulate Rank's view in *The Trauma of Birth* that he was pointing, as he told his American audiences, to "an unconscious absolutely inaccessible to any *intellectual* grasp" (Rank 1996:223; italics in the original).

In *Psychology and the Soul*, Rank (1930) suggests that the existential unconscious "holds more than past reality: it contains something unreal, extrasensory, formerly attributed to the soul" (3). The existential unconscious is beyond language, beyond science, beyond rationality. It is ineffable. It is "the abstract, the unfathomable, and the esoteric" (23).

"[W]e all seem to recoil" from the existential unconscious, said Rank (1941a) in *Beyond Psychology*, a recoil that "leads to an over-estimation of the rational mind, i.e. some kind of understanding which would calm the fear" (277).[2]

Neither mother nor father, said Rank, is the primary cause of our deepest suffering. It is ordinary living—*mere consciousness*—that is painful. In *The Courage to Create*, Rollo May (1975) calls the anguish of this experience, without exaggeration, "the terror of human consciousness" (30). Many others have felt this terror.

In *The Varieties of Religious Experience*, William James (1902) describes a moment in his life "when suddenly there fell upon me without any warning, just as if it came out of the darkness, a horrible fear of my own existence. . . . and

I became a mass of quivering fear. After this the universe was changed for me altogether" (157).

Echoing James, Rank, and May, Ernest Becker (1973) in *The Denial of Death* writes of "the terror of the world, the feeling of overwhelming awe, wonder, and fear in the face of creation—the miracle of it . . . the fact that there are things at all" (49).

Were we to rip away all our psychological defenses, all our cultural symbols, all our religious beliefs, all our ideologies, were we to let truly and profoundly sink into our hearts and minds the awesome incomprehensibility of the strange *consciousness of living* forced on us, without our consent, would we not be terrified?

In his therapeutic practice, Rank focused on helping suffering human beings find the courage and creative will to overcome the *Urangst* attached to the consciousness of living. "What they need," Rank (1936a) proposed in *Will Therapy*, "is an emotional experience which is intense enough to lighten the tormenting self-consciousness" (74).

Not anti-intellectual, Rank also emphasized: "If I have at one time designated consciousness when it goes beyond a certain breadth or depth as destructive, . . . now while still maintaining this, I would exclude expressly intelligence, which represents exactly the factor that can realize the conscious surplus constructively if one succeeds in putting it at the service of the will" (250).

With the trauma of separation at birth, my feeling of Oneness with the ALL is lost, according to Rank. All is profoundly cracked. While I live, it is only the glue of art or love that can bind my broken parts together, make me feel whole again, if only for a fleeting moment. I = pain.

Only through a return to a feeling of Oneness, first experienced in the womb, can we be "delivered from [our] isolation and become part of a greater and higher whole," says Rank (1932a) in *Art and Artist* (86).

Our creation of a neurosis, in these terms, is an unsuccessful attempt to solve the "part-whole problem," Rank (1936a:189) observes in *Will Therapy*—the anxiety of feeling separateness and loneliness, and simultaneously the guilt-fueled search to return to a feeling of connection and wholeness, of Oneness. Experiencing wholeness in relation to another is the primary step toward healing.

As anxiety-ridden persons, we often hurtle from one extreme to the other, unable to find a constructive balance on the continuum between individuation and merger, separation and union, differentiation and connectedness, I and Thou, part and whole:

> Here psychotherapy enters as a binding function . . . which offers to the patient in the person of the analyst, the "thou" from whom he had estranged himself in

self-willed independence. That this "thou" then so easily becomes the "all" for the patient . . . constitutes the most difficult aspect of the neurotic type, which is formed on the all or none psychology so that either aspect has for him a death meaning, that is, tends to unleash fear [*Angst*]. (219)

It does not seem possible, says Rank, for us to eradicate our two "ultimate" anxieties—*Lebensangst* and *Todesangst*—which appear to be a burden carried out of the womb by every new arrival on the planet.

Sometimes it is our fear of living—the anxiety of becoming and being ourselves, separate and different from everyone else—that has the upper hand. At other times, it is our anxiety at the prospect of death—our fear of merging into the other, into the collective, and losing our dearly bought individuality—that predominates. The eternal conflict between our wish for and fear of separation, and our wish for and fear of union, has no final solution.

We must solve, unsolve, and resolve this problem continuously throughout life, at every developmental stage, "from birth, via childhood and puberty to maturity and from there downward through old age to death" (190), which is simultaneously the final separation and the final union. "It can only be a matter of balance between the two, which, however, is not attained once and for all but must be created anew and ever anew" (129).

Whereas there is no final solution to this lifelong dilemma—the "part-whole problem" (189)—some solutions are healthier than others. No one has expressed the searing tension between the will to separate and the will to unite more keenly than Ernest Becker (1973), whose *The Denial of Death* captures the largest—*macrocosmic*—meaning of separation and union for Rank:

> On the one hand, the creature is impelled by a powerful desire to identify with the cosmic process, to merge himself with the rest of nature. On the other hand, he wants to be unique, to stand out as something different and apart . . . . As Rank put it, man yearns for a "feeling of kinship with the All." He wants to be "delivered from his isolation" and become "part of a greater and higher whole." (151–152)

> . . . You can see that man wants the impossible: He wants to lose his isolation and keep it at the same time. He can't stand the sense of separateness, and yet he can't allow the complete suffocation of his vitality. He wants to expand by merging with the powerful beyond that transcends him, yet he wants while merging with it to remain individual and aloof, working out his own private and smaller-scale self-expansion. (155)

On a *microcosmic* level, however, our *Urangst* can be made more bearable, according to Rank, in an empathic relationship with another person who accepts our uniqueness and difference, and allows for the emergence of our creative urge—without too much guilt-feeling or anxiety for separating from the other.

Living fully requires individuating and connecting, without succumbing to the anxiety that leads us to shuttle endlessly from one pole to the other. Creative solutions for living emerge out of the fluctuating, ever-expanding and ever-contracting, space between separating and uniting, autonomy and connectedness, I and Thou, will and love.

Art, music, poetry, dance, literature, and all other creative endeavors, says Rank in *Art and Artist* (1932a), "originate solely in the constructive harmonization of this fundamental dualism of all life" (xxii).

Like anxiety, the creative urge itself seems to divide into two emotional currents: "[W]ill and guilt," argues Rank (1936b) in *Truth and Reality*, in one of his most important learnings, "are the two complementary sides of one and the same phenomenon" (61). In *Civilization and Its Discontents*, Freud (1930) had written that "the sense of guilt [is] the most important problem in the development of civilization" (134). Rank agreed, but saw guilt in a much deeper light than Freud, who framed guilt only through his Oedipal lens as sexual transgression.

One can never speak of willing without guilt-feeling, for they are of a single piece, infusing and shaping each other. Although Rank adopted Nietzsche's term "will," he opposed Nietzsche's attack on Judeo-Christian morality. There is no going "beyond good and evil." For Rank, willing and guilt-feeling are inextricably linked, like day and night.

It is the never-ending ebb and flow of these emotional currents, for good or evil, that gives music, color, poetry, and drama to our existence, a hymnal of creativity and suffering, joy and sorrow. If freedom is doing whatever we want, not every want will do. Freedom and responsibility are the same.

Willing and guilt-feeling define the greatness and limits of a flesh-and-blood mortal, who is both creator and creature, artist and worm, whose awareness of being alive is split, writes Rank (1936b) in *Truth and Reality*,

wavering between his Godlikeness and his nothingness, whose will is awakened to knowledge of its power [but] whose consciousness is aroused to terror before it. The heroic myth strives to justify this creative will through glorifying its deeds, while religion reminds man that he himself is but a creature dependent on cosmic forces. (61)

On a *macrocosmic* level, our consciousness of living—the dim awareness that we are alive for a moment on the planet Earth, a speck of Nothingness located somewhere in the unfathomably vast universe—gives us "the status of a small god in nature," according to Ernest Becker (1973):

> Yet, at the same time, as the Eastern sages also knew, man is a worm and food for worms. This is the paradox: he is out of nature and hopelessly in it; he is dual, up in the stars and yet housed in a heart-pumping, breath-gasping body that once belonged to a fish and still has the gill marks to prove it. . . . Man is literally split in two: he has awareness of his own splendid uniqueness in that he sticks out of nature with a towering majesty, and yet he goes back into the ground a few feet in order blindly and dumbly to rot and disappear forever. It is a terrifying dilemma to be in and to have to live with. (26)

Because of this great conflict between our Godlikeness and our Nothingness, "I," even with my powerful creative will, am not master in my own house. I am simultaneously a *maker of destiny* and an *object of fate*, a creator of art and a creature of cosmic forces forever beyond my ken, a master and a servant.

For everyone—artist and non-artist alike—our acts of willing are never "free," argues Rank (1996) in his American lectures.

Although a necessary part of growth, separating and individuating have an emotional price: "The more we individualize ourselves—that is, remove and isolate ourselves from others—the stronger is the formation of guilt-feeling that originates from this individualization, and that again in turn unites us emotionally with others" (236). Willing, in short, is always relational.

Guilt-feeling "springs from our own willing," observes Rank in *Will Therapy* (1936a:71). Willing = guilt-feeling. To say, "*I am*" is also to say "I am, to some degree, in debt, to some degree beholden to cosmic forces beyond my control." Only when willing and guilt-feeling are in balance—a balance that we must constantly adjust and re-adjust as our life unfolds—can the dance of creativity and connection, will and love, begin anew.

The human being who has *failed to separate* and individuate also feels guilt—a kind of thrown-back responsibility or debt to life—for remaining embedded in "the Other," submerged in the womb, "being buried alive" (209).

Not an ordinary sense of obligation, Rank is pointing to a much deeper guilt-feeling than the Oedipal or pre-Oedipal guilt uncovered by psychoanalysis. Guilt-feeling is not just our feeling of committing wrong against another, a residue of our sexual wishes, or fear of punishment.

For Rank, this feeling is guilt for self-betrayal: for refusing the burden of consciousness, for *denying* our vital need for growth.

A crisis "seems to break out at a certain age when the life fear [*Lebensangst*] which has restricted the [I's] development meets with the death fear [*Todesangst*] as it increases with growth and maturity," writes Rank (1936a) in *Will Therapy*. "The individual then feels himself driven forward by regret for wasted life and the desire still to retrieve it." He adds:

"But this forward driving fear is now death fear, the fear of dying without having lived, which, even so, is held in check by fear of life" (265).

The fear of dying correlates with "unused life, the unlived in us" (211). The more our life is "unlived," maintains Rank, the more we will fear dying. We cannot avoid life even by throwing it away.

Paradoxically, the greatest artists—those rare human beings, whether painters, dancers, scientists, musicians, writers, philosophers or other especially creative persons, who experience and express "difference" (or creative willing) to the *ultimate*—feel the most profound uneasiness for taking on the largest burden, creating a whole world in their own image, for rivaling the primal life force of the universe, for "negotiating" as mere mortals "with the problem of the Beyond," as Rank (1932a) says in *Art and Artist* (49n).

In a macrocosmic sense, the greatest artists struggle with all their emotional energies and creativity to wrest a sliver of meaning out of, what theologian Rudolf Otto (1924) in *The Idea of the Holy* calls, the *mysterium tremendum et fascinosum* (12–24), the awesome, terrifying, fascinating mystery of creation.[3]

They absorb into themselves, as a personal problem to be solved, nothing less than the *entire universe*. With an eye fixed on all of existence, the great artist, says Rank (1936b) in *Truth and Reality*, "creates a whole world in his own image, and then needs the whole world to say 'yes' to his creation, that is, to find it good and thus to justify it" (134).[4]

But what mortal's "creation of an own individual cosmos" (25) can rival the trillions of galaxies in the universe, the brilliant blue skies and waters of the Aegean, the giant redwoods of California, the vast mountain ranges of the Himalayas, the awesome beauty of a single rose?

The responsibility for creating "a new cosmos" is too much to bear on one person's shoulders, no matter how large. Even human genius is not enough for such a grandiose project, which accounts for the profound and honest humility of scientists of monumental stature like Isaac Newton, Albert Einstein, Marie Curie, and Rachel Carson. Rank's view that the *highest* form of creativity leaves guilt-feeling in its wake is found nowhere else in the psychoanalytic literature.

Why do the greatest artists, scientists, and creators often say they feel over-whelmed, uneasy, dissatisfied with their creative productions—"a queer divine

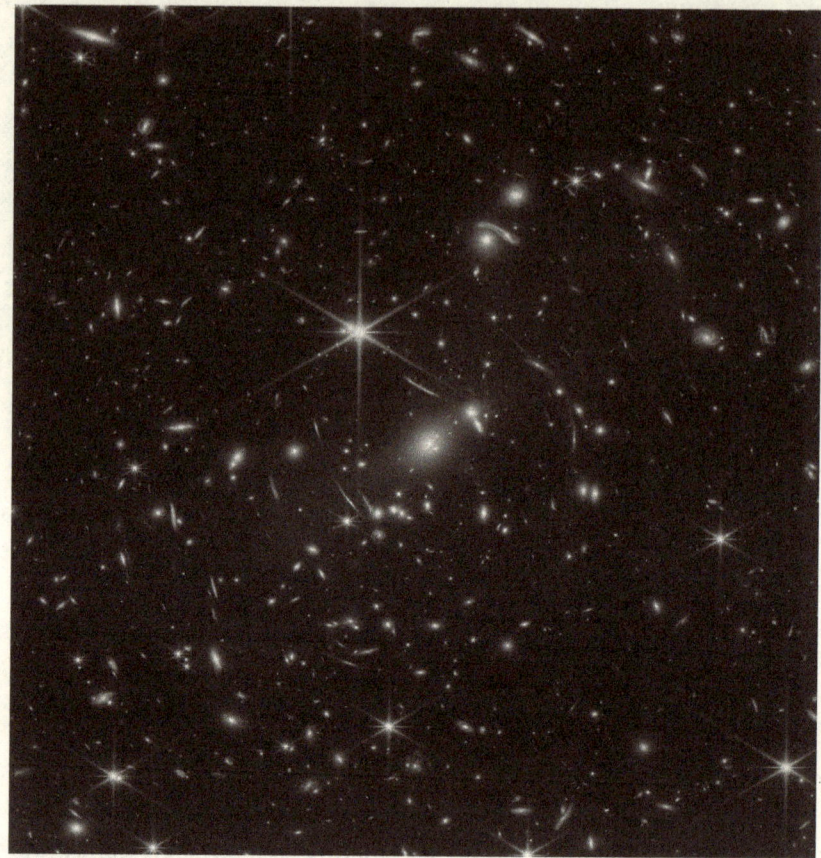

Figure 13.2 NASA describes the Webb Telescope's "First Deep Field," galaxy cluster SMACS 0723, as "approximately the size of a grain of sand held at arm's length, a tiny sliver of the vast universe."
Credit: NASA, ESA, CSA, STScI

dissatisfaction," according to Martha Graham (quoted in De Mille 1991:264)? In *Truth and Reality* (1936b), Rank answers, perhaps in part autobiographically:

> The creative type must constantly make good his continuous will expression and will accomplishment and he pays for this guilt toward others and himself with work which he must give to the others and which justifies himself to himself. Therefore, he is productive, he accomplishes something because he has *real* guilt to pay for, not *imaginary* guilt like the neurotic, who only behaves *as if* he were guilty but whose consciousness of guilt is only an expression of his *will denial*, not of creative accomplishment of will, which makes one *truly* guilty. (132; italics added)

By the most intense act of creating, the greatest artists strive toward spiritual freedom and the illusion of immortality, to make themselves independent of the compulsions of sex and death, of the inexorable will of Mother Nature—reaching toward the fantasy of *causa sui*: self-causation, pure independence.

But the project to create oneself—to be one's own parent, so to speak—is confronted with the existential limits mandated by biology, because bodily destruction and death await us all, artist or neurotic, hero or coward, master or servant.

Neither a prophet of pain-free self-actualization nor an advocate of pure "free will," Rank (1932a) analyzes the dialectic between freedom and determinism, willing and guilt-feeling, independence and dependence, most acutely in his masterpiece, *Art and Artist*:

> [M]an's acceptance of his dependence on nature is more *honest*, while freedom ideology, beyond a certain point, presumes the negation of that dependence and is therefore, also in a deeper sense, *dishonest*. This fundamental dishonesty towards nature then comes out as the *consciousness of guilt*, which we see active in every process of art. . . . the more strongly man feels his freedom and his independence, the more intense on the other hand is the consciousness of guilt, which appears in the individual partly *restrictive*, partly *creative*. . . . (328–329; italics added)

Our guilt-feeling, therefore, is not merely a fear of punishment by a higher authority such as parents or God. Like anxiety, our guilt-feeling is existential, a given. As the ancient Greek dramatists knew so well, guilt-feeling is double-sided, a *Doppelgänger*, and can never be completely eliminated.

In the deepest sense, guilt-feeling is what defines us as a human being *as long as we live*, grow, and create, or, conversely, as long as we deny and betray ourselves by *failing to live*, refusing to change and develop our potential, unthinkingly remaining embedded in "the Other"—be it the safety net woven by parents, religions, organizations, ideologies, gods, gurus, leaders, or therapists.

For this reason, says Rank (1996) in his American lectures, guilt-feeling—the inescapable complement of creative willing—is an emotional force in many people as powerful as the biological drive of their sexuality:

> Indeed, it is even shown that in many human beings inhibitions manifesting themselves as anxiety and guilt are *stronger* than the drives, that these inhibitions themselves, so to say, operate 'as a driving force' although in a different way from the biological impulses. In a word, we see that the *psychical* has

become a force at least equal to the *biological* and that all human conflicts are to be explained just from this fact. (229; italics in the original)

Even more profoundly, each person must accept and honor this existential pain, a necessary and vital part of the fully alive and functioning person. In their *creative* expression, anxiety and guilt-feeling are not to be condemned or analyzed away merely as an unconscious residue of early upbringing, social oppression, or religious training.

"In no case will one be able to do away with human guilt feeling," says Rank (1936a), whose understanding of anxiety and guilt-feeling in *Will Therapy* is matched only by that of Kierkegaard and Kafka, "but it makes a great difference whether the patient has fear and guilt reactions without visible reason, or whether he experiences guilt-feeling as a result of exercising his own will" (254).

If not too severe, guilt-feeling serves as a *harmonizing* factor between our "will to separate" and our "will to unite," re-attaching part to whole, allowing us to heal our feeling of brokenness, while simultaneously retaining our difference from each other and allowing for the expression of our creative will—all at once.

Guilt-feeling is a bridge, a liminal space, a feeling that attaches I to Thou, Thou to I. In his American lectures, Rank (1996) offers his clearest articulation of what he means by guilt-feeling:

> I think guilt-feeling occupies a special position among the emotions, as a *boundary* phenomenon between the pronounced painful affects that separate and the more pleasurable feelings that unite. It is related to the painful separating affects of anxiety and hate. But in its relation to gratitude and devotion—which may extend to self-sacrifice—it belongs to the strongest uniting feelings we know. As the guilt-feeling occupies the *boundary line* between the painful and pleasurable, between the severing and uniting feelings, it is also the most important representative of the relation between inner and outer, I and Thou, the Self and the World. (158; italics in the original)

Each of us is propelled forward by the urgent need to will—to accept and *be* ourselves, *be* our own difference—but also drawn back from expressing our difference fully by the fear that we'll be cut off from the rest of society and the love and connection that only others can provide.

As we become more aware of our difference from others, beginning to strongly assert this difference threatens separation from existing relationships. The more creative we are, the greater the threat of separation from others.

For Rank, the purpose of the end-setting phase in therapy—which usually takes a number of sessions in order to ease the pain of separating from someone who has listened deeply to us—is to learn how to *will creatively* without suffering too much anxiety and guilt-feeling for asserting our difference from the therapist.

It is only during the end phase of therapy that the "courage to be" (Tillich 1952) could be "willed," says Rollo May (1989) in *The Art of Counseling*: "In counseling I make it a specific practice near the end of the interview to *will courage*, knowing that this courage will carry over into the will of the counselee" (155; italics in the original).

Expressing the same idea, Jessie Taft (1933), perhaps reflecting on her own experience in gaining the "courage to be" while in relationship therapy with Rank, writes:

Therapy is a process in which a person who has been unable to go on with living without more fear and guilt than he is willing or able to bear, somehow gains the courage to live again, to face life positively instead of negatively. How is this possible? If one thinks of an exact scientific answer to this question, I must confess I do not know; that, at bottom, therapy of this kind is a mystery, a magic, something one may know beyond a doubt through repeated experiences but which in the last analysis is only observed and interpreted after the fact, never comprehended in itself or controlled scientifically any more than the life process is comprehended and controlled. (283)

14

I–Thou ... Thou–I

Vital to the process of differentiating ourselves from others, our painful "separating" feelings of defiance and rebellion, anger and hate, must be accepted alongside our pleasurable "uniting" feelings of gratefulness and devotion, communion and love.

In *Will Therapy*, Rank (1936a) urges us to learn how to live creatively with "our split"—the tension we feel between our need to separate and our desire to unite, between *difference* and *likeness*—"which no therapy can take away, for if it could, it would take with it the actual spring of life" (289).

Neither separating nor uniting can be denied if we are to become whole persons. Neurosis, in this sense, is a *partialization* of the human being, an absence of wholeness, an unwillingness to accept the permanence of this ambivalent condition of life, a refusal of the burden of selfhood, a refusal of necessary suffering—"a refusal of life itself" (153).

Each therapeutic hour, according to Rank, is an experience of "living and dying." If we can accept our difference in this microcosm, without too much anxiety or guilt-feeling, then living and loving more fully outside the allotted hour may also be possible for us.

Only through atonement, or, more precisely, *at-one-ment* or being-at-One, can our existential guilt be eased. Existential guilt is the feeling of separation, of loneliness, we carry, usually unconsciously, to one degree or another, for being different from everyone else who has ever lived.

The painfulness of difference, says Rank (1936a) in *Will Therapy*, cannot be solved "in and by the individual himself, but only in relation to a second person, who justifies our will, makes it good, since he voluntarily submits himself to it" (79)—in other words, *accepts* us as we are, a double helix of willing and guilt-feeling, evil and good, joy and sorrow, destruction and creation.

Freud's psychoanalytic technique does not do this, Rank maintains, because it interprets all expressions of willing in the therapeutic hour as "resistance" to the authority of the analyst, who stands in the center of the analysis in spite of his or her so-called "neutrality."

By dismissing the authenticity of the here-and-now relationship, Freud denied the energetic feeling, the creative willing and counter-willing, experienced in the moment by *both* parties.

Otto Rank and the Creation of Modern Psychotherapy. Robert Kramer, Oxford University Press.
© Robert Kramer (2025). DOI: 10.1093/9780197698303.003.0014

"Classical psychoanalysis"—a term coined almost 100 years ago by Sándor Ferenczi to criticize the indifference of analysts toward the suffering of their patients—does not permit a genuine feeling relationship between patient and analyst, I and Thou, Thou and I.

According to Ferenczi (1932), an authentic, empathic relationship creates the "most favorable atmosphere in the analytic situation: desperately rigid clinging to a theoretical approach is quickly recognized by the patients as such, and instead of telling us (or even admitting it to themselves) they use the characteristic features of our own technique, or our one-sidedness, in order to lead us ad absurdum" (1).

Going further, Rank maintained that psychoanalysis, if promoted as an interminable process, results in an endless minuet of projection and identification between a "will-less," virtually impotent patient and an all-knowing analyst who never lets go of his powerful will.

"Many people have had traumatic experiences with psychoanalytic therapy. . . , and they have left treatment feeling fragmented, objectified, and pathologized rather than appreciated, understood, and whole" (Safran et al. 2019:53).

Beginning with Freud, almost all psychoanalysts have insisted that the patient's resistance is "intrapsychic"—that is, resistance to the emergence into consciousness of repressed sexual thoughts, impulses, defenses, or memories.

Although Rank never denied the dynamics of inner conflict, which he saw as the creative tension between willing and guilt-feeling, he observes that Freud tended to label as *resistance* anything that opposed his theory or, what amounts to the same thing, anything that "interfered" with uncovering the Oedipal core of neurosis: fear of the powerful will of the father.

"Where Freud met the will of the other, he called it 'resistance,'" writes Rank (1936a:13) in *Will Therapy*, but this reaction by patients was resistance to *Freud's own will*, says Rank, rather than, as Freud claimed, intrapsychic resistance to accepting interpretations or insight.

Rank turns resistance, which he calls "counter-willing," into a creative factor: "[T]his negative reaction of the patient represents the actual therapeutic value, the expression of will as such" (19). Resistance is "proof, however negative, of the strength of will on which therapeutic success ultimately depends" (10).

Far from trying to overcome resistance, Rank "prize[d]" as an "act of will" (270) all of the human being's creative energies, even when misdirected into neurotic production.

Relationship-based will therapy, rather than "draining" feelings, helps us make deeper contact with ourselves and our ambivalences—i.e., all our emotional experiences, good or bad.

Relationship-based will therapy allows us to own unacknowledged parts of our suffering, own our fear of life and fear of death, letting the pain sit in our laps, rather than displacing or projecting it onto others.

Relationship-based will therapy opens a "space" deep inside us to contain our whole self, both our joys and our sorrows.

Relationship-based will therapy helps us listen more respectfully, more empathically, more lovingly, to *ourselves*, to our own feelings; it helps us accept, to the maximum extent possible, our own time-limited presence on earth, our *difference*.

"I try to bring to fruition the autotherapeutic forces in the neurotic, which hide behind the so-called resistances, and often can only manifest themselves negatively," says Rank (1936a) in *Will Therapy* (220).

All feelings—positive and negative, loving and hateful, constructive and destructive—are expressions of human willing that must be confronted, accepted, and integrated to make a whole person.

The therapist, according to Rank, is an "assistant [I]" (96) who provides a helping relationship in which we may be able to discover or recover our creative will—our "*I am*"—becoming our own therapist, with the ultimate goal of giving rebirth to ourselves as active, ethical agents, now empowered as self-leaders.

We will then be able to accept a maximum amount of responsibility for our own difference, and say "Yes" to the painful obligation of the consciousness of living as well as to the dreaded obligation of dying.

In the life-long, never completed, process of differentiation, we must learn to bear courageously, even affirm, the pain and suffering of our existence. "My formula for greatness in a human being," writes Nietzsche (1887:258), "is *amor fati*"—to love our fate.

Following Nietzsche, Rank (1932a) argues in *Art and Artist* that fate can, indeed, be overcome through the "volitional affirmation of the obligatory" (64)—that is, when we deliberately say "Yes" to the "Must," accepting our will to individuate as well as our will to merge, experiencing both separation and union, at once, without becoming shackled to one pole at the exclusion of the other.

Our will to separate and our will to unite exist simultaneously. Together, they infuse a feeling of wholeness in us. Separating and uniting make each other possible. Love and will, insists Rank, are interdependent. One without the other cannot restore wholeness.

For Rank, the quality of the client-therapist relationship is the most important factor in healing. The therapist does not heal by "re-educating" us— "*Nacherziehung*" as Freud (1916:312) maintained. Instead, the person of the therapist himself or herself is the healing factor in the here-and-now: "[T]he only means of healing which psychotherapy has learned to use is itself a human being, the therapist," says Rank (1936a:4) in *Will Therapy*. The relationship *is* the therapy.

The problem with spending too much time on interpreting the past, observes Rank, is that it allows both patient and therapist to escape the feeling-charged present: the experience of two creative and destructive wills encountering, resisting, trusting, hating, loving, healing, and transforming each other.

For Rank, beginning almost immediately after he started practicing full-time as a therapist, it was self-evident that the analytic relationship is co-created. To claim otherwise, he insisted, is to deny the feelings being experienced at all times by therapist and patient.

Neither aloof nor reluctant to confront patients when he felt it was helpful to promote their growth, Rank did not refrain from offering challenging interpretations to help patients surface, examine, and unlearn values, assumptions, beliefs, or expectations that no longer served them well.

But he insisted that all interpretation is subjective and tentative. Even interpretation of the *present moment* is scarcely valid or reliable while it is being

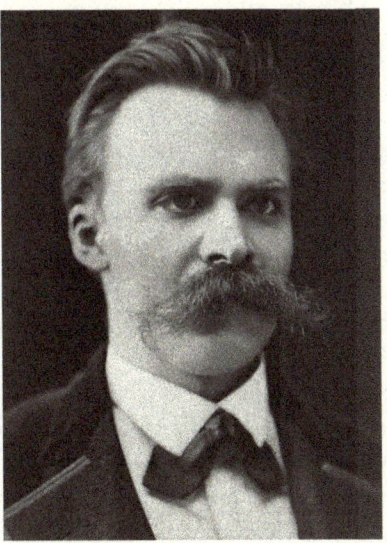

Figure 14.1 Friedrich Nietzsche
Credit: Friedrich H. Hartmann via
Wikimedia Commons

enacted. "[I]t is not a question of whose interpretation is correct," says Rank in a 1930 lecture, "because there is no such thing as *the* interpretation or only *one* psychological truth":

> Psychology does not deal primarily with facts as science does but only with the individual's attitude toward facts. In other words, the objects of psychology are *interpretations*—and there are as many of them as there are individuals and, even more than that, also the individual's different situations, which have to be interpreted *differently* in every single manifestation. (Rank 1996:222; italics in the original)

For human beings, there is no escaping interpretation. The experience of living, philosopher Alfred North Whitehead (1929) had written one year earlier, in *Process and Reality*, is "a complex of failure and success in the enterprise of interpretation. If we desire a record of uninterpreted experience, we must ask a stone to record its autobiography" (15).[1]

One of the greatest learnings of Rank is that the individual and society are not antagonistic, as Freud had insisted, but complementary. There's an eternal oscillation between the need for individuation and the need for attachment, the desire to separate and the desire to unite, independence and dependence, aloneness and intimacy—between the invigorating, creative solitude of freedom and the acceptance obtainable only within community.

Both will and love are essential, at once. This requires an exquisite balancing act, and presupposes that human beings accept the compatibility of what are often seen as irreconcilable or contradictory needs.

The tension between separation and union, difference and likeness, can never be fully resolved. Tension is not the same as opposition. According to Rank, the possibility of healing in relationship therapy means that, perhaps for the first time, clients will experience *being oneself* and *being related*—simultaneously.

What is necessary, suggests Ernest Becker (1968) in *The Structure of Evil*, is learning how to experience "maximum individuality and maximum community at the very same time" (81).

For Freud, on the other hand, the terms "I" and "Thou" were zero-sum. "The therapy of all therapies, the secret of all secrets, the interpretation of all interpretations, in Freud," Philip Rieff (1966) has written, "is not to attach oneself exclusively or too passionately to any one particular meaning, or object" (59).

In his papers on technique, Freud recommended that the analyst's "I" be kept as aloof as possible from the "Thou" in order to receive the maximum amount of "transference love" from patients.

According to psychoanalyst Erich Fromm (1959), love "for Freud, is always a fixed quantity, which can be spent in this or that way, but which is subject to the laws of matter: what is spent cannot be recovered. This lies behind concepts like narcissism, where it is a matter of *either* sending out [love] to the outside, *or* taking it back to my own ego" (99; italics in the original).

Ferenczi and Rank knew, of course, that Freud had attached himself exclusively to one object: the *Urmutter* of psychoanalysis, Amalia, and could never differentiate himself from her.

Moreover, Ferenczi and Rank saw that Freud, trapped tragically like a "small boy" in the pre-Oedipal phase all his life, had manipulated the ecology of the psychoanalytic hour to create the conditions for "transference" in order to attach patients interminably to *one* object exclusively: the analyst.

"Transference," a love lured from patients, sometimes for years, suppresses appearance of a patient's will, or the power of the "real I or self," in Rank's terms. When Freud did see it emerge, he called it "resistance" to accepting insight into the Oedipal unconscious.

Seeking to reduce transference as much as possible, Rank opposed this process of interminable infantilization, which applied most starkly to Freud's female patients, for whom the theory of psychoanalysis allowed *no will* at all.

For Rank, experiencing the creative tension between difference and likeness, autonomy and connection, is the principal task of the human being in the process of becoming a fully mature person, in the process of "the never completed birth of individuality," as he argues in *Truth and Reality* (1936b:24).

Maintaining psychological health, Rank (1932a) writes in *Art and Artist*, is a lifelong process of "seeking at once isolation and union" (86). Independence or autonomy alone is not enough, but neither is total immersion in the other at the expense of affirming one's difference. There is a dialectic, not a conflict, between will and love.

Individual and social life are in peril, according to Rank, if we cannot somehow find creative solutions to integrate "part and whole"—that is, to optimize jointly our two lifelong needs for differentiation and relatedness, assertion and togetherness, selfhood and connection. One must solve, unsolve, and re-solve the "part-whole" problem throughout every stage of life, not just in therapy.

The continuing development of the emotionally mature person proceeds, according to social worker Fay Karpf (1953), in a back-and-forth pattern,

> in terms of relationship and separation by a succession of emotional attachments and dependencies on the one hand and independence seeking separations and detachments on the other hand, with the creation of personality and the emergence of individuality as constantly evolving and

expanding goals. From the primal attachment and separation at birth to the final detachment and separation at death, this process of binding and freeing continues, throughout the entire course of human life. (74–75)

♨

In *Will Therapy*, Rank (1936a) maintains that the experience of living is an ongoing process of "emotional surrender to the present" (40)—to the Now or the New.

"Such a new experiencing, and not merely a repetition of the infantile, represents the therapeutic process . . . thus making possible a connection with the reality of the moment" (56). Transference of feelings from the past is not a means to "cure," as Freud insisted.

The question of experience, says Rank, is not how to understand or speak about the past, which we've already interpreted and reinterpreted a thousand-fold in memory, but how to *live in the present*: our feeling and willing can be experienced only in the present, in our bodies, viscerally. Every moment of our life is unprecedented. "This, then, is the New, which the patient has never experienced before" (92).

Healing, or making whole, comes from mutual recognition not intellectual understanding or insight into the past—Oedipal or pre-Oedipal. "The making-good must be individual, personal, from the analyst as a person to the patient as a person" (84).

It is a feeling experience in the "here and now" (55) relationship with a caring therapist, person-to-person, that is healing. "Not only less theory, but less 'art of interpretation' is necessary" (9).

The "art of interpretation" cannot be avoided, only minimized. At times, an interpretation may spark the surfacing, examining, and unlearning of assumptions or beliefs that are unhealthy or out-of-date. When offered, according to Rank, interpretations are always to be shared tentatively. But interpretations alone are never sufficient, no matter how artful.

Something else must be added if the relationship is to be healing. "In love and through love," argues Rank, "the individual can accept himself, his own will, because the other does" (91).

Against Freud, who allowed only transference interpretations in therapy and insisted that the analyst maintain indifference (*Indifferenz*, in Freud's German, means "uncaring," not "neutrality") to the suffering of patients, Rank had constructed "a Philosophy of Helping" (4).

Although Freud was never able to accept the "caring mother" in himself—or, for that matter, in Rank or Ferenczi—his entire world was "a small island of pain," he once confessed to Princess Marie Bonaparte, "floating on an ocean of indifference [*Indifferenz*]" (Schur 1972:524).

According to Rank, it is not what the client learns from the therapist's "insights" that is healing. All "insights" or "interpretations" are merely speculations or suggestions. Healing comes, rather, from what Martin Buber calls the Ich–Du—I–Thou—relationship. This is a real relationship, an authentic meeting between two embodied human beings, both of whom have a creative will.

"All real living is meeting," writes Buber (1923: 11) in *I and Thou*, and "through the graciousness of its comings and the solemn sadness of its goings, [the I–Thou relationship] teaches you to meet others and to hold your ground when you meet them" (33).[2]

Although Rank does not cite Buber, he observes in a 1927 lecture at the University of Pennsylvania School of Social Work: "One could designate the human emotional life as 'Thou Psychology' ['*Du Psychologie*'] because it determines our relation to fellow men, and at the same time, to reality in general" (Rank 1996:153).

"No less than Buber," writes historian William M. Johnston (1983), "[Rank] glorified interdependence between I and Thou. An I should nourish itself in a Thou. . . . Diligent observer that he was, Rank could praise embeddedness in society without scanting its dangers" (260).

According to psychologist Jean Susan Graham (1960): "Although Otto Rank and Martin Buber spring from radically different backgrounds . . . there is a striking similarity in their underlying philosophies. Both men have been motivated by an unusually profound respect for the integrity of human personality, and a reliance upon the healing, redemptive power of love as a force in molding and directing these personalities" (2).

In his American lectures, Rank argues that the feelings vital to an ethical life—freedom, responsibility, caring, love—get their meaning from the I–Thou relationship. For therapy as in all of life, the value of love, says Rank in a 1927 Penn School lecture, is that it "unites our I with the other, with the Thou, with men, with the world and so does away with all fear."

> What is unique in love is that—beyond the fact of uniting—it rebounds on the I. Not only, I love the other as my I, as part of my I, but the other also makes my I worthy of love. The love of the Thou thus places a value on one's own I. *Love abolishes egoism; it merges the self in the other to find it again enriched in one's own I.* This unique projection and introjection of feeling rests on the fact that one can really only love the one who accepts our own self as it is, indeed will not have it otherwise than it is, and whose self we accept as it is. (154; italics in the original)

Therapist and client, like everyone else, seek to find a constructive balance between separation and union, difference and likeness. In psychological health, the contact boundary that links I and Thou "harmoniously [fuses] the edges of each without confusing them," says Rank in *Art and Artist* (1932a:104).

Joining together in feeling, therapist and client, rather than lose their identities, can experience sublime moments in which they rediscover and recreate themselves in a larger whole that encompasses both of them.

In the simultaneous dissolution of their difference in a greater whole, both surrender their isolation for a moment, only to have individuality returned to them in the next, re-energized and enriched by the experience of "loss."

On a *microcosmic* level, relationship-based will therapy is a process of learning how to give and take, surrender and assert, merge and individuate, unite and separate. Only through a mutually empathic relationship can the "part-whole" problem be solved, albeit temporarily.

"The two selves become one, and the patient can now find in this enlarged self the differentiation necessary for life," writes Rank (1936a:248) in *Will Therapy*. As in the womb, two become one, creating a larger whole.

A hallmark of narcissism is too extreme egoism or too much "partialization": the incapacity to experience the feeling of love or empathy. So obsessed are narcissists by the fear of losing themselves, and their hard-won individuality, that they rarely let "emotion become whole or come up wholly, so that it can only express itself partially" (197).

Unable to solve even for a moment the "part-whole" problem, the narcissist remains agonizingly alone, isolated psychologically from others while physically in their midst.[3]

This compulsive, overconcentration on self prevents the giving up of self. Narcissism, according to Rank, is "cement, as it were, that holds the parts of the [I] together so firmly that they cannot be given out separately" (198–199). Narcissists want to see others who look, think, and feel like them; they can't tolerate difference, diversity, or genuine otherness.

Only through surrender to the wholeness of experience, with simultaneous emotional differentiation of the I, can the obsessively narcissistic person begin to be healed.

Only by reconnecting part to whole, I to Thou, Thou to I, can the compulsiveness of "obsession"—which derives from the Latin, *sedere*: to sit—be integrated into one's own self, be tolerated to "sit" more peacefully, as it were, less destructively, more creatively, on one's own lap.

On a *macrocosmic* level, taking the feeling of being together as far as humanly possible, to the boundary of the spiritual, Rank compares the artist's "giving" and the enjoyer's "finding" of art with the dissolution and rediscovery of the self in mutual love.

"The art-work," says Rank (1932a) in *Art and Artist*, "presents a unity, alike in its effect and in its creation, and this implies a spiritual unity between the artist and the recipient" (113). In art, and its correlative, love, microcosm meets macrocosm, the human meets the spiritual.

At the height of the individuating impulse, the "will to separate," we feel most strongly the longing for attachment, the "will to unite." For the greatest artists, self-actualization, at the peak, mutates into self-transcendence—dissolution of the difference between subject and object, self and universe.

Although the greatest artists begin their creative process by liberating themselves from conforming to the past, escaping from "the anxiety of influence" (Bloom 1973)—eventually the creative impulse merges into a desire for a return to "a larger whole." In human terms, the "larger whole" is the "collective" that alone has the power to immortalize the artist with the approval it grants the artwork (Menaker 1984).

Offering his deepest reflections on "the soul life of feeling and willing," Rank (1932a) observes in *Art and Artist*:

> For this very essence of a man, his soul, which the artist puts into his work and which is represented by it, is found again in the work by the enjoyer, just as the believer finds his soul in religion or in God, with whom he feels himself to be one. It is on this identity of the *spiritual* . . . and not on a psychological identification with the artist that [aesthetic pleasure] ultimately depends. . . . But both of them, *in the simultaneous dissolution of their individuality in a greater whole*, enjoy, as a high pleasure, the personal enrichment of that individuality through this feeling of oneness. They have yielded up their mortal ego for a moment, fearlessly and even joyfully, to receive it back in the next, the richer for this universal feeling. (109–110; italics added)

At optimal moments in therapy, says Rank, both patient and therapist are "artists" who create and recreate each other by uniting their souls in a "greater whole"—which Rank considers to be an experience of love or mutual empathy.

As William James (1902) suggests in *The Varieties of Religious Experience*, "we can experience union with *something* larger than ourselves and in that union find our greatest peace" (515; italics in the original). He adds: "All that the facts require is that the power should be other and larger than our conscious selves" (ibid.).

The I–Thou relationship that Rank advocated for therapists, according to Esther Menaker (1995a), is "fired in the kiln of love" (151). Moreover, if we experience mutual love in our relationships with significant others, we will carry images of each other in our memories as an intimation of immortality:

> While belief in a personal immortality is a matter of faith and lies beyond the realm of our certain knowledge, there is an aspect of immortality that ...

adds greatly to the creation of meaningfulness in life. . . . [It is] the internalization of emotional experience with significant others—preferably with those whom we have admired and to whom we have been attached. These memory images are transmuted to harmonize with the original, constitutionally given nature of the self to form a cohesive whole. Thus the "other" lives on—is immortalized—within ourselves. . . . One can even say, in these terms, that the spiritual dimension in human life is the memory of love. (ibid.)

15

Client-centered therapy

What, exactly, did Carl Rogers learn from Rank during their weekend together in 1936, an encounter that would have epochal consequences for the creation of modern psychotherapy?

Rank mentions his time with Rogers only twice, in correspondence with Jessie Taft, without naming Rogers. "Yesterday," wrote Rank on June 10, 1936, "I gave a general lecture somewhat like for the students in Philadelphia" (Taft 1958:215). He adds: "I announced the books [i.e., *Will Therapy* and *Truth and Reality*, both published by Alfred A. Knopf one month later] and am sure that most of them will get them" (216). A few days later, in another letter, he told Taft: "Rochester was interesting and successful, but I am tired" (ibid.).

And what about Rogers? What was the impact on him? Decades later, Rogers spoke in almost revelatory terms about meeting Rank in person:

> I became infected with Rankian ideas and began to realize the possibilities of the individual being self-directing .... I was clearly fascinated by Rankian ideas but didn't quite adopt his emphases for myself until I left Rochester. But the core idea did develop. I came to believe in the individual's capacity. I value the dignity and rights of the individual sufficiently that I do not want to impose my way upon him. Those two aspects of the core idea haven't changed since that time. (quoted in Kirschenbaum 1979:95)

Asked in the mid-1970s "Were you influenced by Rank?," Rogers answered: "Yes, I was ... [by his] ideas of the relationship and focusing more on the immediate present .... There's no doubt that my 'therapy' was influenced by his thinking" (Evans 1975:28–29). In the same breath, however, without elaborating, Rogers noted that he was not attracted to Rank's "theory" (ibid.).

It's not clear what Rogers meant by "theory," but it's likely that Rank's existential emphasis on guilt-feeling as an inevitable outcome of willing would not have been congenial to Rogers, who wrote little about guilt.

There can be no doubt, however, that Rogers was transformed by Rank's focus on the authenticity of the "here-and-now" relationship. Long before meeting Rogers, Rank had been advocating for the mutual experience of feelings between client and therapist as the healing element, with the therapist serving as empathic "midwife" for the birth of a client's creative will.

Otto Rank and the Creation of Modern Psychotherapy. Robert Kramer, Oxford University Press.
© Robert Kramer (2025). DOI: 10.1093/9780197698303.003.0015

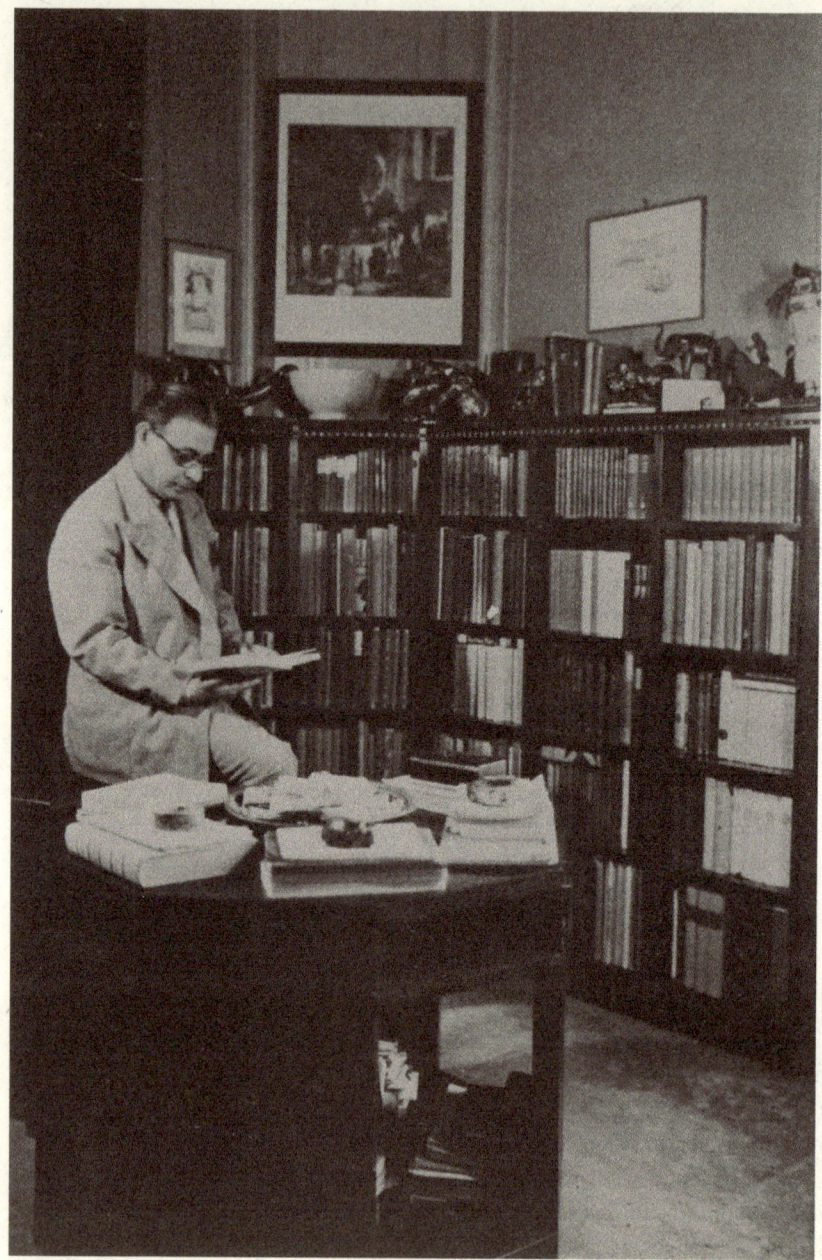

Figure 15.1 Rank in his Paris library, with a portrait of Freud behind him
Credit: Ruhama Veltfort for the Estate of Otto Rank

During his time in Rochester, Rank would certainly have talked about relationship therapy and will therapy, pointing to their equivalence, and explained how his thinking differed from that of Freud. Yet, whatever Rank said, it's likely that Rogers learned more from Rank's soft-spoken, humane way of being—his simple presence—than from Rank's words.

In a 1930 lecture delivered in Washington, DC to participants from fifty-three countries at the "First International Congress on Mental Hygiene," Rank (1996) said:

> The most valuable factor in a gathering of a crowd like this from all over the world lies in the human element, in the meeting of people, in the contact with the personalities themselves and not with their written and read words. So I hope I have been true to the real human spirit of this conference in pushing the personal element into the foreground, not without feeling greatly obliged to the broad-minded attitude of the leaders in Mental Hygiene who offered me the opportunity to do it. (223–224)

It is impossible now, almost a century after Rogers met Rank, to reconstruct exactly what Rank said or did that so moved Rogers in 1936. No record exists. During much of their time together, Rank may have spoken spontaneously, as he often did in the courses he taught at the University of Pennsylvania School of Social Work.

At some point, Rank was probably asked to demonstrate with audience volunteers *how* he conducted relationship therapy, just as Rogers did with client-centered therapy in later years. Each demonstration by Rank would have been tailored to the unique situation, concerns, and emotional needs of his volunteer, so Rogers could have learned no Rankian "technique" to emulate, only a way of being in relationship with clients.

In *Will Therapy*, Rank (1936a) revealed that, in fact, he had no technique: "in every single case, yes in every individual hour of the same case, [it] is different .... My technique consists essentially in having no technique" (148–149).

Perhaps the most vivid impression Rank would have left with Rogers was the one Jessie Taft (1958) reported after her first encounter with Rank in 1924: "He was the very image of my idea of the scholarly German student and he spoke so quietly, so directly and simply, without circumlocution or apology, that despite the strong German accent I was able to follow his argument and I thought to myself, 'Here is a man one could trust'" (x).

In her *Diaries*, Anaïs Nin (1966) conveyed the same impression after her first consultation with Rank in 1933: "I trust him. We are far from the banalities and clichés of orthodox psychoanalysis. I sense an intelligence rendered clairvoyant by feeling. I sense an artist" (286).

As the first practitioner of therapy as a performing art, Rank honored the uniqueness of every client. Each person's life is different. "In each separate case," Rank (1936a) says in *Will Therapy*, "it is necessary to create, as it were, a theory and technique made for the occasion, without trying to carry over this individualized solution to the next case" (6). One client recalls how attentively Rank listened to him:

> I really had great respect for Rank and already admired him for several reasons. One thing was his extraordinary memory; he kept no notes. He would say, "You remember last Wednesday when you told me this or that," and I couldn't.... But he would name the date and quote I had told him, verbatim. So, in many ways, besides being very pleasant to know, he was also one that excited quite a bit of admiration on my part .... He was very quiet, but he made these very sharp penetrating observations. (quoted in Lieberman 1985:272)

How much of Rank, a tangled writer, did Rogers actually read? Nobody knows. "One searches Rogers's writings in vain for even a single quotation from Rank," says Rogers's biographer, "or even for more than three consecutive sentences on Rank's thinking" (Kirschenbaum 1979: 92).

Yet Rogers was so moved by Rank's way of being during his weekend with him in 1936, and later by the lucid writings of Jessie Taft, Virginia Robinson, and Frederick Allen, another prominent student of Rank's, that his views on human nature and the best way to conduct psychotherapy changed radically.

"Relationship therapy," wrote Rogers (1939) three years after meeting Rank, "rests upon the attitude and feeling of the worker, rather than any specific technique" (209), a viewpoint identical to that of Rank (1936a), who describes his practice of helping in *Will Therapy* as "experience and understanding that are constantly converted into skill but never crystallized into technical rules" (149).

Rank improvised in every session. "Rank's approach is impossible to formalize and teach," according to Will Wadlington (2012), "it relies on intuition and experiential knowledge, and comes to light when therapist and client are immersed in the therapy process" (394).

> Rank's insight into psychotherapy process is that what happens spontaneously and cannot be anticipated is often of most interest. Therapy, by its very nature, is situational, styled by and for the client, and non-replicable. If it were able to be performed the same way each time, it would inevitably become stale and irrelevant. (ibid.)

To be in a healing relationship, according to Rank, therapist and client must touch each other's souls, in the here-and-now. Therapy is a creative, feeling process for both parties, a jointly created work of art. No art can be created or appreciated without a deeply feeling person present.

Within the relationship Rank constructed between himself and his client, observes John Suler (1993), the client "simultaneously becomes both the creator and the created" (96). For Rank, therapist and client, drawing on their feelings, were constantly creating and re-creating each other during every session.

Although none of Rank's dense writings capture the artistic, quicksilver nature of his relationship with clients, Rank summed up his approach to therapy with unusual clarity in a 1938 lecture before *Psi Chi*, the psychology honor society, at the University of Minnesota:

> From my own experience, I learned that the therapeutic process is basically an emotional experience—which takes place *independently* of the theoretical concepts of the analyst, a statement that is borne out by the fact that therapeutic results have been attained and achieved by various methods of psychotherapy, based on different theories. Furthermore, emphasis on the emotional experience—instead of on intellectual enlightenment of the patient—brings two essential principles of my dynamic therapy into focus. Firstly, the emphasis is shifted from the past to the *present*, in which *all* emotional experience takes place; secondly, the therapeutic process allows the patient a much more *active* role than being merely an object upon whom the therapist operates, like a surgeon. (Rank 1996:268; italics in the original)

During their weekend together, Carl Rogers would have heard Rank express similar views and probably demonstrate them with volunteers. But it took a considerable period of time for Rogers to grasp the revolutionary nature of Rank's approach, so different was it from anything he had learned during his training in psychoanalysis during his PhD years at Columbia University's Teacher's College.

"It would seem quite absurd to suppose that one could name a day on which client-centered therapy was born," said Rogers, employing Rank's trademark metaphor, birth. "Yet I feel it is possible to name that day and it was December 11, 1940" (quoted in Kirschenbaum 1979:112).

On that day at the University of Minnesota, before *Psi Chi*, at the same place where Rank had spoken in 1938, Rogers presented his paper "Newer Concepts in Psychotherapy." Crediting the thinking of Rank, Taft, Robinson, and Allen, Rogers told his Minnesota audience that "the aim of this newer therapy is not to solve one particular problem, but to assist the individual to *grow*" (113; italics in the original).

Firstly, unlike traditional approaches, this approach does not *do* anything to the individual; instead of "treating" the person as an illness might be treated by a medical doctor, the newer therapy ignites the capacity for self-leadership from *within* a person.

"In the second place, this newer therapy places greater stress on the emotional elements, the feeling aspects of the situation, than on the intellectual aspects .... In the third place, this newer therapy places greater stress upon the immediate situation than upon the individual's past .... Finally this approach lays stress upon the therapeutic relationship itself as a growth experience" (ibid.).

Soon thereafter, Rogers began composing *Counseling and Psychotherapy*, which he published in 1942. "It was in this book," observes Brian Thorne (1992), who was close to Rogers in the last decade of his life, "that the term 'client' first appeared" (13), a term that Rank had been using as early as 1935.[1]

According to a recent history of psychotherapy, "some argue that no single volume influenced the practice of psychotherapy in the United States more [than *Counseling and Psychotherapy*]" (Tallis 2021:273).

Sometime in the late 1930s, Rogers started to formulate the three "core conditions" that he felt were necessary for healing, a "making whole" of the human being. The word *whole* derives from the Old English *hal*, which means "healthy" or "hale"—that is, not broken. The "wholeness" that comes from "healing" is also related to the words *holy* and *holiness*. Healing and wholeness, therefore, are spiritual phenomena.

Deceptively simple to state, but remarkably difficult to practice, Rogers's three core conditions describe how a person could become a "midwife" for the "birth," spiritually, of another person.

"I rejoice," wrote Rogers in the introduction to *Client-Centered Therapy*, "at the privilege of being a midwife to a new personality—as I stand by with awe at the emergence of a self, a person, as I see a birth process in which I have had an important and facilitating part"—the birth of a person—"struggling to be himself, yet deathly afraid of being himself" (Kirschenbaum & Henderson 1989b:3–4), Rogers's translation of Rank's *Lebensangst* and *Todesangst*, life fear and death fear.

How could a therapist become a "midwife" for the birth of a new person? Rogers identifies three conditions, each of which must be demonstrated in the therapist's way of being when in relationship with clients:

- congruence;
- unconditional positive regard; and
- empathic understanding

First, and most important, the helper must be authentic, fully present in the here-and-now, with no pretense of emotional distance, no professional facade— *congruent*. "It is only as he is, in this relationship, a unified person, with his experienced feelings, his awareness of his feelings, and his expression of those feelings all congruent," wrote Rogers, "that he is most able to facilitate therapy" (quoted in Kirschenbaum 1979:196).

Often misunderstood as simply a passive reflection of the client's feelings, Rogers's way of being authentic demanded a wholesome self-assertion of the helper's own feelings, own creative will—own *difference*. A colleague remembers admiringly Rogers's personal strength and "will power" (398), a powerful sense of will that shines through all of Rogers's dialogues with Martin Buber, Paul Tillich, B.F. Skinner, Gregory Bateson, Michael Polanyi, and Rollo May (Kirschenbaum & Henderson 1989a).

Obviously, affirming one's own will does not mean that helpers burden clients with their problems or blurt out all their feelings impulsively. The client, not the therapist, is at the *center* of therapy. Nevertheless, for Rogers, in his "directive nondirective way," as his close friend Tom Greening (1995:4) once shrewdly described him, fully accepting a client never meant denying the helper's *own* feelings, being overly permissive, or becoming weak and ineffectual.

Accepting the reality of another person's feelings did not mean approving of how they think or act. No "gentle Jesus," Rogers was a "very strong and controversial man" who consistently strove to behave in a respectful but "confident, direct, and self-assertive manner" (Kirschenbaum 1979:186), according to the testimony of close associates.

"The therapist encounters his client directly," says Rogers, "meeting him person to person. He is *being* himself, not denying himself" (Kirschenbaum & Henderson 1989a:12; italics in the original).

Second, the helper must communicate "unconditional positive regard" for the uniqueness of the other person. Rogers defines this as "caring for the client as a *separate* person, with permission to have his *own* feelings, his *own* experience" (quoted in Kirschenbaum 1979:199; italics added)—Rogers's translation of Rank's psychology of difference.

The perceptions of the client are not distortions of a "transferred reality" that only "experts" on the unconscious have the vision to see clearly. The interpretations of Freudian analysts would often make patients feel that their emotional experiences were unreal—infantile fantasies transferred onto the analyst from the past. In the case of women who vigorously challenged these interpretations, Freudian analysts often left them with the impression that they suffered from maladjustments such as "penis envy."[2]

Rogers believed that transference, as Ferenczi and Rank had maintained, is mostly a creation of the psychoanalyst's emotional distance. Transference—lured by the analyst's indifference to the suffering of the patient—is not a means to healing.

For analysts to provoke transference, by claiming to be "neutral," can only lead to desperate pleas by the patient for love, or any sign of affection or recognition, from the analyst, who, by refusing to "gratify" the patient, distorts the actual, here-and-now relationship into a tortured, interminable experience of "power over."

"The concept of 'transference,'" according to Rollo May (1983), "has often been used as a convenient protective screen behind which both therapist and patient hide in order to avoid the more anxiety-creating situation of direct confrontation" (160).

What Freud called transference, says Rogers, "disappears when the feelings are expressed in a client-centered climate" (Kirschenbaum & Henderson 1989b:131). He adds:

> To deal with transference feelings as a very special part of therapy, making their handling the very core of therapy is, is to my mind, a grave mistake. Such an approach fosters dependence and lengthens therapy. It creates a whole new problem, the only purpose of which appears to be the intellectual satisfaction of the therapist—showing the elaborateness of his or her expertise. I deplore it. (134)

As a practical matter, Rogers frankly admitted that "unconditional positive regard" was "a matter of degree in any relationship," and that he himself sometimes experienced "only a conditional positive regard—and perhaps at times a negative regard, though this is not likely in effective therapy" (225n).

Third, the helper must demonstrate genuine understanding for the client's feelings. This requires empathic listening, a form of non-possessive love that the ancient Greeks called *agape*—to distinguish it from *eros*, a grasping possessive love that insists on its own desires being met.

In dialogue with Paul Tillich, Rogers defines *agape* as "a listening to oneself, as well as a listening love for the other individual" (Kirschenbaum & Henderson 1989a:78).

In a 1980 essay entitled "Empathic: An Unappreciated Way of Being," Rogers recalls a social worker on his Rochester staff named Elizabeth Davis, who had been taught by Rank at the University of Pennsylvania School of Social Work. Davis "helped me to learn that the most effective approach was to listen for the feelings, the emotions.... I believe she was the one who suggested that the best response was to 'reflect' these feelings back to the client" (Rogers 1980:137–138).

In another interview Rogers reiterated: "And one of the things she taught me was to focus on the feelings that were being expressed and to respond to those feelings" (Rogers & Russell 2002:113).

Responding meant that Rogers would need to listen to his own feelings while he was listening to those of his client. By so doing, Rogers, like Rank, used *himself* as an instrument to register the feelings of his clients. Feelings, for both Rank and Rogers, were always experienced viscerally. Neither saw a need to distinguish between feelings and emotions.

In the context of empathic listening, one of Rogers's favorite words was "visceral," a word he used 24 times in his 1951 work *Client-Centered Therapy*. "Put another way, I have learned," wrote Rogers, "that my total organismic sensing of a situation is more trustworthy than my intellect. . . . It is fallible, I am sure, but I believe it to be less fallible than my conscious mind alone" (Kirschenbaum & Henderson 1989b:23–24).

The way of being with another person that is termed "empathic" has several facets, according to Rogers (1980):

> It means entering the private perceptual world of the other and becoming thoroughly at home in it. It involves being sensitive, moment to moment, to the changing felt meanings which flow in this other person, to the fear or rage or tenderness or confusion or whatever, that he or she is experiencing. It means temporarily living in the other's life, moving about it delicately without making judgments; it means sensing meanings of which he or she is scarcely aware, but not trying to uncover totally unconscious feelings, since this would be too threatening. (142)

Rogers also made it clear that empathy—giving oneself freely to another person—did not mean losing oneself in the other. As Rank had insisted, maintaining the separateness of the helper is essential for permitting the separateness of the client. By not losing oneself in the other, the potential of emotional burnout for the helper is minimized.

In fact, only by being separate could empathy be offered. "When I can freely feel this strength of being a separate person," said Rogers, "then I find I can let myself go much more deeply in understanding and accepting [the client] because I am not fearful of losing myself" (Kirschenbaum & Henderson 1989b:121).

Within a short time of his encounter with Rank, Rogers began to rail against the absence of authenticity, unconditional positive regard, and empathy on the part of psychoanalysts. Lack of these core conditions for healing was positively harmful, according to Rogers. In turn, Freudians condemned Rogers for adopting Rank's "anti-Oedipal" ideas and, thereby, denying "the unconscious."

"And even if Otto Rank was no longer welcomed among the psychoanalytic establishment," writes Howard Kirschenbaum (2007), "Rogers readily acknowledged that 'Especially are the roots of client-centered therapy to be found in the therapy of Rank, and the Philadelphia group [of social workers] which has integrated his work into their own'" (279).

Neither Rank nor Rogers ever excluded the possibility of unconscious factors affecting the perceptions of either party in the therapeutic relationship. The helper, according to Rank and Rogers, accepts the client's feelings as reflecting the constantly fluctuating conditions of the moment, whether or not the client's perceptions agree with the helper's view.

There are no objective psychological facts for Rogers, as for Rank, only subjective interpretations. And the client, not the helper, is the "expert" on interpreting the meaning of the feelings emerging inside or outside the consulting room.

"Each person is an island unto himself, in a very real sense, and he can only build bridges to other islands if he is first of all willing to be himself and permitted to be himself," said Rogers. "So I find that when I can accept another person . . . then I am assisting him to become a person" (Kirschenbaum & Henderson 1989b:22).

The key to healing, concluded Rogers, is the experience of being in relationship, fully separate yet simultaneously connected with another—in other words, *integrating difference and likeness.*

Only by accepting our own difference and having it accepted by another can we discover the creativity and courage to change. The word *change* derives from the Latin *cambire*, which means "to exchange," or "to give and take"—reflecting the *relational* aspect missed by the word *change* alone.

Beyond the three core conditions of congruence, unconditional positive regard, and empathy, technique was irrelevant, insisted Rogers. Of course no mortal can always be completely authentic, accepting, and empathic. Therefore, Rogers visualized the core conditions, which are met to a lesser or greater degree, as located on a continuum. And the art of the helper, Rogers believed, consists entirely in moving further and further along the continuum, getting better and better at *being* or *performing* these conditions—not just espousing them.[3]

Modest about his therapeutic prowess, Rogers, who was never convinced that he fully met his own conditions, thought it fortunate that "imperfect human beings can be of therapeutic assistance to other imperfect human beings" (Rogers 1959:215).

He confessed that, in certain cases, even empathic listening would not be enough to promote healing. Like Rank, Rogers failed to help some clients but, also like Rank, he valued "not knowing" as an opportunity for learning more about the art of therapy. Rogers was comfortable in "accessing his own ignorance" (Schein 2009: 91) and learning from his failures. The possibility of transformation rested on the *client's* frame of reference, concluded Rogers, not the therapist's:

> I have learned, especially in working with more disturbed persons, that empathy can be perceived as lack of involvement; that an unconditional positive regard on my part can be perceived as indifference; that warmth can be perceived as threatening closeness; that real feelings of mine can be perceived as false. (Rogers 1967a:93)

Nevertheless, there were moments when Rogers was at his best, when he felt most deeply connected to his clients and, simultaneously, to himself. What might the "feeling experience" of being in relationship with Rogers have been like, from a client's frame of reference, when the client perceived him as genuinely authentic, respectful, and empathic? In *On Becoming a Person*, Rogers (1961) provides a moving account:

> For the client, this optimal therapy would mean an exploration of increasingly strange and unknown and dangerous feelings in himself, the exploration proving possible only because he is gradually realizing that he is accepted unconditionally. Thus he becomes acquainted with elements of his experience which have in the past been denied to awareness as too threatening, too damaging to the structure of the self. He finds himself experiencing these feelings fully, completely, in the relationship, so that for the moment he *is* his fear, or his anger, or his tenderness, or his strength. And as he lives these widely varied feelings, in all their degrees of intensity, he discovers that he has experienced *himself*, that he *is* all these feelings. He finds his behavior changing in a constructive fashion in accordance with his newly experienced self. He approaches the realization that he no longer needs to fear what experience may hold, but can welcome it freely as a part of his changing and developing self. (185; italics in the original)

Echoing Rank's Nietzschean philosophy of life in *Art and Artist*—"the volitional affirmation of the obligatory" (Rank 1932a: 64)—Carl Rogers came to define the fully functioning person as one who deliberately says "Yes" to the "Must."

By doing so, the person affirms the loan of life, a loan that is fated to be repaid in full at the end, returned, as Rank (1936a) said in *Will Therapy*, to "the ALL" (219). Such a person, concluded Rogers, in words that resonate with those of

Rank, "voluntarily chooses and wills that which is also absolutely determined" (Kirschenbaum & Henderson 1989b: 418).

In sum, then, what was Carl Rogers's message to the countless social workers, counselors, and therapists who were drawn to his ideas?

"I can state the overall hypothesis in one sentence," said Rogers (1961) in *On Becoming A Person*. "If I can provide a certain type of relationship, the other person will discover *within* himself the capacity to use that relationship for growth, and change and personal development will occur" (33; italics added).

16

The daimonic, counter-willing, and an "other world"

Striving to draw out the power of each person's creative will, Otto Rank would certainly have endorsed Rogers's "overall hypothesis." If asked, however, he might have urged a crucial addition: the centrality of confrontation in therapy as in life.

The rumbling of the daimonic, according to Rank, can usually be heard when two wills—two powerful, creative, and destructive subjectivities—discover, test, love, hate, and heal each other, inside or outside the consulting room.

As Rollo May observed long ago, the daimonic is perhaps the single aspect of human nature that Rogers was never able to integrate fully into his therapy. A student of ancient Greek culture and myth, May knew that the term "daimon" was employed by writers such as Homer, Hesiod, and Plato as a synonym for *theos*, god. For both Rank and May, the energy of the primal life force, the will, is "godlike" when expressed creatively, but also contains within itself destructive aspects. In *Love and Will*, May (1969) explains:

> The daimonic is the urge in every being to affirm itself, assert itself, perpetuate and increase itself. . . . Aggression, hostility, cruelty [are] the reverse side of the same assertion which empowers our creativity. All life is a flux between these two aspects of the daimonic. We can repress the daimonic, but we cannot avoid the toll of apathy and the tendency toward later explosion which such repression brings in its wake. (123)

During the late 1960s, May saw the destructive consequences of the power-lessness felt by millions of Blacks, women, and young people across America. Their primal life force had been stifled. The daimonic was exploding in inner city riots, protests by feminists against patriarchy, and demonstrations on college campuses, where students were raging against the Vietnam War.

After *Love and Will*, May's subsequent book, published in 1972, *Power and Innocence: A Search for the Sources of Violence*, was fiercely critical, writes his biographer Robert Abzug (2021), "calling for individualistic, pseudoinnocent America to wake up to its own daimonic essence, its capacity for evil as well as

Otto Rank and the Creation of Modern Psychotherapy. Robert Kramer, Oxford University Press.
© Robert Kramer (2025). DOI: 10.1093/9780197698303.003.0016

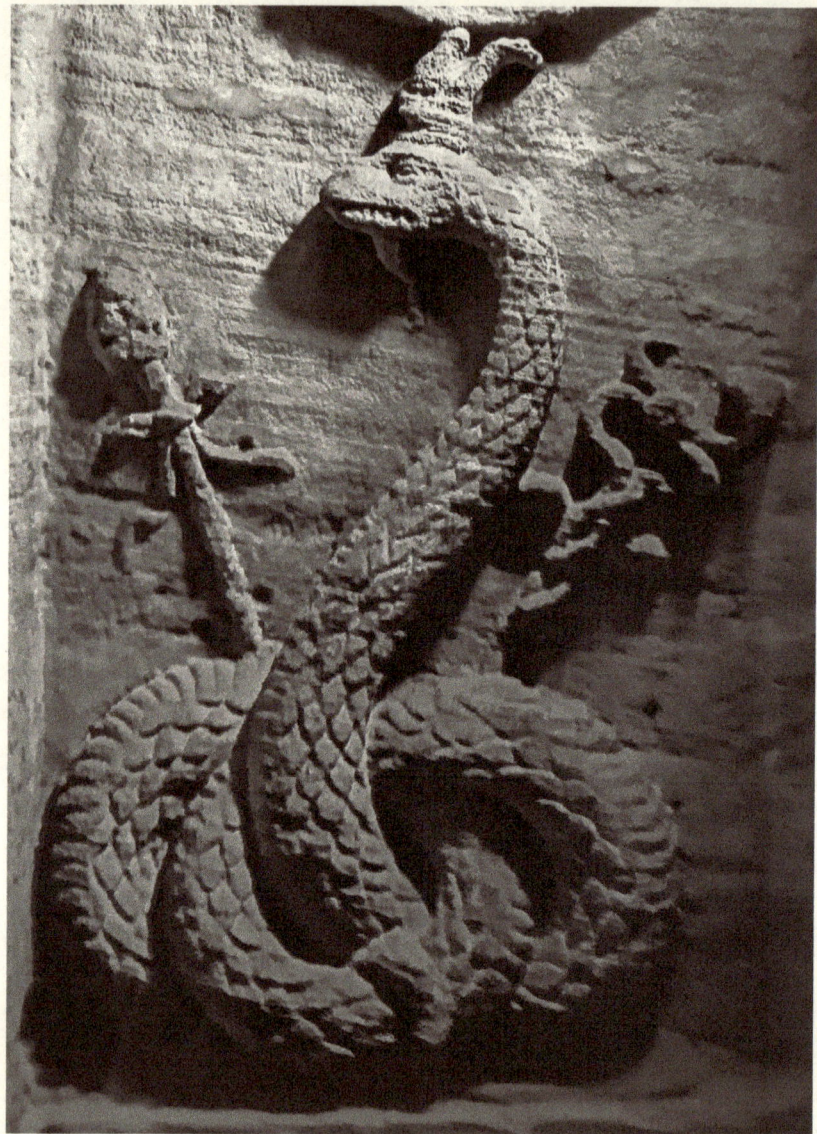

Figure 16.1 *Agathos daimon,* a deity of ancient Egyptian-Greek religion
Credit: Carole Raddato via Wikimedia commons

good" (294). May's *Power and Innocence* foreshadowed the Rankian thesis of Ernest Becker's *Escape from Evil* published three years later.

"The future," asserts May (1972) in *Power and Innocence,* echoing Rank's argument that creativity emerges from holding and living within the tension between difference and likeness, "lies with the man or woman who can live as an individual, conscious *within* the solidarity of the human race. He then uses the tension between individuality and solidarity as the source of his ethical creativity" (254; italics in the original).

Frustrated that Carl Rogers was uneasy about accepting what Rank had dubbed the counter-will—and that May was calling the daimonic—May wrote Rogers an open letter: "If the daimonic urge is integrated into the personality, which is, to my mind, the purpose of psychotherapy, it results in creativity" (Kirschenbaum & Henderson 1989a:240)—that is, the liberation of the constructive or positive will.

May always distinguished the demonic—a term he reserved for Freud's "death drive," the *Todestrieb*—from the daimonic, which, like Rank, he insisted had a positive, healthy, "godlike" side.

Rogers, wrote May in his open letter, had confused the *daimonic* with the *demonic*. "I find it important that the patient be able to take a stand against me," May told Rogers. "This means that aspects of evil—anger, hostility against the therapist, destructiveness—need to be brought out in therapy" (246). But Rogers was always uncomfortable with the daimonic element in human nature when it surfaced during therapy.

"I do not have a Pollyanna view of human nature," argued Rogers (1961). "I am quite aware that out of defensiveness and inner fear individuals can and do behave in ways which are horribly destructive, immature, regressive, anti-social, hurtful" (27). Yet Rogers was never willing to draw out the daimonic within his clients, a powerful force lying just underneath the surface of their inhibitions, symptoms, and anxieties, always ready to erupt inside the therapy room.

May's supportive position on releasing this powerful force was also rejected by Freudian psychoanalysts who evaluated expressions of the daimonic by their patients as refusal to accept the analyst's interpretations, a "resistance" stemming, they maintained, from the self-destructiveness of the *Todestrieb*.

The daimonic is especially prominent during the end phase of therapy, according to Otto Rank and Rollo May, when patient and therapist are often locked in a conflict of will and counter-will—a symbolic "battle," said Rank (1936a) in *Will Therapy*, with only slight exaggeration, "of life and death" (251).

It's worth recalling how Rank helped Henry Miller unlearn his "terrible timidity" during a single therapeutic encounter in 1933, a blazing hour that Miller, in a long letter to Anaïs Nin, had said "rained blood." Afterwards, Miller reported that he felt his experience with Rank to have been "a brilliant, an artistic cure.... Cured I was of certain terrible timidities.... What I needed was the high challenge, the acid test, and I got it. . . . I felt my wrist stronger, firmer, my aim more accurate, a deadly aim.... it remains a fact that I conquered" (Stuhlmann 1979:108).

In *Will Therapy*, Rank (1936a) explains: "In the simplest formulation derived from my experience, the end phase . . . can be represented as a battle for life heightened to the utmost between two individuals, one of whom must die that the other may live" (251).

There can be no doubt that in this duel the *patient must remain victor* if he is to feel himself healed, that is, capable of living, and the danger of the therapist lies in the fact that he himself instinctively wants to be victorious, that is, to live and not be killed. (251–252; italics added)

[The patient's] restoration to health consists essentially in the freeing of the creative powers, which must be first released in the therapeutic process in an aggressive way before they can be applied to the constructive governing of life. (253)

Applying Rank's birth metaphor, existential therapist Irvin Yalom reports that, during the end phase, and even earlier, he encourages his clients to acknowledge the "intrauterine kicks of [their] inborn will" (Yalom & Elkin 1974:226), just as Rank and May did.

The "will conflict" between therapist and client, said Rank, is an *external* representation of an *internal* battle roiling within the client's psyche. Rank saw signs, most vividly during the end phase, of an internal battle emerging from within the souls of many of his clients.

They were struggling between the *will to separate* from their own self-concepts, values, beliefs, expectations, and taken-for-granted assumptions—as culturally conditioned to conform to familial, group, religious or other allegiances—and become independent, and the equally strong *will to stay merged* in the womb of therapy, remaining dependent, "unborn" as fully realized, self-empowered, self-reliant persons.

"The [I] needs the Thou in order to become a Self," writes Rank (1941a) in *Beyond Psychology*. "The tragic element in this process is that the [I] needs a Thou to build up an assertive self *with and against* this Thou" (290; italics added).

A close friend of Abraham Maslow's, Colin Wilson (1972) offers a keen appreciation of Rank's achievement, which, he maintains, was even more revolutionary than that of William James, the greatest American exponent of the will before Rank:

[I]t would not be paradoxical to say that psychoanalysis, in its therapeutic consequences, is an involuntary proof of the existence and strength of the will, and that this was and is its only therapeutic value. . . . [T]he real benefit a patient derives from being psychoanalyzed is that the clash with the psychoanalyst revives his deflated and passive will.

The sick patient has a will-to-health, says Rank, which he has allowed to collapse under the pressure of anxieties; when he goes to the analyst, it has often become a mere spark. Successful therapy, says Rank, consists of carefully blowing this spark into a bonfire.

This was the most revolutionary assertion that had ever been made in psychology; even [William] James had not penetrated to this amazing and simple truth, although he had come very close. (101)

Patients experience a will conflict with the therapist to a lesser or greater degree, depending on the intensity of their passions. In some cases, according to Rank, there is little conflict of wills by patients with their therapist. No patient is like any other. But signs of the daimonic often surface during the end phase, especially with highly creative people.

After therapy is over, not all patients will become as creative as were, for example, Jessie Taft, Virginia Robinson, Anaïs Nin, and Henry Miller—but they all now have the potential for more fully realizing the power of their own wills, integrating their ambivalences about union and separation, likeness and difference, more creatively than they had been capable of doing before experiencing will therapy.

There "is a general life principle," says Rank (1936a) in *Will Therapy*, citing the Russian psychoanalyst Sabina Spielrein, "on the basis of which no creating is possible without destruction, and no destroying without some kind of new creation" (178). For Rank (1936b), neurosis, as we have seen, is a distortion of the godlike energy of the "cosmic primal force" (10), the life-affirming energy of creative willing.

The appearance of neurosis, although self-destructive, is not a derivative of Freud's *Todestrieb*, a demonic theory which, according to Rank, Freud had invented in 1920 in *Beyond the Pleasure Principle* to justify the failure of psychoanalysts to help patients get better. "Both patient and therapist are at once creator and creature," Rank (1936a) insists in *Will Therapy*.

The patient . . . must also become creator; while the therapist plays not only the creator role, but at the same time, must serve the creative will of the patient as material. . . . This also describes the moment in the therapeutic experience when the time for separation has come, the critical moment between fate and self-determination. (125–126)

The creative power of a patient's positive will cannot be released merely through the giving of interpretations, according to Rank, no matter how compelling or insightful. The daimonic, therefore, must be always affirmed by the therapist, especially as the relationship enters the end phase, when the "intrauterine kicks of [their] inborn will" often show signs of expression.

"Prizing" the combative counter-will of patients, as Rank advocated, was a radically new perspective, never countenanced by Freud or by psychoanalysts, many of whom saw signs of counter-willing as "resistance" to their interpretations. Even today, some White training and supervising analysts continue to press their psychology of likeness onto Black, indigenous, and other analysts of color who, in resisting this pressure, demand, instead, acceptance and affirmation of their difference (American Psychoanalytic Association 2023).

The purpose of scheduling the end phase in therapy, according to Rank (1936a), is to *gradually* unleash the power of creative willing for the patient "without permitting the will justification in the projection or the rolling off of responsibility in the identification" with the therapist (112). When the time for separation from the womb of therapy comes, and the intrauterine kicking increases, the birth of self-determination is near.

It's hard to imagine Carl Rogers, who never felt entirely comfortable in accepting his client's angry or hateful feelings toward him, encouraging the daimonic force that Otto Rank, Rollo May, and Irvin Yalom insist is essential for change in therapy—the counterpart of the creative will.

One can only speculate as to why Rogers, a deeply cultured person who understood full well the evils that humanity has inflicted on itself and the planet, minimized the daimonic or, as May notes in his open letter, confused it with the demonic, Freud's death drive.

To be sure, Rogers always saw the anger, hatred, and rage that emerge at times, like volcanic eruptions, within the crucible of the therapeutic encounter. But perhaps Rogers's own strong need for acceptance and love from patients clouded his vision of the daimonic, leading him to downplay the power of anger within himself and his clients.

"I find it difficult to be easily or quickly aware of angry feelings in myself," Rogers admitted. "I deplore this, and am slowly learning in this respect" (Kirschenbaum & Henderson 1989b:348). And even more revealingly, in his autobiography, Rogers (1967b) confessed that empathic understanding—love— was what he himself had always been seeking: "I have since become keenly aware that the point of view I developed in therapy is the sort of help I myself would like" (368).

A highly sensitive person, Rogers saw that clients, from their side, may attempt, intuitively and spontaneously, to "cure" the therapist's emotional suffering with their own help, their own love, their own empathic understanding. Therapists are human, too.

Naturally, therapists appreciate the genuinely loving feelings they receive from their clients in response to the caring and empathic listening they offer (Searles 1975). But taken to the extreme, argued Otto Rank, a client's "love" or empathy for her therapist may end up unintentionally forfeiting the client's dearly bought, still fragile, sense of independence.

Ferenczi and Rank were the first analysts to recognize the mutuality of an authentic therapeutic encounter. Feelings of appreciation, generosity, and empathy—love—flow back and forth between therapist and client, as do feelings of anger, resentment, hate, and even boredom.

Like Ferenczi, Rank did not disdain the healing he obtained from the love he felt coming from his clients. He acknowledged it. In the therapeutic relationship, experiencing empathy, believed Rank, is a mutual process of giving and receiving love. To be a force for healing, empathy cannot be one-sided.

In learning how to feel their emotions—and, thus, to will—clients were also learning how to give and receive love, as Phoebe Crosby affirmed in the journal she kept of her therapy in 1927 with Rank. Let's look again at how Crosby described her *simultaneous* experience of likeness and difference during the end phase:

> *Separation.* The next step in loving. Loving and leaving. You do not really love unless you are able to "leave" the beloved. And leaving can be terribly destructive unless at the same time, you are able to love the thing you leave.
>
> It was nearly time for the analysis to end. The two months allotted to it were almost over. I had learned at great cost to love myself and Rank and now I had to leave him.
>
> One thing that helped was that I realized that this was no strange thing that was being suddenly thrust upon me. He had been preparing for it almost from the beginning, with as I now saw it, incredible skill. He had known all the time that it would be like this. I had not known, now I did. We were doing it together. (Crosby & Janus 2017:452)

At times, each participant in a healing therapeutic relationship will experience the other's love, a moving experience for both of them. But Rank never forgot that the goal of deepening a therapeutic relationship is, paradoxically, the client's separation, and the therapist's affirmation of the client's *difference*.

Immersed in the feeling-charged field of the relationship, Crosby recognized that Rank had been preparing for separation from the very beginning, so she did not show any signs of the conflict of wills that Rank said often emerges during the end phase. Some births are easier than others. For each person, as we have seen, Rank created a new therapy. No end phase is like any other: each person is unique.

In the therapeutic setting, love and separation are bound together. Just as there is a daimonic side to the creative will, there is a daimonic side to love, said Rank in *Will Therapy*. To continue forever loving or identifying with "an all-pardoning" (Rank 1936a:31) therapist may end up infantilizing clients, inhibiting their creativity, keeping them attached to the therapist by guilt-feeling. Clients may react "as if [they] could not desert the therapist because the latter would suffer too much" (119).

In a recent account, Carina Schorske (2023) recalls the guilt she felt at the prospect of leaving her psychoanalyst:

> I knew that the "transference" was working. . . . I had promised myself that I would stay in analysis for two years; after that, I was free to leave if I felt like it. As the secret deadline approached, I chafed more and more against the frequent meetings, growing jealous of my time. . . . Dr. S knew better than to pressure me to stay, but she did not fulfill my fantasy of a reparative final session. . . . When I left her office, tears blurred my vision, and the clouds above Central Park looked like faces pushing against fabric. I'd been afraid of disappointing Dr. S—and then I did. (52)

If the therapist's *own* need for healing or love "leads to misunderstanding or, more correctly, misinterpreting the situation, then emerges the so-called 'counter-transference,'" says Rank (1996) in his American lectures (178). "This consists in the analyst going *beyond* the identification necessary for understanding the patient. The analyst, in his turn, now projects onto the patient, who identifies with this projected part of the analyst's ego" (ibid.; italics in the original).

However, Rank did not see this process of "projective identification" by the therapist as supporting patients in discovering their own source of power: "One cannot help them by driving them back to the old identifications or by offering them new possibilities of identification. One has to help them to get *beyond* the deadlock in their personality and in the process find their *own* self" (196; italics in the original).

For self-leadership to emerge during the end phase of therapy, the patient must be able to find the courage and creative will to "destroy," metaphorically, the therapist-midwife and the therapeutic relationship, and differentiate from both without suffering too much guilt and anxiety.

A parallel process is taking place *inwardly*, said Rank, as patients, consciously or unconsciously, are battling their will to stay embedded in the womb of therapy and their will to be reborn. By projecting this inner battle *outwardly*, patients feel relieved, according to Rank, when therapists unprotestingly accept and, even more so, value their need to separate—that is, when they celebrate their difference.

Essential to the differentiation of self from non-self, and to furthering individuation, counter-willing, said Rank (1936a) in *Will Therapy*, is "proof, however negative, of the strength of will on which therapeutic success ultimately depends" (10).

Despite the different value they placed on the daimonic, it is to Carl Rogers, and before him, Otto Rank, "the precursor of client centered practice" (Thorne 1992:58), that therapists owe the great idea of offering "a certain type of relationship" (Rogers 1961:33) to clients as a way of helping them find a vital balance between part and whole, individuation and connection, difference and likeness.

By their teachings, and even more by their way of being with others in relationship, Rank and Rogers opened the way for countless other helpers to "prize the new," as Rank (1936a) wrote in *Will Therapy* (148), to prize, through empathic understanding, the spiritual rebirth of their clients.

"So I have come to prize these learnings," said Rogers (1995), adopting Rank's metaphor, which Rogers used often, "because they seem to lead to the development of separate, unique, and creatively different personalities" (19).

It is only through the experience of being in an authentic relationship, insisted Rogers (1959), that the person "accepts others as unique individuals different from himself, prizes himself, and prizes others" (207).

Advocating Rank's psychology of difference, Rogers (1978) asserted that, in the ideal society, "The natural human tendency to care for another would no longer be: 'I care for you because you are the *same* as I,' but instead, 'I prize and treasure you because you are *different* from me'" (9; italics added).

In relationship therapy, the spiritual boundaries of two human beings touch each other as they share the empathic feeling of being together while, at the same time, recognizing each other's difference. But what, exactly, do we mean when we speak of the spiritual—as opposed to the merely human—core of the therapeutic relationship?

Nearing the end of his life, Carl Rogers experienced something close to an epiphany. Sharing mutual, deeply empathic feelings with countless clients had brought him, without his full awareness, to the border of, what he now called, "the transcendent, the indescribable, the spiritual" (Rogers 1986:199).

All along, it seems, Rogers had been "negotiating" in his uncompromisingly secular way "with the problem of the Beyond" (Rank 1932a:49n)—an "other world" than the ordinary one we live in each day. To Jessie Taft, as a Christmas gift, Rank (1938) once inscribed a copy of Shakespeare's *Sonnets*: "This book has as much a touch of the 'other world' as anything can have in this world."[1] Like Rank, Carl Rogers concluded late in life, after having practicing therapy for half a century, that there was, indeed, an "other world."

Two decades after Rank's *Beyond Psychology* appeared, in *On Becoming a Person* Rogers (1961) pointed to "the 'out-of-this-world' quality which many therapists have remarked upon, a sort of trance-like feeling in the relationship from which both client and I emerge at the end of the hour, as if from a deep well or tunnel" (202).

Until the last few years of his life, however, Rogers was reluctant to make his "concluding unscientific postscript" explicit, for fear, perhaps, of having his spiritual longings confused with the dogmatism of Christianity that he had rejected in his youth (Kirschenbaum 2007).

But, by the late 1970s, partly in response to coping with the long illness of his wife, Helen, Rogers began posing his greatest challenge to mainstream psychology: "Is this the only reality?" (Kirschenbaum & Henderson 1989b:370). Or, more poignantly: "Do we need 'a' reality?" (420).

> I would like to make this a bit more personal. I have never had a mystical experience, nor any type of experience of a paranormal reality, nor any drug-induced state that gave me a glimpse of a world different from our secure "real" world. Yet, the evidence grows more and more impressive (371).

> Perhaps in the coming generations of younger psychologists, hopefully unencumbered by university prohibitions and resistances, there will be a few who will dare to investigate the possibility that there is a lawful reality which is not open to our five senses; a reality in which present, past, and future are intermingled, in which space is not a barrier, and time has disappeared; a reality which can be perceived and known only when we are passively receptive, rather than actively bent on knowing. This is one of the most exciting challenges posed to psychology. (373)

Although remaining agnostic, Rogers (1986) came to speak glowingly of this "other-worldly realm" in mystical terms such as "the transcendent, the indescribable, the spiritual" (199). This was a realm that Rogers had turned away from in the 1920s when he abandoned his religious studies at Union Theological Seminary for a career in counseling and scientific research on improving psychotherapy outcomes.

It was *within* the therapist-client relationship that Rogers was finding the most compelling data to support his hypothesis of a realm "beyond" psychology. An "other world" had always been there, hidden in what was closest and most familiar to Rogers: the mutually empathic relationship between client and therapist.

"I am compelled to believe," wrote Rogers one year before he died, "that I, like many others, have underestimated the importance of this mystical, spiritual dimension" (ibid.).

Although never devaluing science, he now acknowledged that there was a spiritual core to practicing psychotherapy. Without embarrassment, he had come to see himself as a mystic. "I feel as though I am somehow in tune with the forces in the universe," Rogers told theologian Paul Tillich, "or that forces are operating through me in regard to this helping relationship" (Kirschenbaum & Henderson 1989a:74).

Feeling nebulous sensations in his body that he couldn't explain by means of the rational categories of conventional psychology, Rogers had begun to channel something larger, much larger, than himself and his client.

"It is like listening to the music of the spheres," wrote Rogers (1980) in *A Way of Being*, "because beyond the immediate message of the person, no matter what that might be, there is the universal ... the universe as a whole. So there is both the satisfaction of hearing this person, and also the satisfaction of feeling one's self in touch with what is universally true" (8).

As he listened, with awe, to the keynote of the universe, Rogers found himself feeling, viscerally, a "transcendent awareness of the harmony and unity of the cosmic system, including humankind" (133). He was "tuning in to a potent creative tendency which has formed our universe, from the smallest snowflake to the largest galaxy" (134), a cosmic primal force similar, he suggested, to "the mystic's experience of union with the universal," a union in which a "person feels at one with the cosmos" (128).

Art Bohart (2003) says that Rogers "originally discussed an *actualizing tendency* in living things and later expanded this idea by suggesting that it was merely an individual form of a broader tendency found in the universe at large" (111; italics in the original), a tendency virtually identical to the "cosmic primal force" that Rank had termed the "creative will" in *Truth and Reality* (1936b:10), and that William James (1902) had called "cosmic emotion" in *The Varieties of Religious Experience* (78).

Deeply moved by his feeling of cosmic union—on both microcosmic and macrocosmic levels—Rogers quotes a woman who'd participated with him in one of the many "person-centered" community workshops he conducted in the last decade of his life. In a remarkably compelling account of a *simultaneous* experience of likeness and difference, she told him:

I found it to be a profound spiritual experience. I felt the oneness of spirit in the community. We breathed together, felt together, even spoke for another. I felt the power of the "life force" that infuses each of us—whatever that is. I felt its presence without the usual barricades of "me-ness" or "you-ness"—it was like a meditative experience when I feel myself as a center of consciousness, very much a part of the broader, universal consciousness. And yet with that extraordinary sense of oneness, the separateness of each person present has never been more clearly preserved. (quoted in Rogers 1980:129–130)

In *Beyond Psychology*, Rank (1941a) observed that "psychology is searching for a substitute for the cosmic unity which the man of Antiquity enjoyed in life and expressed in his religion, but which modern man has lost—a loss which accounts for the development of the neurotic type" (37). To begin to heal the pain of existential suffering, maintained Rank, one must re-experience, at least momentarily, this cosmic unity—a sense of Oneness in which the separateness of each person is simultaneously retained.

Human beings, according to Rank and Rogers, are able to live in the spirit, connecting the personal to the universal, the microcosm of the individual psyche to the macrocosm of the universe, by deep sharing within an I–Thou relationship.

"When I am at my best," wrote Carl Rogers (1986), just months before he died in 1987, "when I am somehow in touch with the unknown in me, when perhaps I am in a slightly altered state of consciousness in the relationship, then whatever I do seems to be full of healing. Then simply my *presence* is releasing and helpful. . . . At those moments it seems that my inner spirit has reached out and touched the inner spirit of the other. Our relationship transcends itself and becomes a part of something larger. Profound growth and healing and energy are present" (198–199; italics in the original).

In light of Rogers's turn toward spirituality, mysticism, and cosmic union, I want to explore a question whose implications for therapy are truly astonishing. A question whose implications Otto Rank understood in all his writings beginning as early as 1924 with *The Trauma of Birth*, but most profoundly in *Art and Artist* (1932a), *Will Therapy* (1936a), *Truth and Reality* (1936b), and *Beyond Psychology* (1941a).

The question is this: In a cosmic sense, what does it mean for a human being to serve as "midwife" for the emergence of "a new personality" (Rogers in Kirschenbaum & Henderson 1989b:4)?

What does it mean to be born, much less reborn? To come alive? To be "conscious of living"? To be fully present in the here and now? What does it mean "to develop" a human being—to make visible that which is invisible, like a photograph developing out of its chemical solution?

In the process of exploring this question, I will, at the same time, be reflecting more deeply than I have before on what Rogers meant when he crafted his therapeutic credo in these hauntingly Rankian terms: "I stand by with awe at the emergence of a self, a person, as I see a birth process in which I have had an important and facilitating part"—the birth of a person—"struggling to be himself, yet deathly afraid of being himself" (Kirschenbaum & Henderson 1989b:3–4).

17

Empathy and *agape*

From Biblical times through the Crusades to current events in the Middle East, the history of religion gives bloody proof that belief in "God" inhibits, as much as promotes, expression of spirituality. But Otto Rank did not want to throw out the baby of spiritual experience with the bathwater of religious dogma.

Without opposing science or advocating religion, either Western or Eastern, Rank (1932a) wrote lyrically in *Art and Artist* of how mutual empathy allows mortals to "negotiate," if only fleetingly and metaphorically, "with the problem of the Beyond" (49n.)—the "other world" that Rank alluded to in his birthday inscription to Jessie Taft.

In the jointly created—and endlessly recreated—"moment" of empathy between lover and beloved, I and Thou, client and therapist, separateness is dissolved only to be rediscovered, enriched, and renewed. "*Love abolishes egoism,*" said Rank (1996) in his American lectures, "*it merges the self in the other to find it again enriched in one's own I*" (154; italics in the original). I can only love the one who truly accepts me as I am, and whose self I accept in like manner.

"What is unique in love is that—beyond the fact of uniting—it rebounds on the I," continued Rank. "Not only, I love the other as my I, as part of my I, but the other also makes my I worthy of love. The love of the Thou thus places a value on one's own I" (ibid.). Only through mutual recognition is healing, or becoming whole, possible.

That we can also "masochistically" love someone who rejects us is evidence, Rank thought, for the irrepressible human urge to lose our separateness, reduce the pain of our difference, and merge with another—even when such love is one-sided or chimerical.

Rank did not ignore the darker side of love, what D.H. Lawrence (1920) once called the "yoke and leash of love" (241). This is love as uncritical obedience; love as willing bondage; love as the green-eyed monster, jealousy; love as transference.

As psychoanalyst Clara Thompson observed, Rank and Ferenczi were the first to discover the importance of being real persons in therapy. Transference, wrote Thompson, whose own analyst was Ferenczi, "became more precisely defined as only the irrational attitudes felt and expressed toward the analyst" (quoted in Lieberman 1985:237).

Otto Rank and the Creation of Modern Psychotherapy. Robert Kramer, Oxford University Press.
© Robert Kramer (2025). DOI: 10.1093/9780197698303.003.0017

Like Ferenczi, Rank distinguished transference love from the deep sharing possible in genuine, mutual loving. Transference, Rank (1936a) said in *Will Therapy*, is "an attempt of the individual to personify his will in the other and so to justify it instead of denying it.... 'Being in love' [with the analyst] is the continuation of the unreal will justification in God through the earthly deification of a real person whose will must be as like ours as possible" (85).

This is not a healthy expression of creative willing, nor does it accept the difference of "the other." Only a differentiated human being, maintained Rank, can experience a mature, loving relationship with another differentiated human being. Carl Rogers agreed.

"If transference attitudes are defined as emotionalized attitudes which existed in some other relationship, and which are inappropriately directed to the therapist," wrote Rogers (1951) in *Client-Centered Therapy*, "then transference attitudes are evident in a considerable proportion of cases handled by client-centered therapists" (218). But the illusory nature of transference, according to Rank and Rogers, can be rectified by the authenticity, respect, and empathy shown by the therapist.

In his therapeutic practice, Rank minimized transference by creating a real relationship, while recognizing that transference, nevertheless, will often surface in the irrational projections of patients onto him.

Unfortunately, in *The Denial of Death*, Ernest Becker (1973) conflated Freud's insistence on fostering transference from his patients with Rank's altogether different idea. Becker describes "Transference as Fear of Life" and "Transference as Fear of Death" (144–150), yet nowhere in Rank's chapter entitled "Life Fear and Death Fear" in *Will Therapy* (1936a:168–188) can one find the word "transference."

Rank saw *Lebensangst* and *Todesangst* in existential terms, as the anxiety of living and dying on a speck of cosmic dust called the planet Earth, an *Urangst* felt to one degree or another by all *self-conscious* human beings.

Writing in the early 1970s, Ernest Becker was unaware of Ferenczi's critique in his *Clinical Diary* of how Freud "lured transference" to get love from his patients. (The *Clinical Diary* was published only in 1988.)

Although Becker (1973) misread Rank on transference, he was optimistic in *The Denial of Death* about the healing possible within Rank's relationship therapy, which offered "intense experience in the present moment that is now freer of prefixed perceptions, new possibilities of choice and action" (270), and the birth of the creative will. While cautioning against seeing therapy as promising "perfect freedom," Becker argued, along with Rank, that therapy can

> give great gifts to tortured and overwhelmed people and even added dignity
> to anyone who values and can use self-knowledge. Psychotherapy can allow

people to affirm themselves, to smash idols that constrict the self-esteem, to lift the load of neurotic guilt—the extra guilt piled on top of natural existential guilt. It can clear away neurotic despair—the despair that comes from a too-constricted focus for one's safety and satisfactions. When a person becomes less fragmented, less blocked and bottled up, he does experience real joy: the joy of finding more of himself, of the release from armor and binding reflexes, of throwing off the chains of uncritical and self-defeating dependency, of controlling his own energies, of discovering aspects of the world, intense experience in the present moment that is now freer of prefixed perceptions, new possibilities of choice and action, and so on. (ibid)

According to Rank, the dependence and subjection of transference love in psychoanalysis is an *unhealthy* solution to the "part-whole" problem, a too-extreme unburdening of responsibility and selfhood—which led female patients, in particular, to feel disempowered.

In psychoanalysis, the patient "makes a god for himself as he yields himself to the deified loved one," said Rank in *Will Therapy* (1936a:86)—referring to the analyst, whose aloof, unfeeling behavior provokes and lures transference from patients, making detachment from the person of the analyst virtually impossible and analysis interminable.

Although traces of transference linger in our relationships, the real love obtainable in a mutual relationship, and the sublime, "other-worldly" pleasure we experience in surrendering willingly to the beautiful in art, allows us, asserted Rank (1932a) in *Art and Artist*, a more creative solution to the "part-whole" problem than transference to an all-powerful analyst: the "dissolution of ... individuality in a greater whole" (110). But what, precisely, is this "greater whole"?

Echoing Martin Buber, in *The Trauma of Birth* (1924) Rank cited the mystic "who cries out in blessed ecstasy: The [I] and the You [*das Ich und das Du*] have ceased to exist between us, I am not I, You are not You, also You are not I; I am at the same time I and You, You are at the same time You and I" (177). Following the wisdom of the "philosophical mystics," Rank called this experience "the *unio mystica*, the being at one with the All" (176)—being "in tune" with the universe.

And in *Will Therapy* (1936a), he emphasized that the *Urangst* that clients feel during the separation (or rebirth) phase of relationship therapy is existential: "Birth fear remains always more universal, cosmic as it were, loss of connection with a greater whole, in the last analysis with the 'all'" (175).

Rank maintained that the healing nature of a mutually empathic relationship *affirms* difference but, paradoxically, also "leads to the *release* from difference, to the feeling of unity with the self, with the other, with the cosmos" (82; italics added).

Only through empathic identification with an "other" can the pain of separation be eased. If we truly open our hearts, moreover, we may find that there is a *macrocosmic* level of empathy as well as a *microcosmic*—or merely human—form. In *Art and Artist* Rank (1932a) writes:

> This identification is the echo of an original identity, not merely of child and mother, but of everything living—witness the reverence of the primitive for animals. In man, identification aims at re-establishing *a lost identity*: not an identity which was lost once and for all, phylogenetically through the differentiation of the sexes, or ontologically in birth, but *an identity with the cosmic process*, which has to be continually surrendered and continually re-established in the course of self-development. (376; italics added)

In the most profound sense, then, our experience of dissolution in art or love—that is, temporarily "surrendering" our identity to "find" it again later,

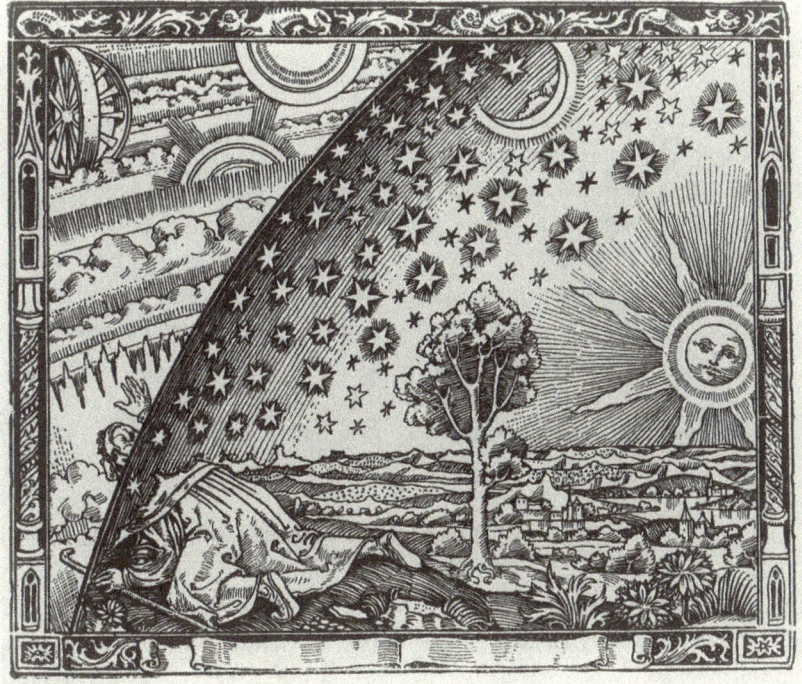

Figure 17.1 A man crawls out from under the world to wonder at "the Beyond," a *terra incognita*

Credit: Unknown artist. Published in Camille Flammarion, *L'Atmosphère: Météorologie Populaire* (1888)

enriched as a by-product of the experience of merger—brings us, asymptotically, to the border of the ineffable, an "other world," a wordless region, beyond "the passing identification of two individuals" (113). It brings us to the Beyond.

This approach is asymptotic. We can never actually cross over into the Beyond, for how can human consciousness ever know that which is utterly different from itself? In a macrocosmic sense, empathic understanding brings us to the border, one might say, of the "unthought known" (Bollas 1987), the border of a *terra incognita*—unthinkable because it is shrouded in darkness.

Yet, if we surrender with all our heart and soul to the experience of mutual empathy—real love—the outlines of the unthought, elusive, and forever unreachable, may nevertheless somehow be dimly "known."

In *Art and Artist*, Rank (1932a) suggests that this transcendent feeling of empathy implies not only a "spiritual unity" between artist and enjoyer, I and Thou, Thou and I, but also an identity with the ALL that once was but is no more. In art and love, difference meets likeness, microcosm meets macrocosm.

Of the uncanny feeling of Oneness we experience in surrendering ourselves—giving up temporarily the burden of our difference—to "the other," in art or love, Rank says:

> [It] produces a satisfaction which suggests that it is *more* than a matter of the passing identification of two individuals, that it is the potential *restoration* of a union with the Cosmos, which once existed and was then lost. The individual psychological root of this sense of unity I discovered (at the time of writing *The Trauma of Birth*, 1924) in the prenatal condition, which the individual in his yearning for immortality strives to restore. Already, in that earliest stage of individualization, the child is not only factually one with the mother but beyond all that, one with the world, with a Cosmos floating in mystic vapours in which present, past, and future are dissolved. The individual urge to *restore this lost unity* is (as I have formerly pointed out) an essential factor in the production of human cultural values. (113; italics added)

Is it conceivable that a search for this lost unity—an "other-worldly" identity, an identity not merely with the human mother who bore us but an even larger identity that echoes, pre-verbally, mystically, with everything in the macrocosm—is what Carl Rogers was hinting at when he wrote, in almost the same terms as Rank, of investigating the possibility of "a reality in which present, past, and future are intermingled, in which space is not a barrier, and time has disappeared" (Kirschenbaum & Henderson 1989b:373)?

In *Love and Will* Rollo May (1969) observes that by surrendering our difference in the experience of love we are temporarily thrown into a "void." In love, according to May, we approach the ultimate but veiled boundary of existence, the nonexistent geography of the Unknown and Unknowable:

> When we love, we give up the center of ourselves. We are thrown from our previous state of existence into a void; and though we hope to obtain a new world, a new existence, we can never be sure.... To love completely carries with it the threat of annihilation of everything. This intensity of consciousness has something in common with the ecstasy of the mystic in his union with God: just as he can never be *sure* God is there, so love carries us to that intensity of consciousness in which we no longer have any guarantee of security. (101; italics in the original)

When we experience mutual empathic understanding, is it possible that the unthought we dimly "know"—the lost feeling of unity with the macrocosm we hope, perhaps unconsciously, to restore—is so strange and fantastic that it is entirely beyond reason?

When we fall into the void of love, are we somehow reminded of what Rogers (1986) came to call, with awe and humility, "the transcendent, the indescribable, the spiritual" (199)? In the empathic moment of love or art, do we come face-to-face, at least fleetingly, with the *mysterium tremendum*? But what, exactly, is this "tremendous mystery" that awes, humbles, fascinates, and seduces us, all at the same time—a mystery at once daimonic and godlike?

D.H. Lawrence proposed that the ultimate mystery is none other than the existence of the human being—a mystery beyond all scientific understanding. The human being is an inexplicable "gap" in causality, a "difference" that materializes from Nothing and Nowhere, created out of the void, in defiance of reason and science.

As Rank wrote to Taft (1958), Lawrence "was the greatest psychological philosopher since Nietzsche ... certainly greater than Freud" (175). "Whence," Nietzsche had wondered, "comes this uncanniest of all guests"—the human being? (quoted in Taylor 1987:36).

In *Psychoanalysis and the Unconscious*, Lawrence (1921) argues that science will never be able to answer Nietzsche's question:

> There is in the nature of the infant that which is utterly unknown in the natures of the parents. Something which could never be derived from the natures of all the existent individuals or previous individuals. There is in the nature of the infant something entirely new, underived, underivable, something which is, and which will forever remain, *causeless*. And this something is the unanalyzable, undefinable reality of individuality. Every time at the moment of

conception of every higher organism an individual nature incomprehensibly arises in the universe, out of nowhere. Granted the whole cause-and-effect process of generation and evolution, still the individual is not explained.... There is no assignable cause, and no logical reason, for individuality. On the contrary, individuality appears in defiance of all scientific law, in defiance even of reason. (214; italics in the original)

Because scientific understanding cannot explain the arrival on the planet of a single rose, much less a new human life, "[a]n inexplicable 'remainder' had therefore to be admitted," said Rank (1932a) in *Art and Artist*, "but this remainder embraced no more and no less than the whole problem of artistic creativity" (63).

This, then, is the New, which has never before materialized: a new creation that has arisen incomprehensibly—"a miracle," as Hannah Arendt (1998) observes in *The Human Condition* (178).

"Who," Carl Rogers once asked, "can bring into being this whole person" (Kirschenbaum & Henderson 1989b:370)—a person for whom "each moment would be new" (413)?

The "natural-scientific" or "biological-sexual" explanation of human birth, explains Rank (1932b) in *Modern Education*,

does not satisfy the child in the least, and if we want to be honest we have to admit also that it does not satisfy ourselves and it only seems to satisfy because we know we have no other reply. Perhaps this explains why the adult seems to suffer from the sexual problem as much as the child: because the biological solution of the problem of humanity is also ungratifying and inadequate for the adult as for the child. The religious solution was and still is so much the more gratifying because it admits *the Unknown*, indeed recognizes it as the chief factor instead of pretending an omniscience that we do not possess. (Rank 1932b:44; italics in the original)

Lebensangst, the fear of life, is not experienced as ordinary fear of an object, like fear of mother or father; it is, as Rank (1996) suggests in his American lectures, a "cosmic fear" (223)—or what William James (1902) in *The Varieties of Religious Experience* calls "the fear of the universe" (158), the fear of being no more than a particle of dust blowing in the wind, a Nothingness engulfed by the immeasurably vast spaces of the ALL.

Biological explanations for how human beings arrive on the planet, observes Rank (1932b) in *Modern Education*, do not reduce our *Lebensangst*, which begins in childhood:

We might give the correct biological answer to the child's concrete question as to the arrival of a little brother or sister, but we do not thereby touch the child's fear of life that is behind this question, and which cannot be explained causally because it is rooted in the fear of the Unknown and Unknowable.... But this craving for the truth is rather a fanaticism for reality than a real love of truth and hence stops short before the admission of the truth concerning our lack of knowledge. (46–47)

Neither anti-science nor a religious believer, Rank concluded that science, for all its magnificent contributions to improving the lot of humanity, curing diseases, and discovering the principles of quantum physics, has nothing to say about beginnings or endings—*alpha* or *omega*. No matter how much science unravels the secrets of biology, chemistry, physics, or the brain, it will never have one word to say about what it means for a human being to exist—*for anything to exist.*

Rank did not discover the existential unconscious. Long before Rank, the Romantic poet Samuel Taylor Coleridge (1831) had asked a question that was already known to the pre-Socratic philosophers:

Hast thou ever raised thy mind to the consideration of EXISTENCE, in and by itself, as the mere act of existing? Hast thou ever said to thyself, thoughtfully, IT IS! Heedless in that moment, whether it were a man before thee, or a flower, or a grain of sand? Without reference, in short, to this or that particular mode or form of existence? If thou hast indeed attained to this, thou wilt have felt the presence of a mystery, which must have fixed thy spirit in awe and wonder. (450–451; capitalization in the original)

What do we know of the two darknesses that engulf us—the oblivion before our arrival on the planet and the oblivion after our departure? Nothing. "For, after all, what is man in nature?," wondered Blaise Pascal (1670), mathematician and mystic. "A nothing in comparison with the infinite, an absolute in comparison with nothing, a central point between nothing and all. . . . He is equally incapable of seeing the nothingness from which he came, and the infinite in which he is engulfed" (52). Thunderstruck at finding himself *alive* and *conscious* in the cosmos, Pascal asks:

When I consider the short extent of my life, swallowed up in the eternity before and after, the small space that I fill or even see, engulfed in the infinite immensity of spaces unknown to me and which know me not, I am terrified and astounded. . . . Who put me here? (57).

According to philosopher Michel Foucault, self-consciousness discovers "both in itself and outside itself, at its borders yet also in its very warp and woof, an element of darkness, an apparently inert density in which it is embedded, an unthought which it contains entirely, yet in which it is also caught" (quoted in Sass 1992:329–330).

Caught in the darkness of the unthought known, like a deer in a car's head-lights, is our *consciousness of living*—the beam of light shining, for the briefest of moments, on the here-and-now.

"In infinite time, in infinite matter, in infinite space," wrote Tolstoy in *Anna Karenina*, "is formed a bubble-organism, and that bubble lasts a while and bursts, and that bubble is I" (quoted in Morson 2023:40).

To be fully conscious that *I am alive* is to experience "fear and trembling," in Kierkegaard's terms, an existential *Angst* in the face of the terrifying vast-ness of the cosmos, the ALL, whose scope cannot be grasped, or even imagined, by the human mind. "Full humanness means full fear and trembling," argued Ernest Becker (1973) in *The Denial of Death*, "at least some of the waking day" (59).

The vexed problem of the consciousness of living—being fully present, here-and-now, on the planet Earth—may be condensed into one, almost unanswer-able, question: How do we muster the courage from within to say, "'Yes' to this force, this internal 'must,'" asked Rank (1936b) in *Truth and Reality*, in full awareness of the suffering, bodily decay, and death that existence has in store for us? (107).

"How are [we] able to live in a world where we are all alone," wondered Rollo May, "where we all die?" (quoted in Rabinowitz, Good, & Cozad 1989:439). How do we find the courage to choose that which is also absolutely determined: our lives?

The father of existential philosophy, Kierkegaard, whose writings Rank had studied before he met Freud (Taft 1958:37), once asked perhaps the most absurd, yet most comical, question of all:

Who am I? How did I come into the world? Why was I not consulted?. . . . And if I am to be compelled to take part in it, where is the director? I should like to make a remark to him. Is there no director? Whither shall I turn with my complaint? . . . How did it come about that I became guilty? Or am I not guilty? Why am I then so called in all human tongues? (Kierkegaard 1843:114–115)

Thrown out of the womb into life, screaming, kicking, and mewling, how do we find the courage to deliberately affirm "the existence forced on us by fate" asked Rank in *Art and Artist* (1932a:65), affirm the godlike but anguished exis-tence forced on us—without our being consulted—as a gift from "the Beyond,"

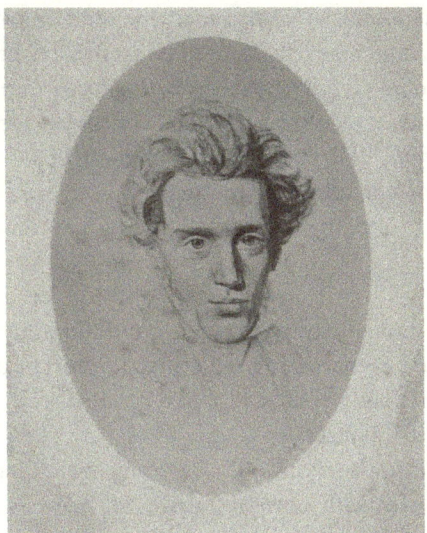

Figure 17.2 Søren Kierkegaard

Credit: Peter Most. Digital Collections, Royal
Danish Library

a gift that, according to Kierkegaard and Rank, makes us feel eternally guilty, eternally in debt?

The idea of "fate," wrote Rank (1936a) in *Will Therapy*, "perhaps rests on the fact of our biological existence" (122), a fact so improbable, so unfathomable, that it passes all human understanding.

In existential suffering, our living energy, continued Rank, "manifests itself as *being* fate" (124; italics added), a denial of freedom and responsibility, a living death—a condition in which, as William James (1902) noted in *The Varieties of Religious Experience*, we "hug the safe shore, and do not tempt the deeper raptures" (140).

Hugging the safe shore, according to Rank, is the outcome of a too-extreme experience of *Lebensangst* and *Todesangst*.

Although the individual is "at once creator and creature," said Rank (1936a) in *Will Therapy*, when we do not accept the burden of our difference "the creative expression of will is a negative one, resting on the denial of the creator role" (123).

On the other hand, the greatest artists, scientists, and philosophers seem to come closest to living fully, "making fate" rather than "being fate" (124), refusing to hug the safe shore, expressing their passions fully, yet not being overwhelmed by the terror of not-knowing where we come from, what we are doing here, and where we are going.

They take into themselves all of existence, and then throw it out again in the creation of a new cosmos, now refashioned in their own image, living themselves out purposefully and powerfully in the "deeper raptures" of creative production.

"The most that any of us can seem to do," concluded Ernest Becker (1973) in *The Denial of Death*, "is to fashion something—an object or ourselves—and drop it into the confusion, make an offering of it, so to speak, to the life-force" (285).

⁂

In his titanic, superhuman struggle to wrest meaning out of the *mysterium tremendum*, Sigmund Freud came to interpret all mortals as "like," reducible to the same unconscious sexual and destructive desires, to the "repetition compulsion" of biological drives.

Against the "repetition compulsion," Otto Rank argued for the expression of our creative urge, our equally powerful "drive" for *newness* and *difference*, for creative production not just sexual *re*-production—a lifelong, never-completed process that is balanced precariously on the boundary of Nothingness and nonbeing.

In a strange twist, Freud's "fear of the unconscious, that is, of the life force itself, from which we all seem to recoil, [led him] to an over-estimation of the rational mind," observed Rank (1941a:277) in *Beyond Psychology*. It led Freud to the supremely positivist view that rational understanding would calm the *Urangst* expressed so poignantly by such existential thinkers as Pascal, Kierkegaard, Coleridge, and William James.

Ridden with guilt and the fear of death, Freud, who is reported to have thought about death every day of his life (Schur 1972), seems to have swung back and forth, eternally, from all to nothing and nothing to all.

To relieve his anxiety, Freud projected his infantile psyche onto the whole world, insisting on interminable analysis for everyone, thus creating a vast Freudian cosmos in which everyone on the planet Earth was a magnified reflection of himself, someone who could never heal his own suffering.

The paradox of Freud "betrays itself," said Rank (1941a) in *Beyond Psychology*, "in the basic axiom of psychoanalysis, a mechanistic theory of life according to which all mental processes and emotional reactions are determined by the Unconscious, that is, by something which in itself is unknown and undeterminable" (13).

When Freud prophesied that *wo Es war, soll Ich werden*—where It was there I shall become—he was, in a sense, overvaluing both unconscious, "the It," and conscious, "the I."

"The over-valuation of the unconscious," pointed out Rank (1932a) in *Art and Artist*, "would then be explained by a more or less strong feeling of guilt, such as is felt by every productive type; and the over-valuation of the conscious would be due to a desire to magnify and exalt oneself—as the other is due to the ... tendency to minimize" (424).

We should not be too surprised to discover that Freud, one of the most creative writers of all time, grasped only too well both the grandiosity and the absurdity of his *causa-sui* project. "Mocking laughter or immortality or both" (Freud & Ferenczi 1993:243) would be the verdict of posterity, predicted Freud—with uncanny accuracy on each count.

According to historian William M. Johnston (1983), "Freud embraced a limited therapeutic nihilism, concluding that sometimes neither nature nor therapy can foil the will to die" (248)—*thanatos*. As Rollo May (1969) observed in *Love and Will*, there is no *agape* in Freud, no possibility of mutual love, no empathic understanding, only *eros* and *thanatos*—sex and death.

Unlike Freud, in *Beyond Psychology* Rank (1941a) saw *agape*—the self-transcendence that is possible in mutual love—as the healing factor not only in relationship therapy but also in the face of death.

Agape, argued Rank, "can overcome the fear of death, for [paradoxically] it is the most positive expression of it. In the yielding love emotion," he continued, "the individual voluntarily accepts the dissolution of the Self by freely submitting to something bigger than the [I] and also bigger than the other person, the Thou. Thereby the individual conquers death, and with it sex, in a willing surrender to the bigness of nature" (197)—a willing surrender to the mystery, awesomeness, and miracle of EXISTENCE.

In *Beyond the Pleasure Principle*, Freud (1920) declared that "the aim of all life is death" (38). On September 23, 1939, the Jewish Day of Atonement, *Yom Kippur*, Freud, aged 83, committed physician-assisted suicide, enacting his own *Todestrieb*, the death drive he claimed was universal.

One month later, Otto Rank, aged 55, was hospitalized with kidney trouble. He died of reaction to an antibacterial drug that was in use before the discovery of penicillin. The last word he was heard to say on his deathbed was "*Komisch*"— comical, strange, peculiar (quoted in Lieberman 1985:389).

Epilogue

"I was born beyond psychology"

To account for the arrival on the planet of a new human being, molecular biology asserts, with experimental proof, that sexual intercourse causes two sets of germ cells—called "mother" and "father"—to fuse their nuclei and melt down into Nothingness. From the ruins of these germ cells emerges something never before seen, like the phoenix arising from its ashes to start another life: a new germ-plasm.

The human being, insisted Sigmund Freud (1914), is nothing but "an appendage to his germ-plasm" (78). Rank agreed. For nature, observes Rank (1941a) in *Beyond Psychology*, "the whole individual—man or woman—is nothing but a sex-cell" (227). While this coincides with Freud's view, Rank adds a twist in the next sentence, based on his psychology of difference: "Man's need to *differentiate* himself as an individual . . . from his purely biological function precipitated the split between him and nature, from which he suffers, but which has enabled him to achieve human culture" (227; italics added).

As a biologist of the mind (Sulloway 1979), Freud made sex the cause of everything, including culture, creativity, and art. But how, wondered Rank, does one build a bridge between a biological impulse common to all men and women and the production of Beethoven's *Ode to Joy*, an astonishing and never-to-be-repeated masterpiece? Did Martha Graham give birth to her dazzling dances, full of passionate intensity, or was her art brought to life by an impersonal "compromise formation" of biological vectors, intrapsychic forces, and defense mechanisms?

"One is almost tempted to say," Rank (1932a) muses in *Art and Artist*, "that the sexual act was made 'creative' by comparison with the generation of fire, and not that the generation of fire needed to be sexualized" (174). New life is the mating of two mysteries, or more precisely, two sets of trillions of mysteries each, going back to the emergence of the first germ-plasm. Each new arrival on the planet is an "unthought known," leaping out of its chemical soup from Nowhere and Nothing.

In *Feminine Sexuality*, psychoanalyst Jacques Lacan (1985) observes that something irreducible—about which we know nothing—goes "beyond" the

Otto Rank and the Creation of Modern Psychotherapy. Robert Kramer, Oxford University Press.
© Robert Kramer (2025). DOI: 10.1093/9780197698303.003.0018

orgasmic fire. Always leaving an inexplicable remainder, *jouissance* (French, *jour*, "to come") cannot be translated, according to Lacan, who defines himself as a "mystic":

> There are men who ... sense that there must be a *jouissance* which goes beyond. That is what we call a mystic. ... What was tried at the end of the last century, at the time of Freud ... was an attempt to reduce the mystical to questions of fucking. ... Might not this *jouissance* which one experiences and knows nothing of, be that which puts us on the path of ex-istence [Latin, *ex-sistere*: "to come forth"]? (147)[1]

In Lacan's terms, "the real is a 'beyond,'" remarks theologian Mark Taylor (1987:92). "That which sends Being and beings," adds Taylor, "is not completely revealed in the missionary act" (45).

"Too limited a meaning has been placed upon the sexual experience," Rank once told Anaïs Nin (1966). "In psychoanalysis we still see the consequences of this, in the fallacy that because sex is obviously biologically fundamental, it must also play the leading role" (292). Too *limited* a meaning? Was Rank joking? Ernest Becker (1982) explains:

> You don't know where you came from—oh, I know, you say "the sperm and egg." Sperm and egg!. ... Idiot answer. It's not an answer at all, it's merely a description of a speck in a causal process that is a mystery. We don't know where babies come from. You get married, you're sitting at a table having breakfast— there are two of you—and a year later there's somebody else there. And if you're honest with yourself, you don't know where they come from. (12)

According to Rank, Lacan, and Becker, sexual conception is preconceptual: before thought, words, speech, or language. Sexual conception is before Oedipus, before pre-Oedipus. Mystery remains. A "*breakdown*," writes psychoanalyst D.W. Winnicott (1989) mystically, "*has already been experienced*" (90; italics in the original) but cannot be remembered "because the patient was not there for it to happen to" (92).

Arriving on the planet "is more nearly about BEING," insists Winnicott (1986), capitalizing the word "BEING" for effect, "than about sex" (35). In *The Trauma of Birth*, as Winnicott knew, Rank had confronted the ontological, or better, the pre-ontological, mystery of BEING itself: the ineffable difference between nonexistence and existence.

"[H]uman existence," according to philosopher Costica Bradatan (2023), "is something that happens, briefly, between two instantiations of nothingness.

Nothing first—dense, impenetrable nothingness. Then a flickering. Then nothing again, endlessly" (1). We cannot eff the ineffable.

At the moment of conception, we are "lifted," in the apt metaphor of the poet E.E. Cummings (1991), "from the no of all nothing" (663). Adds author Gore Vidal (1993): "The creation of a work of art, like an act of love, is our one small 'yes' at the center of a vast 'no'" (20). To overcome death—the vast "no"—the artist says "yes" to the "must," argues Rank in *Art and Artist.*

"A certificate tells me that I was born," observes Lacan (1981) of the document displaying the Name-of-the-Father and the Name-of-the-Mother. "I repudiate this certificate" (viii). At the same time, with unusual humility, Lacan (1989) confessed that he was not his own. "I am not the cause of myself" (13), he admits, calling into question Freud's *causa-sui* project. "The creator," according to Lacan, "is something greater than me. It is my unconscious . . . beyond me" (quoted in Clark 1988:35).

In *The Ego and the Id* (1923a), Freud wrote that "the property of being conscious or not is in the last resort our one beacon-light in the darkness of depth-psychology" (18). At the end of his life, in *An Outline of Psycho-Analysis*, Freud (1940) conceded that the starting point of psychoanalysis is a "fact without parallel, which defies all explanation or description—the fact of consciousness" (157).

Early on, Freud (1915) adopted the term "depth-psychology," claiming that he'd gone below the "psychology of consciousness" (173) to explore the sexual "depths" of the psyche. That we are conscious of our own existence, countered Rank, is far more enigmatic than anything to be found in Freud's sexual unconscious.

Although we are thrown into the world at birth and thrown out at death, not only do we forget that we are born to die, we also forget that we are living. Life is a loan from "the beyond" (60), observes Rank (1924) in *The Trauma of Birth*, and death the repayment. One cannot refuse the loan, life, in order to escape payment of the debt, death.

Fascinated by art and artists, Rank was too absorbed in questions of creativity and inhibition of will to reduce the incalculable variety of human beings to one common denominator, biology, to Freud's psychology of likeness. Each person is unique, even if sexuality is common to all of us.

"Will people ever learn," asks Rank (1941a) in *Beyond Psychology*, "that there is no other equality possible than the equal right of every individual to become and to be himself, which actually means to accept his own difference and have it accepted by others?" (267).

But what is difference? According to Rank, difference is how women and men experience the exhilaration of being present, fully alive and conscious, awestruck at the mystery and wonder of existence, never ceasing to create something new out of Nothingness—bringing new life, new ideas, new energy, new knowledge, and previously unimagined ways to transcend anxiety, alienation, and existential loneliness, and overcome death.

"I was born beyond psychology and want to die beyond it," Rank jotted on a note dated July 1939, a few months before he died, "but first and foremost, I want to live beyond it—and formerly it has been in my way" (Rank 1939). There is something beyond psychology. Beyond psychoanalysis. Beyond sex. There is difference.

Individual human beings, men and women—with feeling, willing, creative minds—construct the time-defying symbols of culture, according to Rank, to give us hope that our lives have meaning. "We live in utter darkness about who we are, and why we are here," writes Ernest Becker (1973) in *The Denial of Death*, "yet we know it must have some meaning" (156).

Both joy and sorrow are real; all feelings need to be embraced and integrated to make us whole, according to Rank. It is only when we experience and express our feelings fully, that we affirm our aliveness, our uniqueness, our difference. Feelings, according to poet E.E. Cummings (1965), *constitute* our difference:

> Almost anybody can learn to think or believe or know, but not a single human being can be taught to feel. Why? Because whenever you think or you believe or you know, you're a lot of other people: but the moment you feel, you're nobody-but-yourself.
>
> To be nobody-but-yourself—in a world which is doing its best, night and day, to make you everybody else—means to fight the hardest battle which any human being can fight; and never stop fighting. (335)

All willing, all creativity, all art, involves feeling. As long as we are feeling, willing, creative minds who live and breathe on this planet, as long as we make art, music, and science, as long as we sing and dance and write poetry and make love, human existence is just as enchanting, just as awe-inspiring, just as exhilarating, as it is terrifying. "There is no cure for birth and death," proposes philosopher George Santayana (1922), "save to enjoy the interval" (97).

In *The Trauma of Birth*, Rank planted the first seed of what would later become his psychology of difference, arguing that birth is not only a *trauma* but also a *triumph*.

According to Rank, difference has two sides. Difference brings with it the consciousness of living and suffering; but difference also brings with it the possibilities of reconnecting simultaneously to others and the macrocosm. By surrendering to the majesty of Beethoven's *Ode to Joy*, we rediscover our likeness to all humanity, and feel again, viscerally, our godlike place in the ALL.

"Rank looms too big," argues Anaïs Nin (1966) in her *Diary*, "with his talk about cosmological knowledge, his nonconformism, his subtlety, his paradoxes. Listening to him, I can perceive the brilliant philosopher and the dangerous enemy of Freudism" (326).

To be persons of value and dignity on the planet, human beings throughout history have taken enormous pleasure in the "defiant creation of meaning," asserts Ernest Becker (1973:7) in *The Denial of Death*—no matter how dizzying it is to look into the void of Nothingness. "I can't go on," says Samuel Beckett (1994). "I'll go on."

"The creative person," explains Becker (1973), "becomes then, in art, literature and religion the mediator of natural terror and the indicator of a new way to triumph over it. He reveals the darkness and the dread of the human condition and fabricates a new symbolic transcendence over it. This has been the function of the creative deviant from the shamans to Shakespeare" (220).

Difference, in addition to carrying with it *Lebensangst* and *Todesangst*, the fear of life and the fear of death, is also a powerful source of creative energy—a primal force coursing through the macrocosm and, simultaneously, through each human being's "soul life of feeling and willing" (Rank 1936a:231). Each human being's soul life is a microcosm of the whole, a whole that can be rediscovered in authentic relationship.

Difference propels us continually to create new forms of music, art, dance, literature, poetry, philosophy, religion, and culture as vehicles for cosmic heroism, to tirelessly find yet more imaginative ways to transcend death.

Difference is the ecstasy of being alive. "We ought to dance with rapture," declares D.H. Lawrence (1932), "that we should be alive and in the flesh, and part of the living, incarnate cosmos" (190).

According to philosopher André Malraux, "The greatest mystery is not that we have been flung at random among the profusion of the earth and the galaxy of the stars, but that in this prison we can fashion images of ourselves sufficiently powerful to deny our nothingness" (quoted in Friedman 1967: 17).

The cosmic mystery of life's effusion of creativity reveals itself again and again, at the arrival of each new flower, each new poem, each new scientific discovery, each new child on the planet.

"The never completed birth of individuality," Rank (1936b) exults in *Truth and Reality*, corresponds "to a continued result of births, rebirths and new birth, which reach from the birth of the child from the mother, beyond the birth of the individual from the mass, to the birth of creative work from the individual and finally to the birth of knowledge from the work" (24–25).

"We are born with the capacity to be born again and again," adds philosopher Sam Keen (2006), expanding on Rank's idea. "What must we say about a universe that has given birth to at least one creature whose nature is to be reborn?

Does it not suggest that something wild and unpredictable at the heart of things makes despair an indulgence, a premature closure of possibilities?" (29).

In *Civilization and Its Discontents*, responding to Romain Rolland, a despairing Sigmund Freud (1930) vehemently denied ever experiencing the "oceanic feeling," a feeling that suggests the experience of mother and fetus in the womb: part-in-whole, whole-in-part, "two-in-one"—a *Doppelgänger* experience.

Unwilling or unable to exorcise the power of his mother over himself, Freud was forever immersed, with his eyes wide shut, in the oceanic womb of Amalia Freud, like a fish who doesn't know it's in water. "How tempting to any man harboring such latent potential for terrors and rages [must] be the mystical vision of regaining total bliss—of the ocean as womb!," writes psychoanalyst Selig Harrison (1979). "And psychoanalysis . . . may have been born of Freud's resolute determination to resist just that temptation" (418–419).

In contrast to Freud, Otto Rank, like Romain Rolland, celebrated the oceanic feeling, the *fons et origo* of all feeling, all relationship. At age 20, one year before he met Freud, Rank (1904), wrote exuberantly in his journal: "I can now approximately picture the growth of the child in the mother's body, also the emotions and sensations of the mother. . . . I often do not know at all for a long time that I am carrying something around with me . . . like an embryo" (n.p.). Anaïs Nin (1966) recounts the rest of the story, as Rank told it to her:

> He was already exploring the possibility of a memory of the body, a visceral memory in the blood, in the muscles, long before consciousness, as a child's first awareness of pain or pleasure, a memory of actual birth. A memory which started with birth itself. The experience of birth. Emotions formed like geological strata, from purely animal experiences. Birth, warmth, cold, pain. (278)

Who can deny that mother and fetus are viscerally One in the womb, a relationship obvious to any woman who has ever been pregnant?

If we use our imagination and "existential empathy" (Vanhooren 2022), as Rank did, we may be able to intuit that the fetus's discovery of its first object—mother—comes at the precise moment of birth, when arrive, all at once, the multiple traumas of blinding light, freezing cold, pangs of hunger, existential loneliness, pain and difference, as well the beginnings of *Lebensangst* and *Todesangst*, all of which are registered in the body's implicit memory, pre-verbally, for the rest of life.

How can the anguished experience of being expelled into the world not be felt as traumatic—an "original wound"—by the tiny, vulnerable being, who risks

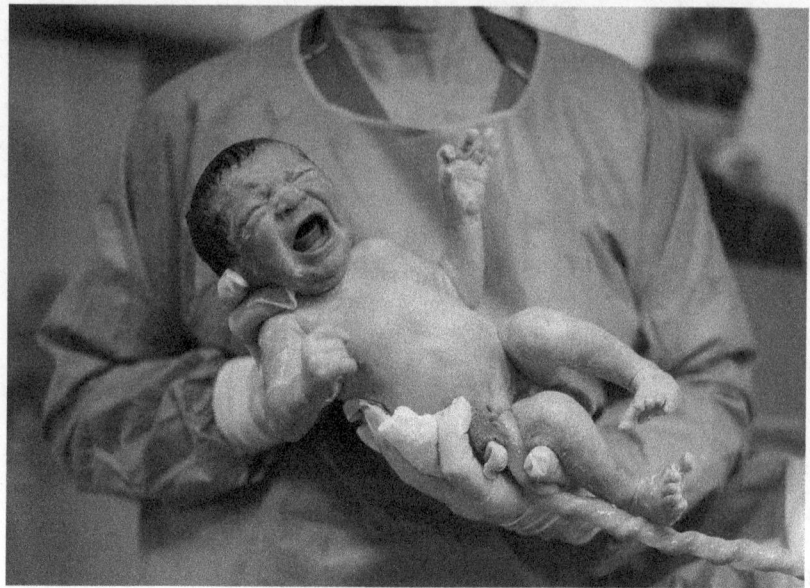

Figure E.1 The trauma of birth
Credit: Photo by Hannah Barata via Pexels

death at the moment of expulsion from the all-embracing "oceanic feeling" of warmth into dry, cold air, gasping for breath? Birth is a matter of life and death for both mother and child.

In *The Trauma of Birth*, "Rank's willingness to empathize," observes Frank Tallis (2021), "to imagine what it is like to experience the symbiotic bliss of the womb, followed by expulsion, represents not only an impressive act of identification, but also an early example of the raised consciousness that mobilized for natural childbirth in the 1970s and ultimately made obstetrics a more humane profession" (52–53).

In "Birth Memories, Birth Trauma, and Anxiety," Winnicott (1949) describes birth as the primal trauma. Prenatal and birth memories remain in the body. "The feeling one gets," asserts Winnicott, once called a *Rankschüler*, a member of Rank's school of thought, is "that the child's body knows about being born" (180). Strongly resonating with Rank's views, he adds: "I do find in my analytic and other work that there is evidence that the personal birth experience is significant, and is held as memory material" (177).

The physiological trauma of birth has long been denied by medical doctors because of the lack of complete myelination in the central nervous system of the fetus before birth. But the amygdala, now shown to be the seat of anxiety, is already active in the womb (Ulfig et al. 2003).

Hugo Lagercrantz, professor of pediatrics at Stockholm's Karolinska Institute, reports that the fetus mobilizes very high levels of catecholamines (stress hormones) during birth, confirming Rank's intuition that there's a *physiological* as well as a *psychological* trauma of separation at birth. "When I showed the results to my colleagues in adult medicine," Lagercrantz (2016) writes, "they did not believe me. [But] the levels [of stress] were even much higher than in adults during severe stress, like running a marathon or during childbirth" (57–58).

In *Brain Sciences*, a team of cognitive neuroscientists (Lang et al. 2020) has shown that memory traces can be formed *in utero*—the autonomic and neuronal responses of newborns to prenatal stimuli and their mother's voice. These traces exist as embodied memories in the periphery of the newborn's awareness. Traces of the trauma of separation at birth, Rank had predicted a century earlier, stay in the implicit, unconscious memory of the newborn's body.

The fragile newborn is flooded with overwhelming amounts of stress hormones at the moment of birth, a level of stress greater than it will ever experience as an adult. For all of us, life, one might say without too much exaggeration, is a post-traumatic stress disorder—an existential, not a psychiatric, condition.

The experience of *agape* at the core of empathic healing in relationship therapy, according to Rank, allows us to rediscover, to feel again in our bodies, even if only temporarily, the *unio mystica*, the "being at One" with the universe.

"We can empathize with 'the other,'" explains Esther Menaker (1995a), pointing to the visceral feeling of Oneness we experienced in the womb, "because once we were one with the other" (110).

By releasing the power of our creative will, Rank's relationship therapy can help us find the courage to affirm, deliberately, the existence forced on us by *das Es*—"the It"—to choose that which is also absolutely determined: our lives. Only by means of an authentic, mutually empathic relationship can human beings transcend their painful difference and experience together the sacrosanct primal life force of the universe.

"[We] have yielded up [our] mortal ego for a moment, fearlessly and even joyfully, to receive it back in the next, the richer for this universal feeling," writes Rank in *Art and Artist* (1932a:110). "[I]t is more than a matter of the passing identification of two individuals," he adds, "it is the potential *restoration* of a union with the Cosmos, which once existed and was then lost" (113; italics in the original).

In the empathic "meeting" of I and Thou, Thou and I, always fleeting and elusive, we may, even if only for an instant, surrender our lonely burden of difference, surrender to the indescribable, to the awesome splendor and vastness of creation—and, if recognition is mutual, receive ourselves back, renewed by our temporary brush with the numinous.

Throughout his many years of practicing relationship therapy, Rank came to understood that he was negotiating with "the Beyond." Negotiating, on a microcosmic level, by means of the countless births he midwifed, the countless differences he prized empathically. But also negotiating, in a macrocosmic sense, by means of his appreciation of the potential for self-transcendence possible in love and art, where microcosm meets macrocosm.

♭

"Rank inaugurated a paradigm shift in the psychological understanding of mysticism," asserts psychoanalyst Dan Merkur (2010). "The psyche was mystical from birth to adulthood" (55).

The word "mystic" comes from the Greek, *muein*, which means to "shut up" about things we don't know, closing the eyes or lips. *Muein* is also related to "mute" and "mystery."

But what *is* the mystical? In philosopher Ludwig Wittgenstein's terms, anyone who maintains that the universe exists—meaning simply the *matter* of the universe—is a mystic. *That* the physical universe exists is the mystical. "It is not *how* the world is that is mystical," says Wittgenstein (1921) in his *Tractatus*, "but *that* it is" (187; italics in the original).

According to science writer George Musser (2023), author of *Putting Ourselves Back in the Equation*, none of the equations of physics accounts for the existence of matter. Just as there is a "hard problem" of *consciousness*, as philosopher David Chalmers (1995) said, there is also a "hard problem" of *matter*. Neither problem is solvable by science. We are all mystics when it comes to grappling with the mystery of consciousness and matter.

Wittgenstein characterizes the mystical as an experience of the universe *sub specie aeternitatis*, "under the aspect of eternity." Many sentences in the *Tractatus* are infused with Wittgenstein's mysticism, from the first—"The world is all that is the case"—to the last: "Whereof we cannot speak—thereof we must remain silent." As Goldsmith and Laks (2019) observe:

> "*We must remain silent*": much of the *Tractatus* is about what we must be silent about. The phrase "remain silent" is a poor translation from the German *schweigen*; in German, *schweigen* is a verb, much like the French verb *se taire*. . . . The silence that Wittgenstein insists on is not the silence that comes from turning a cold shoulder to things, but the silence that we feel when we enter an imposing cathedral. (389–390; italics in the original)

Life is an infinitesimal moment of sound, a holiday on Earth, sandwiched between two eternities of silence.

Outside the therapy room, mysticism is much more prevalent than we might realize, perhaps nowhere more surprisingly than in politics, war, and nationalism.

As we saw in Chapter 4, political theorist Jean Bethke Elshtain (2015) suggests that dying in the name of the nation-state is a "mystical" act (n.p.). Believers in the immortality of the nation-state are, therefore, mystics. According to Elshtain, during times of war, even mothers and women, spurred on by "political plague-mongers" (Becker 1975:93), will often share with men a savage, murderous blood lust, which leads many, whether male or female, to embrace a "dying-centered" mysticism.

Echoing Rank and Becker, political theorist Jennifer Mitzen (2006) explains why the many "holy wars" being fought today are so intractable: "The sense of being part of a greater whole, i.e. the 'we' dimension of their relationship, remains implicit or submerged, making this type of conflict particularly difficult to overcome" (360). Without access to a "greater whole" there is little possibility of achieving peace.

"While there is a yearning to be part of a larger political or religious ideology," according to psychologist Scott Barry Kaufman (2020), "the realization of this yearning is often built on hate or hostility for the 'other,'" as Rank first observed, "rather than pride and deep commitment for a cause that can better humanity" (xix).

Before the difference of the "other" can be accepted, one's own difference must be affirmed. "For only inasmuch as the individual accepts himself," argued Rank (1941a) in *Beyond Psychology*, "can he accept others as they are and in that sense 'love' them. The nonacceptance of the other, manifesting itself through assertion of difference in hatred, springs from the nonacceptance of the self, conceived of as being bad and therefore rejected. Thus self-hatred is the basis for hating others and the world at large" (191).

Rank maintained that there is a much healthier, more creative, form of mysticism than one that is "dying-centered." The alternative form of mysticism is rooted in awe and wonder at "the marvel of creation itself" (250), the miraculous existence of the universe; it is "creation-centered," in theologian Matthew Fox's terms.

According to Fox (2014), "Rank is a creation-centered mystic of the highest order. The via positiva—a rediscovery of the awe and wonder, the delight and joy, of existence itself—is the basic cure for self and society's tiredness and pessimism. A new falling in love with life is the medicine prescribed by Rank and other creation-centered mystics" (143).

Philosopher Hannah Arendt (1998) observes in *The Human Condition* that each person "is unique, so that with each birth something uniquely new comes into the world. With respect to this somebody who is unique it can truly be said," as does Rank, "that nobody was there before" (178).

Like Rank, therefore, Arendt must be considered a creation-centered mystic. "The birth and death of human beings are not simple natural occurrences," she argues, "but are related to a world into which single individuals, unique, unexchangeable, and unrepeatable entities appear and from which they depart" (96-97).

Since we are all mystics, in Wittgenstein's sense, the only question, then, is: What is *life-enhancing* mysticism?

"Dying-centered" mysticism is promoted by genocidal leaders like Vladimir Putin, who dreams of becoming the "master of a fraction of a dot," in Carl Sagan's memorable phrase.

"Dying-centered" mysticism is rooted in the imaginary. If you die at the behest of a toxic leader who wants to sacrifice your life in order for him to rule "a fraction of a dot," your coffin will be tightly wrapped in a flag, symbolizing the immortality promised by the nation-state, a promissory note that cannot be fulfilled.

As Arendt (1973) notes in *The Origins of Totalitarianism*, although we are all born tiny, vulnerable human beings, "The world found nothing sacred in the abstract nakedness of being human" (299). She is alluding, of course, to the nakedness of the newborn. "How should one be able to deduce laws and rights," asks Arendt, "from a universe which apparently knows neither the one nor the other category"? (298). Therefore, the superordinate goal of politics, urges Arendt with all the passion she can muster, is to institute these laws and rights for all human beings without exception.

For Arendt, acceptance of *natality* as the first principle of politics is the only philosophy that can save nation-states from the "dying-centered" politics that Arendt watched, in horror, destroy Europe during the Second World War (Diprose & Ziarek 2018).

The mystery of human existence begins with a cleavage in a blastocyst smaller than the period at the end of this sentence. The blastocyst is the stage of development when the embryo begins to separate into two compartments, one that will become the placenta and another that will become the baby (called the inner cell mass).

This *Ur*-separation precedes the physical passage of the fetus nine months later through the maternal birth canal. The birth trauma, speculates Rank (1924) in *The Trauma of Birth*, making "an asymptotic approach" (7) to the boundary of the metaphysical, is "derived from the germ plasm" (188).

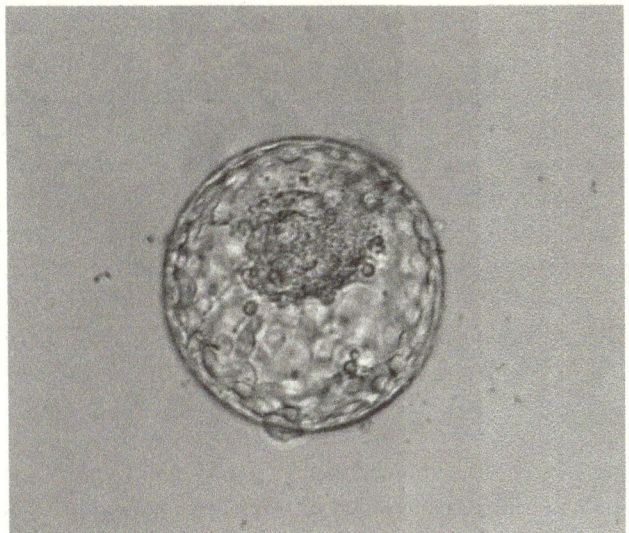

Figure E.2 Human blastocyst within the zona pellucida

The absolute Nothingness of the existential unconscious is a beyond, "the 'thing-in-itself,'" observes Rank, "the only transcendental, and therefore impenetrable, reality" (178).

The existential psychiatrist Ludwig Binswanger (1963) spoke of three interacting elements in every human being's life: the *Umwelt* or "physical" world; the *Mitwelt* or "interpersonal" world; and the *Eigenwelt* or "personal" world. To this list, Rank might have added a fourth: the *Nichtswelt* or the "Nothingness" world.

"Anxiety is the existential awareness of nonbeing"—of Nothingness—proposes theologian Paul Tillich (1952) in *The Courage to Be* (35). But what does it mean to be "aware of nonbeing"? Perhaps only the greatest of artists—writers like Samuel Beckett, who was deeply influenced by Rank—can offer us a glimpse, but only through a glass darkly, of the *Nichtswelt*.

"Beckett may well have been startled by the convergence between his and Rank's conceptions of a prenatal and posthumous timelessness fused in the mind: 'the darkened mind gone wombtomb' and 'the umbra of grave and womb where it is fitting that the spirits of his dead and his unborn should come abroad,'" says literary scholar Angela Moorjani (2004:173), quoting from Beckett's echoes of Rank.

"For Rank," adds Moorjani, "this phantasy in which a progression toward death is identical to a regression to the womb, or where the future after death is also conceived as a return to a past before birth, is an attempt at healing the trauma of separation at birth" (ibid.).

"I'm no intellectual," Beckett revealed. "All I am is feeling" (quoted in Smith 2010:196), resonating with Goethe, Rank, E.E. Cummings, and all other artists for whom *Gefühl ist alles*. Beckett deliberately, silently, evokes "an emotional state in which . . . *nothingness may be felt without being known*" (207; italics added).

The first therapist-artist, committed with Jessie Taft and Virginia Robinson to fostering gender, racial, economic, and social justice, Otto Rank taught that the creative will of clients emerges from being together in an authentic, respectful, empathic relationship.

Born beyond psychology, creator of modern psychotherapy, an advocate for women's self-leadership, Rank was deeply gratified that the University of Pennsylvania School of Social Work had adopted his ideas on relationship, ideas that his one-time mentor, Sigmund Freud, had repudiated as strongly as he repudiated the feelings and creative will of women. "I am sure the School has a unique function to perform," Rank wrote to Virginia Robinson nine days before he died in October 1939. "I am naturally proud of whatever I may have contributed to its present status and future significance. . . . [I]t is still nice to hear that the help I could give to some people has borne fruit" (quoted in Taft 1958:266).

Unfortunately, he did not live to learn of the enormous impact his thought would have on Carl Rogers, whose model of therapeutic healing is today practiced by countless social workers, counselors, and therapists worldwide.

Recalling his transformative encounter with Rank almost four decades earlier, Rogers (1973) told Virginia Robinson: "[T]here are many people who have been influenced by [Rank's] thinking, and this will undoubtedly be true in the future" (95).

To be born twice is surely no more miraculous than to be born once. I cannot but help feel, therefore, that long after Otto Rank died, his spirit was alive in the mind, heart, and soul of Carl Rogers.

Chronology of Rank's life and work

1884 Born in Vienna, April 22.

1904 At age 20, writes in his journal: "I can now approximately picture the growth of the child in the mother's body, also the emotions and sensations of the mother. . . . I often do not know at all for a long time that I am carrying something around with me . . . like an embryo."

1905 Sends Freud a manuscript entitled *The Artist*, using the word *artist* in as comprehensive a sense as Freud had used the word *sexuality*.

1906 Accepts Freud's offer to be secretary of the Vienna Psychoanalytic Society; is adopted by Freud as a "foster son" and becomes a regular visitor to *Berggasse 19* for intimate conversations with "the Professor" and meals with the Freud family.

1906 Is asked by Freud to devote himself to the nonmedical side of psychoanalysis, eventually becoming the first "lay analyst" in the world.

1907 Publishes *The Artist*, the first psychoanalytic work not written by Freud.

1909 Publishes *The Myth of the Birth of the Hero*, presenting a copy to Freud with the inscription: "Dedicated to the father of this book in thanks from—the mother."

1911 Helps Freud edit and revise the third edition of *The Interpretation of Dreams*.

1911 Publishes *The Lohengrin Saga*, for which he later receives a PhD from the University of Vienna, the first dissertation ever published on a psychoanalytic theme.

1912 Publishes *The Incest Theme in Literature and Legend: Fundamentals of a Psychology of Literary Creation*, a 685-page study of incest throughout world literature.

1912 Becomes the youngest ring holder of the Secret Committee—Abraham, Ferenczi, Sachs, Jones (and, later, Eitingon)—formed by Freud as a Politburo to defend psychoanalysis against "heretics" like Adler and Jung.

1912 Co-founds with Freud and serves as the main editor of *Imago* and *Internationale Zeitschrift für Psychoanalyse*, the two leading journals of psychoanalysis.

1913 Publishes, with Sachs, *The Significance of Psychoanalysis for the Human Sciences*.

1914 Contributes two essays, on literature and myth, to the fourth edition of *The Interpretation of Dreams*, his name now appearing (until 1929) below Freud's on the title page.

1914 Publishes *The Double*, an existential study of multiple identity, guilt, narcissism, the fear of death, the soul, and the desire for immortality.

1916–1918 Serves as editor-in-chief of *Krakauer Zeitung*, the official army newspaper in Poland.

1918 Marries Beata (Tola) Minzer, twenty-three, in Poland.

1919   Returns to Vienna to edit *Imago* and *Internationale Zeitschrift* and is asked by Freud to become managing director of the *Verlag*, the newly created international psychoanalytic publishing house, and vice-president of the Vienna Psychoanalytic Society.

1919   Helene, his only child, is born.

1920   Begins full-time practice as a lay analyst and conducts training analyses for visiting American psychiatrists, becoming the "one-man training institute of Vienna," according to Franz Alexander.

1921–23   Drafts with Ferenczi, now his best friend, *The Development of Psychoanalysis*, which advocates the healing effect of the "here-and-now" experience of feelings between analyst and patient over intellectual understanding of the past.

1923   Is informed, immediately after diagnosis, of Freud's life-threatening cancer of the jaw.

1923   Jousts, in "David and Goliath" letters exchanged with Freud, over the origins of the super-ego.

1924   Publishes *The Trauma of Birth*, focusing on the primary role of the powerful mother in the child's psychic life, relegating the powerful father to a secondary place.

1924   Publishes, with Ferenczi, *The Development of Psychoanalysis*, criticizing the "fanaticism for interpreting" among analysts; "The actual analytic task [of healing]," they argue, "was neglected." The arid requirement for emotional distance had led to "an unnatural elimination of all human factors in the analysis."

1924   Sails for the United States in April and lectures on his new "pre-Oedipal" theory and short-term therapy before the American Psychoanalytic Association and other audiences.

1924   From the United States, in an August letter, denies Freud's charge that he has "eliminated the father. That's not so, of course, and cannot be: it would be nonsense. I've only attempted to assign him the correct place." The will of mother comes first in our earliest psychic life, insists Rank, then the will of father.

1924   Confesses in December to an "Oedipal neurosis" occasioned by "the trauma of the Professor's critical illness," but, even while apologizing in a letter to the Secret Committee for creating dissent in the inner circle, refuses to abandon his new pre-Oedipal theory.

1925   In a January talk at the New York Psychoanalytic Society, reiterates: "The only real new viewpoint in [my] contribution [is] the concept of the pre-Oedipus level."

1925   On returning from New York, visits Freud regularly for months, trying to reconcile their differences; Freud gives Rank the impression that he will re-organize the Secret Committee, returning Rank to a leadership role; Rank writes letters to Freud expressing deep gratitude to his beloved "Professor."

1925   To Ferenczi, Freud confesses that he is still "boiling with rage" about Rank, and compares his emotional state to "an absolutism moderated by treacherous assassination;" Freud confides to Ferenczi that he has decided to write a manuscript demolishing Rank's anti-Oedipal theory.

1926   Confronts Freud face-to-face over his "treacherous assassination," published in the form of a book entitled *Inhibitions, Symptoms and Anxiety*,
and accuses Freud of not having "any more insight than a small boy";
enraged by Rank's effrontery, which threatens the validity of the Oedipal insights of his self-analysis, Freud calls Rank a *Hochstaplenatur*—an
imposter by nature.

1926   In response to Freud's public attack on him, moves to Paris with his wife,
Tola, and young daughter, Helene, to start a new practice of psychotherapy, severing all ties with Freud and the Secret Committee, and recanting
his "Oedipal neurosis."

1926   Delivers a series of lectures before the New York School of Social Work,
based on volume 1 of his forthcoming work *Genetische Psychologie*
(1927), whose opening sentence reads: "This book is a direct continuation . . . of my new vision in psychoanalytic theory and therapy." With
the publication of this book, Rank invents modern object relations theory
and therapy.

1926   In his New York lectures, accuses Freud of repressing the powerful will
of mothers: *"The 'bad mother' he has never seen, but only the later displacement of her to the father, who therefore plays such as omnipotent part
in his theory. . . . The 'strict mother'* thus forms the real nucleus of the
super-ego."

1927–38   Collaborates with Jessie Taft and Virginia Robinson at the University
of Pennsylvania School of Social Work, teaching his mostly female students that, by drawing on the power of their "creative will," they can
become leaders of social change; moreover, through building authentic,
empathic, and respectful relationships with their clients, they can lead
them to lead themselves, helping them become self-empowered in the
process.

1927   At the Penn School, defines love in terms of the I–Thou, Thou–I
relationship: "The love of the Thou . . . places a value on one's own I. *Love
abolishes egoism, it merges the self in the other to find it again enriched in
one's own I*. . . . [O]ne can really only love the one who accepts our own
self as it is, indeed will not have it otherwise than it is, and whose self we
accept as it is."

At the same lecture, defines guilt as lying on the boundary "between
the severing and uniting feelings; [therefore,] it is also the most important
representative of the relation between inner and outer, I and Thou, the
Self and the World"—and the relation between love and will.

1929–31   Asserts in *Will Therapy* (translated into English by Jessie Taft in 1936)
that the tension between likeness and difference, love and will, union and
separation, connection and individuation, can never be resolved but is
the source of creativity.

1930   Publishes *Seelenglaube und Psychologie* (Soul-Belief and Psychology),
drawing on Bohr's "theory of complementarity," Einstein's "theory of
relativity" and Heisenberg's "uncertainty principle" to demonstrate that
quantum physics has proven that human beings lie beyond predictability
and cannot be explained by the Newtonian theories of psychoanalysis.

1930 In a Washington, DC, lecture, attended by a large international audience, says that while he has stopped calling himself a psychoanalyst, "I am no longer trying to prove that Freud was wrong and I am right. . . . It is not a question of whose interpretation is correct—because there is no such thing as *the* interpretation or only *one* psychological truth."

1930 Is removed by the American Psychoanalytic Association from its list of honorary members, immediately after the Washington, DC, lecture, on a motion by President A.A. Brill, seconded by Vice-President Harry Stack Sullivan; as a result, re-analysis by Freudians of his psychiatrist trainees is required for them to retain membership in the American Psychoanalytic Association.

1932 Publishes *Art and Artist*, showing that only the "human creative impulse" can harmonize "the fundamental dualism" of life and death, a dualism Rank explores along many lines: the wish for—and fear of—separation; the wish for—and fear of—union; the lifelong oscillation between life fear (*Lebensangst*) and death fear (*Todesangst*); independence and dependence; likeness and difference; and, most importantly, the "will-guilt" problem.

1932 Publishes *Modern Education*, concluding that "psychoanalysis is as conservative as it appeared revolutionary; for its founder is a rebellious son who defends the paternal authority, a revolutionary who, from fear of his own rebellious son-ego, took refuge in the security of the father position."

1936 Meets a young Carl Rogers during a weekend workshop in Rochester, NY, and influences Rogers to abandon Freudian technique for relationship therapy. Shortly thereafter, Rogers becomes the first humanistic psychotherapist in the United States. "I became infected with Rankian ideas," Rogers says.

1936 Rollo May begins analysis with Harry Bone (trained by Rank in Paris), and studies Rank's writings on love and will, and life fear and death fear. Shortly thereafter, May becomes the first American-born existential psychotherapist. "I have long considered Otto Rank to be *the* great unacknowledged genius in Freud's circle," attests May in his foreword to *A Psychology of Difference* (published in 1996), a collection of twenty-two lectures that Rank delivered from 1924 to 1938 at universities throughout America.

1936–39 Drafts *Beyond Psychology* (published posthumously in 1941), explaining why he advocates a "psychology of difference" in contrast to Freud's "psychology of likeness";

1939 Divorces Tola Rank and marries Estelle Buel, his secretary, in July.

1939 Dies, at age 55, in New York from reaction to injection of an antibacterial drug, on October 31—one month after Freud's physician-assisted suicide, at age 83, in London, on September 23, the Jewish Day of Atonement, *Yom Kippur*.

1941 *Beyond Psychology* is published privately by friends of Rank, and later by Dover Books in 1958.

1971 Harry Tucker translates Rank's 1925 edition of *The Double*, published by University of North Carolina Press.

1975 David G. Winter translates Rank's 1922 edition of *The Don Juan Legend*, published by Princeton University Press.

1992 Gregory C. Richter translates Rank's 1912 edition of *The Incest Theme in Literature and Legend: Fundamentals of a Psychology of Literary Creation*, published by Johns Hopkins University Press.

1996 Robert Kramer edits Rank's *A Psychology of Difference: The American Lectures*, published by Princeton University Press.

1998 E.J. Lieberman and Gregory C. Richter translate Rank's 1930 book *Seelenglaube und Psychologie* under the title *Psychology and the Soul: A Study of the Origin, Conceptual Evolution, and Nature of the Soul*, published by Johns Hopkins University Press.

2004 E.J. Lieberman and Gregory C. Richter translate the second (1922) edition of Rank's *The Myth of the Birth of the Hero: A Psychological Exploration of Myth*, published by Johns Hopkins University Press.

2012 E.J. Lieberman and Robert Kramer edit *The Letters of Sigmund Freud and Otto Rank: Inside Psychoanalysis*, translated by Gregory C. Richter, and published by Johns Hopkins University Press.

2024 Robert Kramer edits Rank's 1910 essay *A Dream That Interprets Itself*, translated by Gregory C. Richter, and published by Karnac.

Annotated Bibliography of Selected Writings on Rank

1953

➤ Fay Karpf publishes the first book-length study of Rank's work, entitled *The Psychology and Psychotherapy of Otto Rank: An Historical and Comparative Introduction*. Before dying in 1939, Rank told Karpf that "he became acquainted with [William James's] thought" during his student days at the University of Vienna (55n.9). Surprisingly, Rank never cites James in any of his writings, although a copy of *The Varieties of Religious Experience* was in Rank's library at his death.

➤ In *Man's Search for Himself*, Rollo May writes: "In the 1920s orthodox psychoanalysis was bogging down in artificial excursions into the past which lacked reality and dynamic and were in danger of becoming the same deadening intellectual exercises, interesting as archeological explorations but *without power to change anyone's life....* Rank jarred psychotherapy back to reality by showing that whatever is significant in a person's past—such as in early childhood relations—will be brought into his present relationships" (266; italics added). During the late-1930s, May's analyst was Harry Bone, who'd been trained by Rank in Paris. From his experience in therapy with Bone, May discovered "Rank's theory of neurosis as repressed creativity, as well as his emphasis on dialogue in the 'here and now' of the therapeutic session—all of which would become crucial aspects of May's mature approach to therapy" (Abzug 2021:88).

1955

➤ Ruth Munroe publishes a 21-page chapter on Rank in *Schools of Psychoanalytic Thought*. Of one client, a Penn School social worker told Munroe that "he had wanted to be himself—to be different from the others, to be a separate individual. This 'difference,' then, has now become acceptable to him [after therapy]; and so is the 'difference' of the other persons acceptable to him.... The therapist's acceptance of the patient's own way of working on his problem is in effect an acceptance of the patient's will.... Having had his own difference accepted by another (the therapist) he can now accept himself. Thus, in the therapeutic relationship, as in the ideal example cited above, self-acceptance becomes possible through the 'love experience' of being accepted by another person" (580).

➤ Lovell Langstroth publishes *Structure of the Ego: An Anatomic and Physiologic Interpretation of the Psyche, Based on the Psychology of Otto Rank*. A neurologist, Langstroth proposed a "theory of temporal lobe function based on known anatomic facts and connections" (111), showing connections between his theory, which foreshadows modern relational neuroscience, and Rank's writings.

1956

➤ Ira Progoff publishes *The Death and Rebirth of Psychology: An Integrative Evaluation of Freud, Adler, Jung and Rank and the Impact of their Culminating Insights on Modern Man*. Progoff lauds Rank's *Psychology and the Soul* (1930), *Art and Artist* (1932a), and *Beyond Psychology* (1941a), but alleges—incorrectly—that Rank abandoned the irrational in *Will Therapy* (1936a) and *Truth and Reality* (1936b). Rank never abandoned the irrational, which—beginning with *The Trauma of Birth* (1924)—he saw as the wonder, awe, and mystery of existence itself. That human beings exist—that *anything* exists—is beyond the rationality or comprehension of science, according to Rank.

1958

➤ Jessie Taft publishes *Otto Rank: A Biographical Study Based on Notebooks, Letters, Collected Writings, Therapeutic Achievements and Personal Associations*. Taft shares her admiration for Rank as therapist, teacher, colleague, and friend. For readers who want to begin their study of Rank, Taft's deeply felt book, full of examples of Rank's humanity and humor, is highly recommended as a first choice.

1959

➤ In a collection of excerpts from Rank's aesthetic and cultural essays, Philip Freund edits *The Myth of the Birth of the Hero and Other Writings by Otto Rank*, concluding: "Rank did not think that he had come upon the whole truth about man. He wrote often that psychology is still in a very early stage, that it is limited in what it can hope to accomplish, and that it is merely a transitional discipline to the discovery of something that must lie beyond psychology, a faith that vouchsafes us a glimpse of salvation" (xiv).

1964

➤ Floyd W. Matson publishes *The Broken Image: Man, Science and Society*. "Rankian theory," argues Matson, "presents two alternative approaches to the self and the world (of culture): that of unconscious rejection of the self and the acceptance of the culture, or that of conscious acceptance of the self and rejection of the conventional culture. The first route is the familiar one of escape from freedom, the straight and narrow path of least resistance. The second is the way of creative growth and becoming—the road to autonomy. The task of therapy for Rank is primarily to make clear these alternatives and to help in the liberation of the patient's own will for the voluntary act of choice: to be (himself) or not to be" (219).

1968

➤ Erving Polster, a leading Gestalt therapist, publishes "A Contemporary Psychotherapy," a chapter in *Recognitions in Gestalt Therapy*. "Rank brought the human relationship directly into his office," writes Polster. "He influenced analysts to take seriously the actual present interaction between therapist and patient, rather than maintain the fixed, distant, 'as though' relationship [i.e., transference] that had given previous analysts an emotional buffer for examining the intensities of therapeutic sensation and wish. Rank's contributions opened the way for *encounter* to become accepted as a deep therapeutic agent" (6; italics in the original).

1969

➤ Rollo May publishes *Love and Will*, a huge bestseller. "Man's task is to unite love and will," he writes, echoing Rank's writings on the subject. "We have a memory, a 'reminiscence' in Plato's sense, of a time when there was union of ourselves with our mothers in the early experience of nursing at mother's breast. Then we were also at *union with the universe*, were wedded to it and had the experience of '*union with being*.' . . . This is the backdrop of human existence implied in every myth of the Garden of Eden, every story of paradise, every 'Golden Age'—a perfection which is deeply embedded in man's collective memory" (283–284; italics added).

1970

➤ Drawing on Rank's *The Double*, Robert Rogers publishes *A Psychoanalytic Study of the Double in Literature*. "While doubling in literature usually symbolizes a dysfunctional attempt to cope with mental conflict," writes Rogers, "there is nothing abnormal or malign about this phenomenon considered as part of the artistic process" (vii).

1973

➤ Ernest Becker publishes *The Denial of Death*, single-handedly returning the thought of Otto Rank to a central place in the human and social sciences. Since then, over 1,500 experimental studies in "terror management theory" (TMT) have appeared in peer-reviewed journals supporting Becker's applications of Rank's hypotheses on life fear and death fear to explaining human evil.

➤ In "Evading Art and Society," published in *Chicago Review*, literary critic Maxwell Geismar argues that Rank shows "devastatingly why the Freudian schemata could never get at the essence of art and the artist. . . . So the Rankian aesthetics offers a range of insights—and particularly that of psychology and art *within* culture and society—that the Freudian rationale can never match" (91-92; italics in the original).

➤ Albert Schwartz publishes *"The Trauma of Birth* and Rank's Departure from Freud" in *Review of Existential Psychology and Psychiatry*. Rank gave "anxiety *existential* status," writes Schwartz, "his concept of primary and universal birth-anxiety moved him closer to the tradition of existential Christian theologians like Kierkegaard who claimed a primary ontological status for Angst" (80; italics in the original). According to Rank, observes Schwartz, "men create culture, that is to say, symbolic constructs, in order to recreate in the external world the condition of primal unity and the illusion of immortality they once experienced and the memory of which they preserve in their unconscious minds. . . . Historical change can then be pictured as a grandiose cosmic drama motivated by two contradictory desires acting at the same time: a desire to recreate the condition of the fetus in the womb by projecting a symbolic 'womb' onto the world under the guise of culture and a desire to deny the separation from the womb by disguising this grand symbolic covering in ideal, non-bodily forms" (82–83). For a similar argument, see Langman (1961), "The Estrangement from Being: An Existential Analysis of Otto Rank's Psychology," in *Journal of Existential Psychiatry*.

1974

➤ Paul Roazen publishes *Freud and His Followers*. Contradicting Ernest Jones, who alleged that Rank was "psychotic," Roazen writes: "Rank was peculiarly suited, from Freud's point of view, to be his ideal successor. Freud's own sons were not suitable, since their lack of creativity made them unfit to uphold the immortality Freud felt to be his. . . . Rank had entered Freud's circle with only his native abilities, and Freud was able, metaphorically, to give him birth. Freud felt that his own genius had sprung full-blown and could be traced to no recognizable familial or social past. In Rank, Freud could have a worthy successor, the product of the master's own will" (395).

➤ In "The Spectrum of Loneliness," published in *Humanitas*, Ernest Becker distills his major learnings from Rank. "[T]he problem of loneliness is compounded by a paradox that results from what we must call *the basic ontological motives of the human condition*. These motives are the familiar ones of Agape vs. Eros, the strivings of man in two different directions. Otto Rank summed them up for psychology by designating them as the universal problem of *sameness* vs. *difference*. . . . To fulfill the Agape motive plunges one into the loneliness of non-individuation. To fulfill the Eros motive plunges one into the loneliness of separation. . . . In sum, there can be no cure for a problem that goes this deep into the human condition" (quoted in Liechty 2005:232; italics in the original).

1975

➤ Ernest Becker's widow, Marie, edits and publishes *Escape from Evil*, which Becker considered his magnum opus. "This book also completes my confrontation of the work of Otto Rank," writes Ernest Becker (1975), "and my attempt to transcribe its relevance for a general science of man" (xvii).

➤ In *The Courage to Create*, Rollo May highlights the *Urangst* of Rank's two existential anxieties—life fear and death fear—both of which must be encountered and confronted to live a loving and creative life (18–19).

➤ Donald MacKinnon, director of the Institute of Personality Assessment and Research (IPAR) at the University of California at Berkeley, publishes "IPAR's Contribution to the Conceptualization and Study of Creativity," a chapter in *Perspectives in Creativity*, reporting that Rank's theory of creativity has been validated as a "good fit" (81) by statistical studies conducted by IPAR.

➤ Richard Johnson publishes *In Quest of a New Psychology: Toward a Redefinition of Humanism*, arguing that "The work of Otto Rank represents the first and most important existential approach developed by a practicing psychologist and psychotherapist" (51).

1976

➤ In "Suffering and Charity," published in *Journal of the Otto Rank Association*, Episcopal priest John N. Wall writes: "We cannot give to others, we cannot love others until we love ourselves .... If the [Rankian] therapist can lead a person to this kind of self-acceptance and self-love, then from a Christian perspective, he is serving a priestly function whether he uses Christian language or not" (31).

1977

➤ In "The Will and Empathy in Art Therapy," published in *Journal of the Otto Rank Association*, Josef E. Garai writes that the "peak or cosmic unity" experienced during art therapy by both therapist and client is "similar to that described by artists or innovators who felt it after the completion of a truly great work of art or some creative accomplishment.... It almost seems as if the boundaries separating life from death, mortality from immortality, personal space from global space, present time from infinity, and individual destiny from universal fate were becoming penetrable and irrelevant" (37).

➤ Rollo May publishes a revised edition of *The Meaning of Anxiety*, which originally appeared in 1950. "Many readers," he concludes, "will find Rank's terminology and his dualistic mode of thought uncongenial. But it would be unfortunate if this kept anyone from reading him. No one has attacked more insightfully two basic aspects of the problem of anxiety—namely the relation between anxiety and individuation, and anxiety and separation" (153).

1978

➤ Philip K. Jason publishes "Doubles/Don Juans: Anaïs Nin and Otto Rank" in *Mosaic: An Interdisciplinary Critical Journal*, exploring how Nin, in her fiction, uses Rank's concept of the Double. Nin came to see Rank as her own alter-ego, her

double. "Once Rank entered Nin's life," writes Jason, "he quickly became a dominant figure. . . . As their relationship continued, Nin's awe and respect for Rank
grew. She perceived in him an artistic spirit, a philosopher, a metaphysician—
someone far different from a mere scientist-psychoanalyst" (85).

1979

➤ In *Faces in a Cloud: Subjectivity in Personality Theory*, psychoanalysts Robert
Stolorow and George Atwood publish a chapter on Rank "who anticipated the
breakdown of collective supports for the sense of self. . . . [Rank] emerges as a
fascinating figure in the history of psychoanalysis" (132). Stolorow and Atwood
allege—incorrectly—that Rank "conceives of the love relationship as a wholly
narcissistic affair. In fact throughout his entire work we could find only mea-
ger references to mature object love in which the separate individuality and real
qualities of the object are recognized and cherished" (143). Such references can
be found in Rank's American lectures and the accounts reported by his patients
about their experience of will and love, difference and likeness, with him in
therapy.

➤ Jack D. Spiro completes a PhD dissertation at the University of Virginia entitled
Man and Cosmos: The Educational Theories of Otto Rank. "Cultural symbols,"
writes Spiro, "evolve primarily from the will to immortality so that man can differentiate himself from the forces of nature and his purely biological functions. The
purpose of culture is collective survival, and the formation of collective ideologies
is based on the need for perpetuation" (n.p.). Rank's philosophy of education, as
expressed while he was teaching at the Penn School of Social Work, promoted self-
leadership. "To bring about the 'new personality' is one of the primary goals of an
ideal education" (15).

➤ Judd Marmor, past president of the American Psychiatric Association, publishes
"Short-Term Dynamic Psychotherapy" in *American Journal of Psychiatry*, identifying Rank as "the most important historical forerunner of the brief dynamic
psychotherapy movement" as well as "the prime theoretical precursor of the
nuclear importance of separation and individuation in emotional maturation"
(150).

1980

➤ Irvin Yalom publishes *Existential Psychotherapy*, the foundational work on the
subject. "A discussion of the will in clinical work must include the contributions
of Otto Rank, for it was he who introduced the concept of the will into modern
psychotherapy," writes Yalom (293). "I gasped at his prescience when reading his
works, especially his books *Will Therapy* and *Truth and Reality*." Condemned by
Freudians, Rank, concludes Yalom, is "the brooding genius waiting in the wings"
(ibid.).

➤ Keith Sward publishes "Self-Actualization and Women: Rank and Freud Contrasted" in *Journal of Humanistic Psychology*. "In their sharply contrasting images
of 'femininity,' Rank and Freud were, at bottom, espousing two radically different
concepts of self-actualization," concludes Sward. "To Freud, women are essentially

creatures of instinct, destined by nature to function passively as sex objects and caretakers. Writing in the late 1920s and early 1930s, Rank regarded this sex model as patriarchal and reductionistic. It was his position that women as well as men have a drive for self-realization that transcends the socially imposed roles of any specific culture. . . . For these and other 'heresies' Rank was excommunicated by the Freudian Establishment" (5).

➢ Nancy G. Seif completes a PhD dissertation at Yeshiva University entitled *Otto Rank: On Human Evil*. Comparing Rank's thought with that of John Milton in *Paradise Lost*, Seif writes: "In the realm of poetry, Milton delineated the conditions of conflict which made the paradisiacal naivete of Eden impossible for the human being. He illustrated dramatically the irreconcilable, opposing qualities of man's nature: his need for personal freedom and his need for personal limits, his drive toward individualism and his drive toward union. . . . But because the two needs are at once mutually exclusive, an individual is caught up in a perpetual dilemma which generates both self-condemnation and guilt. A person condemns himself because to pursue one essential aspect of himself requires betrayal of the other, i.e., pursuit of his individual strivings is at the cost of his social strivings and pursuit of the social is at the cost of the individual" (1–2).

➢ Anton Zottl publishes the first book-length study in German of Rank's philosophy of educating clients toward self-leadership, drawing on Nietzsche's language of the "Super-Man": *Erziehung zum Über-Menschen: Individualität, Kreativität und Wille bei Otto Rank* (Educating Toward Superior Persons: Individuality, Creativity and Will in Rank).

➢ In *The Psychotherapy Handbook*, Abraham Schmitt publishes a chapter entitled "Will Therapy of Otto Rank." Schmitt concludes that "every act of creativity is a rebirth process, when a person faces his own longing to be *like* humanity, but he realizes that he must assert his *difference* at the possible price of being rejected by others. He must relive the separation experience in every creative act" (702; italics added).

1981

➢ Jon Amundson publishes "Will in the Psychotherapy of Otto Rank: A Transpersonal Perspective" in *Journal of Transpersonal Psychology*, the leading journal of the field. Amundson explores the transpersonal aspects of Rank's thought, which were first noticed by Stanislav Grof, founder with Anthony Sutich and Abraham Maslow of transpersonal psychology in the late 1960s.

➢ The *Journal of the Otto Rank Association* publishes Otto Rank's "Literary Autobiography," his own enumeration of all his writings up to 1930, including reviews, criticisms, and influence on other analysts, such as Freud, Jung, and Melanie Klein. Seeing his life's work as a continuous evolution of his ideas on myth, art, creativity, birth, and individuality, Rank writes: "There is a direct line from *The Myth of the Birth of the Hero* (artistic-creative type) over *The Trauma of Birth* (1923) to the birth of individuality [*Truth and Reality*], 1929" (7). Rank observes that Freud's article on "The Uncanny" (1919), which was inspired by Rank's 1914 work *The Double*, is "an unconscious attempt on Freud's part to substitute my explanation (fear of death) for his old castration theory" (15). In his attack on *The Trauma of Birth*, Freud (1926a) argued in *Inhibitions, Symptoms and Anxiety* that all situations of mortal danger are experienced as castration anxiety, not as fear of death, which he dismissed as a derivative of castration anxiety, and therefore irrelevant (129–130). What Rank calls *Todesangst*—the fear of death—plays no role in Freud's thought, which includes only *Todestrieb*: the biological, self-destructive drive toward death.

1982

➤ In *Otto Rank: A Rediscovered Legacy*, the first comprehensive treatment of Rank's ideas, Esther Menaker sums up Rank's writings on the creative will: "Paradoxically, the fear of death and its counterpart, the wish for immortality, lead to the fullest expression of life in the form of the creative expression of the will. That is not to say that the wish for immortality is the *cause* of creative action and its consequent product, but rather it motivates and mobilizes the striving for the expression of individuality which is a given and is there at the outset" (47; italics in the original).

➤ In *Maps of the Mind*, Charles Hampden-Turner lauds Rank's theory of creativity. "We exist," writes Hampden-Turner, "between the life fear and the death fear" (64). He captures Rank's existential thought in a single sentence: "The true creator must combine the highest level of self-expression with total self-surrender, Eros married to Agape" (67).

➤ Sharon Spencer publishes "Delivering the Woman Artist from the Silence of the Womb: Otto Rank's Influence on Anaïs Nin" in *Psychoanalytic Review*. From the beginning of her therapy with Rank, he "encouraged her to 'write as a woman,'" says Spencer (112). Rank's chapter entitled "Feminine Psychology and Masculine Ideology" (in *Beyond Psychology*) provided "the rationale for his attempt to strengthen Nin's identity as a woman before assisting in the consolidation of her identity as an artist" (114).

➤ Anton Zottl publishes a second book-length study of Rank in German: *Otto Rank: Das Lebenswerk eines Dissidenten der Psychoanalyse* (Otto Rank: The Lifework of a Dissident in Psychoanalysis).

1983

➤ Will Wadlington completes a PhD dissertation at Penn State University entitled, *Otto Rank's Art of Psychotherapy*. He sees Rank as the first "artist of psychotherapy," and examines Rank's approach "in terms of the philosophical presuppositions that ground it, the psychological theory that guides it, and the phenomenological experience it makes possible" (6).

➤ In *Journal of the American Psychoanalytic Association*, Rita Novey celebrates Rank for his pioneering focus on "beginnings and endings" in therapy, but criticizes him for not having a theory of object relations. "I have traced the theories of Otto Rank as they appeared in his major technical writings" (985), writes Novey. She was unaware that in the late 1920s Rank had published (in German) the first theory of object relations in psychoanalysis, long before Melanie Klein and others such as Ronald Fairbairn, Harry Guntrip, and D.W. Winnicott wrote about it (Rudnytsky 1991).

➤ In *The Broken Connection: On Death and Continuity of Life*, Robert J. Lifton concludes that Rank's writings on life fear and death fear offer "at least a possibility of viewing all mental disturbance from the paradigm of death and continuity [of life], and thereby suggesting a beginning basis [for] a comprehensive theory of mental disturbance that connects equally with evolutionary-biological and social-historical dimensions" (180).

➤ In *Freud and Psychoanalysis: An Exposition and Appraisal*, Richard Stevens sums up a key aspect of Rank's therapy: "Through will and counterwill (the ability to say no to oneself and others) a balance can be developed between the needs to belong and to be free. At the core of neurosis is the failure to achieve this integration. In his therapy, Rank was very concerned not to encourage passivity and dependence" (67).

1984

➤ On the centenary of Rank's birth, *American Imago* publishes an issue devoted to the life and work of Rank. In the most important article, Esther Menaker elaborates on "The Ethical and the Empathic in the Thinking of Otto Rank" (343–351).

➤ *Columbia Library Columns*, sponsored by friends of the Columbia University libraries, where Rank's papers are archived in the Rare Book and Manuscript Library, publishes the "Otto Rank Century Issue," containing Rank's never-before-translated 1904 essay, "Diary Leaves of a Stillborn" and two early poems he wrote, "*Weltschmerz*: Lines Before Breakfast" (1903) and "School for Preparing" (1904).

➤ In *Cries of the Wolf Man*, Patrick J. Mahony criticizes Sándor Ferenczi for betraying his best friend, Otto Rank, at the goading of Freud in 1925: "Ferenczi wrote ... 'According to Rank's view, at the deepest instinctual level the biological attachment to the mother regularly dominates the analytical situation, whereas what Freud assigns to the analyst is in essentials the part of the father.' Today psychoanalysts would be more open to Rank on this question and would critically examine Ferenczi's reaction that when he clinically tested Rank's theories, he became suspicious toward patients who accepted them without resistance. Rank's birth-trauma fantasies are not reproductions of the real event of birth but are rather like other unconscious fantasies (the argument curiously resembles the modern debate over the reality of reconstructions)" (138–139).

1985

➤ The University of Chicago Press publishes Dennis Klein's *Jewish Origins of the Psychoanalytic Movement*, which includes the first translation of Rank's 1905 essay, "The Essence of Judaism," written shortly after Rank met Freud. In it Rank states: "[T]he Jews thoroughly understand the *radical* cure of neurosis, better than any other people" (172; italics in the original). At a 1977 psychoanalytic congress held in Jerusalem, Anna Freud admitted, for the first time, that psychoanalysis was a "Jewish science" (quoted in Yerushalmi 1991:100). Rank's exposition of Judaism in the last chapter of *Beyond Psychology* was linked to his critique of Freud's patriarchy: "I have come to the conclusion that the specific Jewish psychology, expressed in Freudian doctrine as a general psychology, is projected in toto upon the woman, who therefore is depicted as enslaved, inferior, castrated, whereas in the psychology of the male the masculine qualities appear exaggerated to the point of caricature in a libidinal superman" (Rank 1941a:287).

➤ In *Bloomsbury/Freud: The Letters of James and Alix Strachey, 1924–1925*, Perry Meisel and Walter Kendrick show the influence of Rank's *Trauma of Birth* on D.W. Winnicott, who was termed a *Rankschüler* (115)—a member of "Rank's school"— by James Strachey, the main translator of Freud's *Standard Edition*.

➤ E. James Lieberman publishes *Acts of Will: The Life and Work of Otto Rank*, the most complete biography of Rank, superseding the books by Fay Karpf (1953) and Jessie Taft (1958). After interviewing 34 persons who knew Rank personally, including many family members, patients, colleagues, and students, Lieberman concludes: "Rank's concerns with birth, death, and immortality—the nature and preservation of the soul—are as fresh [today] as when he wrote his masterworks some fifty years ago" (xvii).

➤ In *My Quest for Beauty*, Rollo May writes: "Rank believed that the goal of psychotherapy was to help the patient learn to create. The neurotic type of person, so Rank wrote in *Art and Artist*, was the '*artiste manqué*', the artist who cannot create any art. All people are struggling to be creative in some way, and the artist is the one who has succeeded in this task of life. . . . What we seek to do [in existential therapy] is to help each patient to become unified in him or herself, so that they can live out their lives with some integrity, some wholeness, some beauty" (35).

➤ Marvin Goldwert publishes "Otto Rank and Man's Urge to Immortality" in *Journal of the History of the Behavioral Sciences*. Rank, he says, "posited the existence of an 'urge to immortality' as man's deepest drive. In his *Psychology and the Soul*, Rank traced the desire for immortality through four historical eras, with particular emphasis on the creativity of the hero and the artist. By the end of his life, Rank had not only repudiated orthodox psychoanalysis . . . he had moved beyond psychology to a religious view of history and nature" (169).

➤ Stanislav Grof publishes *Beyond the Brain: Birth, Death, and Transcendence in Psychotherapy*, observing that "many of Rank's formulations and insights can be of great value when the [psychedelic] process focuses on the prenatal level" (140). *The Trauma of Birth*, he adds, "was a truly remarkable achievement that preceded the LSD findings by several decades" (173).

1986

➤ William T. O'Dowd publishes "Otto Rank and Time—Limited Psychotherapy" in *Psychotherapy*. "To theorize about time-limited therapy without knowing Otto Rank's work," he observes, "is roughly analogous to theorizing about dream interpretation without knowing Freud's" (140).

➤ In "O'Neill and Otto Rank: 'Death Instincts' and *The Trauma of Birth*," published in *Contemporary Drama*, Stephen Watt concludes: "Rank's later thought, which explores the relationship between religious devotion, guilt . . . Agape . . . and neurosis, seems especially well suited to illuminate psychological conflict in O'Neill" (228).

1987

➤ Indiana University Press publishes Valentin N. Volosinov's 1927 study of Freud, a study that strongly influenced the linguist Roman Jakobson. In it Volosinov summarizes *The Trauma of Birth* and states: "Under no circumstances can it be claimed as mere eccentricity. It expresses to the full the spirit of Freudianism today" (62). However, Volosinov did not know of the "David and Goliath" battle between Freud and Rank over the *Trauma of Birth*, and assumed—incorrectly—that Rank's book heralded the future of psychoanalytic theory and practice. Ironically, he was right in the sense that relational psychoanalysis, founded in the 1980s, has adopted many aspects of Rank's relationship therapy.

➤ Kenwyn Smith and David Berg publish *Paradoxes of Group Life: Understanding Conflict, Paralysis, and Movement in Group Dynamics*. While paradox may be a source of conflict and paralysis in group life, Smith and Berg draw on Rank's creative tension between likeness and difference to show that paradox, if accepted, fuels movement and change. Following Rank, they propose that leaders who live *within* the paradox, rather than choose one pole over the other, can be more effective and more creative in implementing change in their groups and organizations.

➤ Paul L. Adams publishes "The Mother Not the Father" in *Journal of the American Academy of Psychoanalysis*. "Rank showed radical feminist attitudes far ahead of his time," writes Adams, "contending that the female is central and superior to male existence, and that women need a psychology that is not warmed-over male biases but truly a 'female psychology'" (465).

1988

➤ In *Freud: A Life for Our Time*, Peter Gay asserts—incorrectly—that Rank rather than Freud dreamt the "David and Goliath dream" (Gay 1988:480). How Gay could have made this blunder is a mystery. The dream reveals Freud's dread that Rank's ideas about the powerful mother threatened his life's work. One might speculate that Gay, an orthodox Freudian, could not bring himself to believe that Rank regularly interpreted Freud's dreams, although Gay had access to the Freud-Rank letters, which demonstrate that Freud trusted Rank to interpret his dreams more than once (Lieberman & Kramer 2012:176–179; 315–323).

➤ Peter Orban publishes "Validating Otto Rank's Work" in the journal *Anaïs*. "Man's psyche," concludes Orban, "thus emerges, as it were, from the attempt to deal with the trauma of birth. In other words, the development of any neurosis commences already with birth" (119).

➤ Harvard University Press publishes the *Clinical Diary of Sándor Ferenczi*, written in 1932. In 1929–31 Rank published the original German edition of *Will Therapy*. Although not citing Rank, Ferenczi (1932) echoes Rank's vocabulary in many passages in his diary, e.g., "imposition of an alien will" (16); "adults forcibly inject their will...into the childish personality" (81); "immensely strong willpower" (97). Referring to his inability to assert his own will in his relationship with Freud, Ferenczi writes: "Instead of asserting *myself*, the external world (an alien will) asserts itself at my expense; it forces itself upon me and *represses the ego*" (111; italics in the original). Ferenczi wonders, "Is the only possibility for my continued existence the renunciation of the largest part of one's own self, in order to carry out the will of that higher power [Freud] to the end (as though it were my own)?... [I]s it worth it always to live the life (will) of another person—is such a life not almost death?" (212). This is Ferenczi's interpretation, applied to his own experiences with Freud, of Rank's dialectic between life fear and death fear. Ferenczi died in 1933, bitter at Freud for running roughshod over him but unrepentant about betraying Rank. "Had the two friends stayed allied, had Ferenczi not turned his back on Rank, it is possible that they could have saved psychoanalysis from Freud's misogyny and therapeutic nihilism" (personal communication, André Haynal).

1989

➤ In "From Life to Diary to Art in the Work of Anaïs Nin," a chapter in *Creative People at Work: Twelve Cognitive Studies*, Vera John-Steiner explores how Nin was "intellectually stimulated and emotionally supported by Rank" (216). According to John-Steiner, Nin's "conflict, when she first sought out Otto Rank, was that she felt oppressed and trapped by her condition as a woman—trained for devotion, service and loyalty . . . and wanting . . . time to maintain her separate identity, her difference" (221). Experiencing Rank's will therapy allowed her to be reborn as a woman and as an artist with a powerful "creative will," for which Nin was eternally grateful.

➤ Rollo May publishes a revision to his 1939 book, *The Art of Counseling*, adding details on how he applied the principles of Rank's relationship-based will therapy in his practice of counseling.

➤ In *The Ability to Mourn: Disillusionment and the Origins of Psychoanalysis*, Peter Homans provides the first in-depth study of Rank's journals or "daybooks" written at age 20 and 21—i.e., just before he met Freud in 1905. These unpublished journals, called *Tagebücher*, concludes Homans, are a "triumphant self-discovery of a genuine self-identity as an artist" (156).

1990

➤ In *The Spectral Mother: Freud, Feminism, and Psychoanalysis*, Madelon Sprengnether demonstrates that Freud's blindness toward the pre-Oedipal mother, as illuminated in Rank's *The Trauma of Birth*, "nearly effaces her"—and all other women—"from the drama of human development" (3).

➤ In *The Neurotic Foundations of Social Order: Psychoanalytic Roots of Patriarchy*, J.C. Smith offers an overview of the underlying causes of male domination in society. "Otto Rank and Ernest Becker," writes Smith, "analyze the hero and the heroic state in terms of a defense mechanism against death. The heroic image constitutes an inflation of the self and a denial of death. The interpretations of Rank and Becker are not inconsistent with those of Jung and Neumann, in that the basic theme of the heroic is the struggle against engulfment and the consequential loss of self by symbiotic merger with the mother/the feminine, or by death" (189).

1991

➤ Ellen Handler Spitz publishes *Image and Insight*, including in it a chapter entitled "Conflict and Creativity: Reflections on Otto Rank's Psychology of Art." She concludes: "Hard-won, his ideas still possess a freshness and power to challenge us as we carry on the tradition of humanistic endeavor to which he also was so profoundly dedicated" (249).

➤ In *The Cry for Myth*, Rollo May extols Rank's feminism: "Disagreeing radically with Freud's broad references to women's problems by the derogatory term 'penis envy,' Rank believed that what motivates a woman is her 'emotional and spiritual . . . craving for expression of her true woman-self in a masculine world which has no room or use for her.' Rank believed that the end result of psychoanalysis should be that the patient fulfill himself and *herself*. Rank used the term 'self-realization' before any of us in America used it. He also emphasized 'identity confusion' twenty years before Erik Erikson used the term, and he regarded sexism, the prejudice against women, as a 'cultural disease'" (289; italics in the original).

➤ Zachary Leader publishes *Writer's Block*, drawing on Rank's thinking in *Art and Artist* about the *artiste manqué* as a fruitful way to characterize writer's block and other inhibitions to creativity.

➤ Peter Rudnytsky publishes *The Psychoanalytic Vocation: Rank, Winnicott, and the Legacy of Freud*. Although Rudnytsky shows that Rank was the first object relations theorist, historian of psychoanalysis Paul Roazen (2001) criticizes Rudnytsky, who is "so involved in object relations thinking that he only sees Rank as a precursor instead of looking at Rank in all his rich individuality" (396).

➤ Irvin L. Child publishes "Rankian Psychology" in the *Corsini Encyclopedia of Psychology and the Behavioral Sciences*, explaining how Ernest Becker interpreted Rank in *The Denial of Death*. "Becker (1973) has presented an explicitly Rankian psychology of the ills of human society. It attempts to answer the question, 'What unsatisfied needs are predominantly responsible for the widespread misery of human beings?' as did Freud's *Civilization and Its Discontents* (1930). Instead of Freud's implausible attribution of human suffering primarily to sexual repression demanded as a precondition of culture, Becker attributes it to the insatiable quest for symbols of immortality, arising from the universal fear of death" (1366).

➤ Phyllis Grosskurth publishes *The Secret Ring: Freud's Inner Circle and the Politics of Psychoanalysis*, the first in-depth study of the letters (*Rundbriefe*) circulated among members of the Secret Committee, Freud's Politburo formed in the wake of Jung's defection in 1913. Rank kept a set in his files, now at Columbia University's Rare Book and Manuscript Library. They've been published in full only in German, in four volumes. See Wittenberger & Tögel (1999–2001).

1992

➤ Luigi de Marchi publishes *Otto Rank: Pioniere Misconosciuto*, the first book-length study in Italian of Rank, the "misunderstood pioneer" of psychoanalysis.

➤ In literary studies published during 1992, Rank is cited as often as Melanie Klein and D.W. Winnicott, and far more often than R.D. Laing, Roland Barthes, or Noam Chomsky (Hudson 1992).

➤ David L. Wolitzky and Morris N. Eagle write "Psychoanalytic Theories of Psychotherapy" in *History of Psychotherapy: A Century of Change*, published by the

American Psychological Association. In it they claim—incorrectly—that "Neutral [in psychoanalytic treatment] means nonjudgmental; it does not mean indifferent or uncaring" (49). This claim contradicts Freud's explicit directive to analysts that they show "*Indifferenz*" (i.e., indifference or uncaring) to the suffering of their patients, an indifference that Rank and Ferenczi challenged, unsuccessfully, in the mid-1920s. It was only after Anna Freud's death in 1982 that mainstream analysts started, slowly and cautiously, to accept that empathy was central to healing.

➤ Mantosh J. Dewan and Sanjay Gupta publish "Congruence Between Hindu Philosophy and Writings of Otto Rank" in *Psychological Reports*. They show "intriguing parallels between some of Rank's basic assumptions and those of ancient Indian thought" (127) and suggest that Rank may have been influenced by Eastern philosophy.

➤ Huston Smith publishes *Forgotten Truth: The Common Vision of the World's Religions*, showing how *The Trauma of Birth* influenced Stanislav Grof's discoveries in psychedelic research, discoveries that the Nixon administration's prohibition of research on psychedelics stopped in its tracks. For an explanation, see Wayne Hall (2022), "Why Was Early Psychotherapeutic Research on Psychedelics Abandoned?" Today, such research is once again legal. Since the early 2000s, researchers at Johns Hopkins University, supported by FDA regulators, have experimented with using psychedelics (such as psilocybin and MDMA) to relieve the existential suffering of dying patients and reduce the anguish of patients with post-traumatic stress disorder, treatment-resistant depression, and anxiety. Meta-analyses of experimental studies have shown strong, statistically significant, positive effects of psychedelics. In 2018 Michael Pollan published *How to Change Your Mind: What the New Science of Psychedelics Teaches Us About Consciousness, Dying, Addiction, Depression, and Transcendence*. It became a No. 1 *New York Times* best-seller. (Pollan mentions Rank's influence on Stanislav Grof on p. 155.)

1993

➤ John Suler publishes *Contemporary Psychoanalysis and Eastern Thought*. Rank, he concludes, uses the term "will" to mean "the 'cosmic primal force' that launches the person toward the actualization of autonomy, psychological well-being, and creativity. . . . Yalom (1980) claims that the most basic goal of therapy is to liberate will, which brings choice and responsibility. It is the will to heal and develop, the will to find the meaning and purpose of one's existence. At the most basic level, it is the will to create one's identity: the willing of the self" (94). Within the relationship Rank created between himself and his client, the client, observes Suler, "simultaneously becomes both the creator and the created" (96).

1994

➤ Taylor Stoehr publishes *Here Now Next*, the first complete account of how social critic Paul Goodman, who is listed only as the third author of *Gestalt Therapy*

(1951), after Frederick Perls and Ralph Hefferline, actually wrote the major part of this now-classic work. While constructing the theoretical basis for Gestalt therapy, Goodman leaned heavily on Rank, whose "formulation [of the here-and-now]," writes Stoehr (1994), "has the therapeutic moment in view more explicitly than any other" (126). Goodman greatly admired Rank's thought, going so far as to describe his writings on art and creativity as "beyond praise" in *Gestalt Therapy* (Perls et al. 1951:395n). "Rank hit on the creative act as psychological health itself," concluded Goodman (236). "Philosophically," Carl Rogers once told Art Bohart (2003), "Gestalt therapy shares much in common with person-centered theory" (123). This is not surprising since both modes of therapeutic practice are rooted in Rank's thought.

➤ In *Work, Death, and Life Itself: Essays on Management and Organization*, organizational theorist Burkard Sievers interprets the widespread loss of meaning in organizations through the lens of the existential philosophy of Rank and Becker, which explains conventional "motivation theories" in management—Frederick Herzberg's hygiene theory; David McClelland's need for achievement and power; and Frederick Taylor's scientific management—as "denials of death." These conventional theories, still taught today in business schools, have become surrogates for the search for meaning, according to Sievers.

1995

➤ Matthew Fox, a post-denominational theologian with a wide following worldwide, publishes "Otto Rank on the Artistic Journey As a Spiritual Journey, the Spiritual Journey As an Artistic Journey," a chapter in *Wrestling with the Prophets: Essays on Creation Spirituality and Everyday Life*, making a case for Rank as "one of the great spiritual giants of the twentieth century. . . . He died a feminist and deeply committed to social justice in 1939. His work, more than any other psychologist's, provides the appropriate psychological basis for Creation Spirituality" (199).

➤ In *The Psychology of Existence: An Integrative Clinical Perspective*, Kirk Schneider and Rollo May point to Rank as the most important pioneer of existential therapy: "First and foremost," they write, "is the existential obligation to Rank. His stress on fundamental life-structures, immediacy and relation, and the artistry of psychotherapy have become the standard components of contemporary existential practice" (81).

➤ Paul Roazen publishes *How Freud Worked: First-Hand Accounts of Patients*. Some of America's "most distinguished writers have been among Freud's most ardent propagandists," writes Roazen. "For example Lionel Trilling, the eminent literary critic at Columbia University, falsely wrote in 1957 of both Rank and Ferenczi in the Sunday *New York Times Book Review*: 'Both men fell prey to extreme mental illness and they died insane' . . ." (272)—a fabrication by Ernest Jones. Ardent propagandists like Trilling tended to pathologize early analysts who went beyond Freud.

➤ In *Misplaced Loyalties*, her autobiography, Esther Menaker writes: "In studying the works of Otto Rank, I learned how well he understood [the] duality in the struggle of the self to separate as an autonomous individual on the one hand and to merge with a person or idea larger than the self on the other. For Rank this was a universal inevitable aspect of human life, a conflict never fully resolved yet one that, if accepted, could be lived with" (14).

1996

➤ Esther Menaker publishes *Separation, Will, and Creativity: The Wisdom of Otto Rank*, the capstone of her 60 years of studying Rank and applying his thinking on the creative will and relationship therapy to subjects such as the need for mutual empathy between therapist and patient; spirituality; and feminism.

➤ Princeton University Press publishes Robert Kramer's edited collection of Rank's American lectures, *A Psychology of Difference*, with a Foreword by Rollo May. "I have long considered Otto Rank to be *the* great unacknowledged genius in Freud's circle," avers May (xi; italics in the original).

➤ In *A Meeting of Minds: Mutuality in Psychoanalysis*, Lewis Aron concludes that Rank "anticipated many of the distinguishing marks of contemporary relational theories" (183).

➤ James Knowlson publishes *Damned to Fame: The Life of Samuel Beckett*. During his therapy with the psychoanalyst Wilfrid Bion, Beckett "came up with some extraordinary memories of being in the womb. Intrauterine memories" (171). Both Bion and Beckett were influenced by *The Trauma of Birth*.

➤ Haim Finkelstein publishes *Salvador Dalí's Art and Writing, 1927–1942*. "In Dalí's autobiography," writes Finkelstein, "Dalí attests to the fact that Rank's *The Trauma of Birth* had corroborated his personal memories of the intra-uterine period, and that 'in there' it was 'paradise.' Whatever credence this attestation should be given, it is probable that by 1930 Dalí would have read the book, which was translated into French in 1928, since there are many references in his writings of the time that clearly bear the stamp of Rank's thought" (289n.22).

➤ Daniel Burston publishes *The Wing of Madness: The Life and Work of R.D. Laing*. In the fall of 1975, writes Burston, Willam Swartley, a leader in primal therapy, spent an afternoon with Laing in London, and reported in a newsletter to the primal therapy community: "Ronnie showed me the galley proofs of his next book [*The Facts of Life*], which will assure him a role in the history of psychotherapy as the discoverer of the 'implantation trauma' (my term, not his), similar to the status of Otto Rank with the birth trauma. . . . Ronnie had a lot of trouble attaching himself to the wall of his mother's uterus eight days after his conception. . . . All that was clear is that Ronnie had such a will to be born . . . that he overcame her strong reluctance to the idea" (126).

➤ David Loy publishes *Lack and Transcendence: The Problem of Death and Life in Psychotherapy, Existentialism, and Buddhism*. "The problem with . . . immortality projects (a term coined by Otto Rank) is the problem with unconscious motivation generally," writes Loy. "When our conscious concerns only re-present what really drives us, they become symptoms and we become compulsive" (3).

➤ Andrew Webber publishes *The Doppelgänger: Double Visions in German Literature*. "Rank's 'Oedipal revolt,'" writes Webber, "was rooted in his objection to the phallocentric strain of psychoanalytic theory" (38).

➤ Jean Lipman-Blumen publishes *The Connective Edge: Leading in an Interdependent World*. "The terror of death compels us to search for leaders, gods, and belief systems—religious, political, scientific, and artistic—to protect us," writes Lipman-Blumen (328), adopting the views of Rank and Becker.

1997

➤ In a *Festschrift* for Paul Roazen, Robert Kramer publishes "Otto Rank and 'The Cause,'" the first exploration of the strong affinities between Rank and Lacan. As early as 1938, in an article for the *Encyclopédie française*, Lacan referring to *The Trauma of Birth*, stipulates that "anxiety is born with life" (quoted in Clark 1988:126).

1998

➤ Over the span of a six years, Johns Hopkins University Press publishes English translations of Rank's *Psychology and the Soul* (in 1998); *The Incest Theme in Literature and Legend* (in 1992); and the second edition, previously untranslated, of Rank's *The Myth of the Birth of the Hero* (in 2004).

➤ Marina Leitner publishes a book-length study in German entitled *Freud, Rank und die Folgen* (Freud, Rank and the Consequences), showing why the conflict between Freud and Rank over *The Trauma of Birth* was a pivotal event in the history of psychoanalysis.

➤ Ernst Falzeder publishes "Family Tree Matters" in *Journal of Analytical Psychology*, writing: "During the last few years, there has been a growing interest in the work of Otto Rank, who for some is 'the most extraordinary catalytic agent that ever hit the psychoanalytic movement.' . . . Recently, Marina Leitner (1997, 1998) has shown that the conflict between Freud and Rank was a key conflict in the history of psychotherapy of the twentieth century, and that many ideas usually attributed to Erich Fromm, Karen Horney, Melanie Klein, Margaret Mahler, Donald W. Winnicott, etc., originate in Rank. Esther Menaker [1982, p. ix] sees in Rank's work the 'missing link in the historical chain of the development of theory and practice within the psychoanalytic movement'" (135).

➤ Ludwig Janus edits a special issue of the German psychoanalytic journal *psychosozial* devoted to rediscovering the value of Rank's ideas for psychoanalysts. Along with numerous publications on Rank's innovations as a therapist, Janus, a medical doctor and a psychoanalyst, has been at the forefront worldwide for over four decades of promoting prenatal and perinatal psychology in medicine.

➤ Echoing Rank's arguments in *The Trauma of Birth*, Peter Sloterdijk publishes the first volume of his trilogy *Sphären* (Spheres), referring to the spherical configuration of a mother's womb. After Jürgen Habermas, Sloterdijk is the leading philosopher in Germany today. *Spheres* "is the philosopher's magnum opus. The first volume was published in 1998, the second in 1999, and the last in 2004. *Spheres* deals with 'spaces of coexistence,' spaces commonly overlooked or taken for granted which conceal information crucial to developing an understanding of humanity. The exploration of these spheres begins with the basic difference between mammals and other animals: the biological and utopian comfort of the mother's womb, which humans try to recreate through science, ideology, and religion. From these microspheres (ontological relations such as fetus-placenta) to macrospheres (*macro-uteri* such as states), Sloterdijk analyzes spheres where humans try but fail to dwell and traces a connection between vital crises (e.g., emptiness and narcissistic detachment) and crises created when a sphere shatters" (Wikipedia entry, "Peter Sloterdijk," n.p.).

1999

➤ Shuli Barzilai publishes *Lacan and the Matter of Origins*, showing how closely Jacques Lacan identified with Rank. "Lacan wanted all his life . . . simultaneously to occupy two positions: both that of beloved son and intellectual companion, held by Rank before his break with Freud, *and* that of independent, ambitious, even renegade, creator held by Rank thereafter" (29; italics in the original).

➤ Martin Halliwell publishes *Romantic Science and the Experience of the Self*, including a 40-page chapter on Rank dubbing him "the creative romantic" in contrast to William James, whom he calls "the pragmatic romantic." Halliwell writes: "Rank's emphasis on emotion over intellect is essentially romantic in orientation and links his early analytic work in *The Artist* and *The Double* with his later humanistic work on patient-centered therapy" (89). He observes that "Rank's will therapy concurs with Jamesian pathfinding: the individual does not get 'well,' but becomes creative" (108).

➤ Roy deCarvalho publishes "Otto Rank, the Rankian Circle in Philadelphia, and the Origins of Carl Rogers' Person-Centered Psychotherapy" in *History of Psychology*. "[T]he professional conflicts between a male-dominated psychiatry and female social workers," deCarvalho concludes, "were crucial in the dissemination of Rank's psychological thought and the early popularity of Rogers" (132).

➤ Paul Roazen introduces a collection of Martin Buber's writings on the "I–Thou" relationship, observing that "Much has recently been written about the necessary reciprocity in the relationship between therapist and patient, although once again Freud himself never made any such concession from the point of view of orthodox theorizing. But his former apostle Otto Rank would use Buber-like language: in 1928, Rank maintained that 'in contrast to I-psychology . . . one might designate ethics as Thou-psychology'" (xxv).

➤ Claude Barbré publishes "Reversing the Crease: Nietzsche's Influence on Otto Rank's Concept of Creative Will and the Birth of Individuality," a chapter in *Nietzsche and Depth Psychology*. Rank's writings, avers Barbré, cannot be understood without grasping the similarities and contrasts between Rank and Nietzsche on the meaning of "will." Nietzsche was contemptuous toward Judeo-Christian guilt-feeling, while Rank saw the relational elements of guilt-feeling as a necessary component of the ethical practice of willing.

➤ Murray Krim publishes "Otto Rank: Unacknowledged Genius" in *Contemporary Psychoanalysis*, comparing Kramer's collection of Rank's American lectures, *A Psychology of Difference*, with Menaker's *Separation, Will, and Creativity: The Wisdom of Otto Rank*, both published in 1996. "Kramer's and Menaker's excellent books," writes Krim, "turn the spotlight on this forgotten genius, too long in the shadows and with much still to teach us. Rank's time has come" (170).

2000

➤ Louis Breger publishes *Freud: Darkness in the Midst of Vision*, showing Rank's crucial importance in Freud's life and correcting errors about Rank in Peter Gay's 1988 biography of Freud.

➤ Leslie Chamberlain publishes *The Secret Artist: A Close Reading of Sigmund Freud*, observing: "When Freud fell into hostile relations with others, he looked away from what he should have seen, namely his own acts of self-repetition and vengeance. He called Rank a confidence trickster, but who exactly was the confidence trickster? To avoid confrontation with the truth, Freud split this fallible part of himself off and called it Rank" (55). The German word Freud used after 1926 to describe Rank as a "confidence trickster" is *Hochstaplernatur*, which means, literally, "an imposter by nature."

➤ Jeremy Safran and J. Christopher Muran publish *Negotiating the Therapeutic Alliance: A Relational Treatment Guide*, extolling Rank's "emphasis on the importance of the will in healthy functioning and in therapeutic change. . . . This perspective recognizes the inherent tension between agency and relatedness" (33).

➤ Todd Dufresne publishes *Tales from the Freudian Crypt: The Death Drive in Text and Context*. Writing of Rank's *The Double*, Dufresne says: "Doubling is among the most pervasive themes of romantic literature, as outlined so well by Freud's student Otto Rank. . . . Fascinated by and fearful of one version or another of the split or altered ego, the double was a psychological problem that plagued the arts in general. But it was also an inspiration for the contemporary theoretical and clinical research conducted on split personalities" (19).

➤ Ravenna Helson and Jennifer L. Pals publish "Creative Potential, Creative Achievement, and Personal Growth" in *Journal of Personality*, writing that, for Rank, "creativity represented an integration of will and counterwill that leads to more personality development than is possible for those who do not achieve this integration" (2).

2001

➤ Elemér Hankiss publishes *Fears and Symbols: An Introduction to the Study of Western Civilization*, affirming Rank's thesis in *The Trauma of Birth* "that the main motive force and goal of culture was to establish 'protective shells' which reproduced the experience of safety of the prebirth intra-uterine state" (30). Hankiss cites a galaxy of writers in literature, sociology, political science, psychology, philosophy, and cultural anthropology in support of Rank's thesis, including Samuel Beckett, Max Scheler, Ernst Cassirer, Géza Roheim, Mircea Eliade, Clifford Geertz, Eric Voeglin, Franz Borkenau, Peter Berger, Rollo May, and Ernest Becker.

➤ Alex Coren publishes *Short-Term Psychotherapy: A Psychodynamic Approach*, observing that "Rank was among the first to espouse a *developmental model for psychoanalysis* rather than one circumscribed by ideas of 'medical cure'. These ideas continue to inform some of the contemporary 'lifetime models' of brief therapy. Rank advocated . . . [o]pen exploration of feelings and thoughts—and their clinical resistances—in relation to the therapeutic dyad" (13–14; italics in the original).

➤ *American Imago* publishes Georg Groddeck's 1926 essay, "Rank in Freud's School." Concerning Freud's oral cancer, Groddeck, father of psychosomatic medicine, writes of Rank's *The Trauma of Birth* that it "is in some ways connected to Freud's recovery. The truth-loving eyes are again staring fearlessly and without turning to stone at the mother-Medusa.... And—must it still be uttered aloud?—that in psychic and physical life (these two are identical for me) there are other things besides just the Oedipus complex. For even conscious life, or what we call thinking, already begins a long time before birth, that is, long before the father's role commences" (843).

➤ Margaret Alic publishes the entry for Otto Rank in the second edition of the *Gale Encyclopedia of Psychology*. Rank, she says, "strongly influenced the development of psychotherapy in the United States. He was the first psychoanalyst to examine mother-child relationships, including separation anxiety. He also was one of the first to practice a briefer form of psychotherapy.... His work, in contrast to orthodox Freudian psychology, emphasized free will, relationships, and creativity" (535).

➤ In "Otto Rank's Art," published in *Humanistic Psychologist*, Will Wadlington describes Rank's understanding of the creative process from the perspective of an artist. He shows that Rank overturned Freud's tendency to pathologize artistic motives and points out that the Double, as described by Rank, can be an inhibiting block to creativity, but also an inspiration and ideal.

➤ Paul Roazen publishes *The Historiography of Psychoanalysis*, arguing that "Rank can be read as having constructed one of the most searching critiques of Freudian thinking, alongside the presentation of his own approach.... Rank was one of the great intellectuals in the history of Freud's following.... Each of Rank's pages are rich in ideas, and repay the attention of both scholars and therapists. As one of the most scholarly of twentieth-century psychologists, Rank's current neglect makes little sense ... and at no time does Rank indulge in the kind of appalling Freud-bashing that seems so popular now. Rank differed from Freud with the most profound respect, as Rank took seriously the injunction that students repay their teachers best by going beyond them" (390–391).

2002

➤ Peter Rudnytsky publishes *Reading Psychoanalysis: Freud, Rank, Ferenczi, Groddeck* alleging that Rank, the most intellectually sophisticated member of Freud's circle, was "anti-intellectual" (66n.6). Rudnytsky maintains that Rank's post-Freudian ideas, except for Rank's invention of object relations theory, are incomprehensible and unscientific. Unaware of the implications of Rank's existential unconscious, Rudnytsky alleges that Rank abandoned "the unconscious in his final period" (86n.1). What Rank abandoned was the glorification by psychoanalysts of "scientific insight" into the Freudian unconscious. No such insight is possible into the existential unconscious, except through a glass darkly, in, for example, the work of Samuel Beckett (Moorjani 2004). Repression of the existential unconscious, forgetting *Dasein*—the ineffable mystery of existence—is precisely the criticism later leveled by Jacques Lacan against American "ego" psychoanalysts (Kramer 1997).

➤ Robert Joel Kamin completes a PhD dissertation at the California School of Professional Psychology at Alameda, entitled, "Otto Rank's Critique of Psychoanalysis in Light of Philosophical Hermeneutics." Kamin writes: "Rank's break from

Freud is generally portrayed as disparaging to Rank, and Rank's post-Freudian ideas are considered incomprehensible and unscientific by traditional psychoanalytic scholars. Even authors more sympathetic to Rank see his early post-Freudian ideas as precursors to modern object relations theory, but see his later concepts as a decline in scientific rigor. In this study, an alternative interpretation is offered, which sees Rank's late ideas as strikingly similar to those of philosophical hermeneutics, as chiefly represented by Hans-Georg Gadamer. Viewed in this way, Rank can be seen as a harbinger of philosophical hermeneutics. . . . In light of these findings about Rank's late concepts, his work in relation to Freud should be re-examined" (1–2).

➤ Matthew Fox publishes *Creativity: Where the Divine and the Human Meet*, drawing on Rank's *Art and Artist* to explore how expression of our creative will can promote ecumenism, ecological and social justice, and a rebirth of the cosmological wisdom of the ancients, which connects the microcosm of the individual psyche to the macrocosm of the universe. "To allow creativity its appropriate place in our lives and our culture, our education and our family relationships," says Fox, "is to allow healing to happen at a profound level" (9).

➤ Linda Pavloski and Scott T. Darga publish Vol. 115 of *Twentieth-Century Literary Criticism*, including 133 pages of essays by scholars on Rank's innovations as a theorist, therapist, and social philosopher.

2003

➤ Bertram Müller publishes "The Influence of Otto Rank's Concept of Creative Will on Gestalt Therapy," a chapter in *Creative License: The Art of Gestalt Therapy*. "Above all," Müller concludes, "therapists in Rank's sense should allow themselves to be shaped by their patients and should let themselves be made into that which the patients want and need" (139).

➤ Rochelle Kainer and Selig Kainer publish "The Anxiety of Influence in the Creation of Theory," a chapter in *Creative Dissent: Psychoanalysis in Evolution*. They criticize Erich Fromm for falsely ascribing to Rank a "Schopenhauerian view of will as evil" (7). On the contrary, they show that Rank clearly rejected Schopenhauer's view. In the same vein, the Kainers criticize Leslie Farber for ascribing "guilt-free" willing to Rank, "despite the extensive attention Rank had paid to the inevitability of the condition of guilt for a human being, who must suffer it if he denies willing, or if the will is obeyed" (ibid.).

➤ Lydia Marinelli and Andreas Mayer publish *Dreaming by the Book: Freud's Interpretation of Dreams and the History of the Psychoanalytic Movement*, containing English translations of the two essays Rank contributed in 1914 to *The Interpretation of Dreams*. For the next 15 years, Rank's name would appear below Freud's on the title page of Freud's greatest work. Beginning with the 1929 edition, the first one published after their 1926 break, Freud ordered the removal of Rank's name and two essays.

➤ Helen Tookey publishes *Anaïs Nin, Fictionality and Femininity: Playing a Thousand Roles*, providing a richly detailed account of how Nin deployed Rank's ideas in the writing of her diary and her fiction.

2004

➤ Angela Moorjani publishes "Beckett and Psychoanalysis" in *Palgrave Advances in Samuel Beckett Studies*. She writes: "The relatively recent discovery ... that Beckett read Otto Rank's *The Trauma of Birth* ... helps shed light on Beckett's fictional and dramatic reenactments of intrauterine existence, expulsion from the womb, and fizzled-out births-into-death that readers have puzzled over for decades" (173). Moorjani shows that Beckett's writings on "prenatal and posthumous timelessness fused in the mind" are refractions of Rank's pre-linguistic, embodied—but always out-of-reach—existential unconscious (a term that she does not use).

➤ Sylvia Lavin publishes *Form Follows Libido: Architecture and Richard Neutra in a Psychoanalytic Culture*. One of the most prominent architects of the 20th century, Neutra "deliberately modeled his role as an architect for residential clients on the analyst working with neurotic patients" (47). The analyst he modeled himself after, writes Lavin, was Otto Rank, whose theory of traumatic separation at birth was central to Neutra's architectural designs, which were meant to heal this trauma. Lavin quotes Neutra: "Survival starts before birth. There, in the womb, it is best insured. After the 'birth trauma' ... we all slip right into the hands of the architect" for therapeutic healing (55), a position that Rank (1932a) justifies in his chapter on "House-building and Architecture" in *Art and Artist* (161–203). On the last page of her book, Lavin (2004) observes that "Neutra's architecture does not dull the mind but instead generates mood. And that's why we like it now" (144).

➤ Martin A. Bergmann, an orthodox Freudian, publishes *Understanding Dissidence and Controversy in the History of Psychoanalysis* alleging—incorrectly—that Rank made "an arbitrary decision to end the analysis in nine months" (26). There is no evidence for this allegation. Bergmann argues that Rank's "anti-Oedipal" theorizing can be explained because "[h]is father was an alcoholic and had a violent temper. When Rank was 16, he and his brother, who was (unfortunately) named Siegmund, decided to break off their relationship with their father" (23). Bergmann is unaware that Rank's brother was named Paul not Siegmund.

➤ Claude Barbré completes a PhD dissertation at Union Theological Seminary entitled "Otto Rank's Psychology of Will and Soul and its Spiritual Implications for Psychotherapeutic Theory and Practice." Barbré's aim "is to prove that Rank's sensitivity to religious experience offers the psychoanalytic practitioner and theorist important areas of clinical assessment often minimized" (2).

2005

➤ In "The Allure of Toxic Leaders: Why Followers Rarely Escape Their Clutches," published in *Ivey Business Journal*, Jean Lipman-Blumen explains why people follow toxic leaders: "Our existential anxiety and hankering for a life of meaning render us supremely vulnerable to leaders who insist that they can make us safe, instill our lives with significance, and ensure our eternal life either physically here or in another world, or symbolically, in the memory of generations yet unborn. As their followers, we work endlessly on what Otto Rank called our 'immortality projects,' be they a Thousand Year Reich or the rollout of next year's innovative product line" (3).

➤ In "The *Birth of Tragedy* and the *Trauma of Birth*," published in *Humanistic Psychologist*, Will Wadlington examines the writings of Nietzsche and Rank through the lens of Harold Bloom's "anxiety of influence."

2006

➤ Under the editorship of Judith Dupont, the French psychoanalytic journal *Le Coq-Héron*, publishes a special issue with the title, "*Otto Rank, l'accoucheur du sujet*" (Otto Rank, midwife of the subject).

➤ Irwin Z. Hoffman publishes "The myths of free association and the potentials of the analytic relationship" in *International Journal of Psychoanalysis*. Echoing Rank's *Will Therapy*, Hoffman creates a "dialectical-constructivist perspective" for psychoanalytic therapy, criticizing "the denial of the patient's agency (i.e., the myth that the patient is not a free agent); the denial of the patient's and the analyst's interpersonal influence (i.e., the myth that the patient and the analyst are largely unaffected by each other's interpersonal attitudes and actions); and the denial of the patient's share of responsibility for co-constructing the analytic relationship (i.e., the myth that the patient does not share responsibility with the analyst for the quality of the analytic relationship)" (44).

➤ Gareth Morgan publishes *Images of Organization*, a best-selling text adopted by many business schools worldwide. Applying the thought of Rank and Becker, Morgan writes that their "perspective suggests that we can understand organizations. . . in terms of a quest for immortality. In creating organizations we create structures of activity that are larger than life and that often survive for generations" (229).

2007

➤ Hans-Jürgen Wirth publishes "Schismatic Processes in the Psychoanalytic Movement and Their Impact on the Formation of Theories" in *International Forum of Psychoanalysis*, explaining how the differences between Freud and Rank over *The Trauma of Birth* contributed to a schism in psychoanalysis that has lasted to the present day.

➤ Michael L. Shuman completes a PhD dissertation in English literature at University of South Florida entitled *"A Woman's Face, or Worse": Otto Rank and the Modernist Identity*. "Rank's perception of the modern landscape," writes Shuman, "whether literary, social, or cultural, at once illuminates and refutes the concept of modernism" (ii) proposed by artists such as D.H. Lawrence, W.B. Yeats, and T.S. Eliot. Shuman argues "that Rank's theories provide not only a method for reading literature but a means for addressing issues critical for our time, including subjectivity, the process of individuation, diversity, and the empowering exercise of creative will" (iii). Rank, he notes, "provides a context for understanding twentieth-century modernist culture as well as a rationale for developing a new concept of humanism and for advancing twenty-first century post-theory literary studies" (ibid.)

2008

➤ Maxine Sheets-Johnstone publishes *The Roots of Morality*, exploring Rank's argument that "immortality ideologies" are our abiding response to the riddle of death. For Rank, as for Ernest Becker, history is a succession of immortality ideologies, beginning with belief in the soul. In a tour-de-force, Sheets-Johnstone compares and contrasts Rank's writings on the universality of soul-belief, introduced in *The Double* (1925) and expanded later in *Psychology and the Soul* (1930), *Art and Artist* (1932a), and *Beyond Psychology* (1941a), with the thinking of three major Western philosophers—René Descartes, Martin Heidegger, and Jacques Derrida.

➤ George Makari publishes *Revolution in Mind: The Creation of Psychoanalysis*, alleging—incorrectly—that Rank "hid" his approach to psychotherapy from Freud. "Otto Rank had reason to hide his new technique, because it would provoke an outcry" (363). But as the letters between Freud and Rank document (Lieberman & Kramer 2012), Rank tried to persuade Freud for two years to accept the pre-Oedipal ideas and approach to therapy he presented in *The Trauma of Birth*. Marina Leitner (1997) observes that Rank published a 230-page book in 1924, never translated into English, providing details of his new approach. This book was the longest psychoanalytic case history ever published. Unaware of this book, Makari (2008) also alleges that "By giving a rapid termination notice to all of his patients, Rank elicited great anxiety and dreams that seemed driven by an infant's yearning to be back in the womb" (354). There's no evidence that Rank ever gave "a rapid termination notice" to any of his patients. To the contrary, as reports by his patients show, Rank worked with each person as a unique human being, weaning them off therapy during the end phase, while exploring with them what they had learned about themselves during the therapy.

➤ Ram Cnaan and colleagues publish *A Century of Social Work and Social Welfare at Penn*. They elaborate on the contributions of Rank, Taft, and Robinson to creating the foundational curriculum of the University of Pennsylvania School of Social Work. Empathically listening to feelings—to the music underneath a client's words—in order to release the self-actualizing potential of the "creative will" for women, minority, and underprivileged clients was the main theme of Rank's lectures on relationship-based will therapy at the Penn School during the late 1920s and 1930s. Just as Rank fought a "David and Goliath" battle for two years with Freud, the faculty at the Penn School engaged in a multi-year battle with Freudian schools of social work in America, who vehemently opposed Rank's "anti-Oedipal" heresies. The conflict was so intense at times that the two groups refused even to sit together at the same dining room tables during professional conferences on social work. Today, however, Rank's ideas on relationship therapy and the self-leadership potential of the "creative will" for clients are commonplace themes in strengths-based social work education (Koenig, Spano & Thompson 2020).

➤ Robert J. Landy publishes *The Couch and the Stage: Integrating Words and Action in Psychotherapy*. Rank, suggests Landy, director of the drama therapy program at NYU, may have influenced the development of psychodrama as an indirect result of publishing *The Double*. "Although there is no evidence of a direct influence, Rank's ideas found new life in the work of such action psychotherapists as Moreno, who developed a psychodrama technique of doubling . . . and Landy, who attempted to conceptualize balance as an integration of role and counter-role" (29)—similar to Rank's argument that healthy psychological balance is an integration of will and counter-will.

➤ In *Irvin D. Yalom: On Psychotherapy and the Human Condition*, Ruthellen Josselson interviews Yalom about Rank's influence on his practice of existential psychotherapy. "I've always been intrigued with Otto Rank's formulation of going back and forth between the poles of life anxiety and death anxiety," says Yalom (114), whose *Existential Psychotherapy* includes many quotes from Rank.

2009

➤ Herman Westerink publishes *A Dark Trace: Sigmund Freud on the Sense of Guilt*, summarizing Rank's 1926 book *Sexualität und Schuldgefühl* (Sexuality and the Feeling of Guilt), never translated into English. "Otto Rank's overview of the debate and his break with Freud was published in the year of the break itself: 1926. The title of this publication says a great deal: *Sexualität und Schuldgefühl*, a collection of articles from the period 1911–1923, which was in fact designed to demonstrate that his ideas had old roots" (208).

2010

➤ In *Contemporary Psychoanalytic Studies: Explorations of the Psychoanalytic Mystics*, Dan Merkur asserts that "[t]he rehabilitation of Rank's reputation and technical innovations within psychoanalysis awaited the rise in the 1980s of the American school of relational psychoanalysis" (53). Merkur reads Rank as a mystic, but claims—incorrectly—that Rank "had no place for oceanic feelings" (70). He concludes that Rank's "concern to extend the concept of the mystical led him to brilliant and enduring contributions on the topics of individuation and the integration of the psyche" (ibid.).

➤ Eric Stein publishes a comprehensive overview of Rank's impact on social work and social welfare: "His use of present moment interactions with clients, his conceptualization of the will, his ideas on the artist type, and his emphasis on the mother-infant relationship predicated on the birth trauma presaged many later theories and influenced generations of social workers and psychologists to the present" (118). Stein concludes: "Rankian psychology has provided a critical base from which generalist and clinical social work theories and practice continue to flourish" (129).

➤ Badia Sahar Ahad publishes *Freud Upside Down: African-American Literature and Psychoanalytic Culture* with a chapter on how Rank's ideas impacted Black writer Nella Larsen in the writing of Larsen's masterwork *Quicksand*. A major figure in the Harlem Renaissance, Larsen is an outstanding exemplar of American modernism. (In addition to Larsen, other Black writers, including Ralph Ellison, Franz Fanon, and Richard Wright, read Rank.)

➤ Hanna Levenson publishes *Brief Dynamic Therapy* as part of the "Theories of Psychotherapy" series published by the American Psychological Association. Rank, she writes, "broke two important psychoanalytic taboos. The first was by setting time limits on treatment initially stemming from the concept of the *birth trauma*. If pathology were not solely due to insufficient resolution of the Oedipal conflict, but also due to earlier developmental issues of separation and individuation, then setting time limits could help patients deal with their separation anxieties. The second major brief therapy influence was Rank's assessment of the patient's motivation to change—his concept of *will*. Resistance was no longer seen as something negative to be overcome by interpretation, but rather in a positive light, as a strength of the individual" (18; italics in the original).

2011

➤ Robert Segal publishes an essay in *Religious Studies Review* on psychoanalytic contributions to the study of religion and immortality. "In Rank's *Psychology and the Soul*," Segal writes, "and in the posthumously published *Beyond Psychology* (1941 in English), the ultimate goal of separation becomes the forging not just of an independent self but of an immortal one. Immortality constitutes the highest form of creativity. The birth of a child signifies one's own mortality: with life looms death. For Rank, as for Freud, the father thus fears the newborn, but as a threat to his immortal self, not to his mortal one. The creative person forges not merely a new identity but an immortal one. Freud's immortality came through psychoanalysis itself" (13).

➤ Will Wadlington publishes a comprehensive account of Rank's theory of creativity in the *Encyclopedia of Creativity*. "Rank spoke with prescience about the future of psychological thought and practice," concludes Wadlington. "Rank's legacy is a creative improvisational approach to life that is constantly being rediscovered" (285).

➤ Masayo Isono completes a PhD dissertation at the Institute for Contemporary Psychoanalysis, in Los Angeles, entitled *Otto Rank: The Creator of a Relation-Based Psychology of the Self: Toward a Theory of Affects*, noting how similar Heinz Kohut's ideas on empathy are to those of Rank. This should not be surprising, she concludes, since Kohut was Carl Rogers's colleague when both taught for many years at the University of Chicago.

2012

➤ Karl Fallend publishes *Caroline Newton, Jessie Taft, Virginia Robinson: Spurensuche in der Geschichte der Psychoanalyse und Sozialarbeit* (Searching for Clues in the History of Psychoanalysis and Social Work), the first study, in German, of the careers of three well-known social workers who were in therapy with Rank. When Caroline Newton returned to the United States after completing her therapy in Vienna with Rank, Freudian analysts blocked her career. A wealthy Quaker and anti-fascist, she eventually found her place in literary history as a friend and patron of Thomas Mann.

➤ In *The Psychology of Artists and the Arts*, Edward W.L. Smith publishes a study of Rank's *Art and Artist*. Smith quotes literary critic Ludwig Lewisohn's summary of Rank's contributions to the study of art and the artist: "[T]he free creative and self-representative character of all art," wrote Lewisohn, "its tendency of liberation from the biological, its self-justification and immortality urge, its need of, and yet resistance to, the collective culture of its age, the artist's conflict within the dualism of creativity and experience, his need of Muse and mate and the difficulty of combining the two, his resistance to his art itself, his desire for fame and his fear of being depersonalized by that essentially myth-making process—all these explorations and revelations made by Dr. Rank I cannot conscientiously call otherwise than literally epoch-making" (136).

➤ Johns Hopkins University Press publishes *The Letters of Sigmund Freud and Otto Rank: Inside Psychoanalysis*, edited by E.J. Lieberman and Robert Kramer, correcting misrepresentations of Rank.

➤ Francisco Obaid publishes a comprehensive account in *The International Journal of Psychoanalysis* (which had dismissed Rank's ideas for almost a century) of the debate between Freud and Rank over the relationship between anxiety and birth.

➤ Mark Franko publishes *Martha Graham in Love and War: The Life in the Work* revealing, for the first time, how strongly Rank's *Art and Artist* and ideas about creative willing inspired Martha Graham, the mother of modern dance.

➤ Under the guest editorship of Judith Dupont, a special issue of the *American Journal of Psychoanalysis* entitled "Recognizing Otto Rank, an Innovator" is devoted to Rank's life and work. Contributors include Judith Dupont ("Are Innovators Trouble?"); E. James Lieberman ("Rankian Will"); Robert Kramer ("Rank on Emotional Intelligence, Unlearning and Self-Leadership"); Yves Lugrin ("The Rank-Ferenczi Relationship, as Seen from France"); Will Wadlington ("The Art of Living in Otto Rank's Will Therapy"); Masayo Isono ("An Exploration in the Will Psychology of Otto Rank: Human Intentionality and Individuality"), and Claude Barbré ("Confusion of Wills: Otto Rank's Contribution to an Understanding of Childism").

➤ Dorling Kindersley (a Penguin/Random House imprint) publishes an international best-seller, *The Psychology Book*, which identifies "unlearning" as one the "great ideas" in psychology, and credits Rank with being the first to apply it in therapy: "Austrian psychoanalyst Otto Rank proposes [in the 1920s] that separation from outdated thoughts, emotions, and behaviors is essential for psychological growth and development" (132).

➤ Stephen Cave publishes *Immortality: The Quest to Live Forever and How It Drives Civilization*. He writes: "The Soul Narrative, which is so successful at satisfying the will to immortality, has therefore provided the principal values of our civilization—even for those who long since abandoned its more mystical overtones. Ernest Becker, following the psychoanalyst Otto Rank, recognized that individualism and the aggrandizement of the self are not only products of this narrative but a continuation of the same quest for immortality. Whether or not we literally believe we have a soul that will go to heaven, the cosmic significance we ascribe to ourselves as unique individuals reassures us that we transcend mere biology . . . not like the anonymous animals that live and die in their millions around us" (154).

2013

➤ In *The Psychoanalytic Review*, Rosemary Balsam shows that Rank, as an early feminist in psychoanalysis, was the first male analyst to see "childbirth as a central bodily female experience" (713).

2014

➤ Gordon Neufeld and Gabor Maté publish *Hold Onto Your Kids: Why Parents Need to Matter More Than Peers*. Heralding Rank's coinage of the term counter-will, they write: "Counterwill is an instinctive, automatic resistance to any sense of being forced . . . In the first part of the twentieth century, Rank had already noted that dealing with counterwill was the parent's most daunting challenge" (74–75).

➤ Matthew Fox publishes "Psychotherapy and the 'Unio Mystica': Meister Eckhart Meets Otto Rank," a chapter in *Meister Eckhart: A Mystic-Warrior for Our Times*, showing striking similarities between Rank's thought and that of the medieval mystic Meister Eckhart. "Rank believed that premodern and ancient peoples," writes Fox, "saw physics (that is, nature, or the macrocosm) and psychology (human nature, or the microcosm) as one. All of life was a celebration of this union of psyche and cosmos. For Rank, people still seek 'an identity with the cosmic process' and rediscovering cosmology provides the surest healing for our deepest woes, which stem from our separation from the cosmos. Rank calls this the *unio mystica* (the mystical union), our 'being one with the All'.... The earliest humans knew all this intimately. . . . Rank instructs us to look to indigenous peoples—in this instance, to the wisdom they derive from animals and the 'reverence' they hold for animals.... Much of the neurosis of our time, Rank feels, is due to the loss of our connection to the cosmos" (145-146).

➤ *Book X* of *The Seminar of Jacques Lacan* is published by Jacques-Alain Miller. "By emerging into this world where he must breathe, first and foremost he is literally choked, suffocated," said Lacan in this seminar. "This is what has been called trauma—there is no other—the trauma of birth, which is not separation from the mother but inhalation, into oneself, of a fundamentally Other environment" (327).

➤ Jack Martin publishes "Ernest Becker at Simon Fraser University (1969–1974)" in *Journal of Humanistic Psychology*, observing that "Rank's emphasis on the power of art and love to heal the brokenness of men and women lifted Becker's sights to a higher place of cosmic creativity and joy. Infused with the exhilarating positive life force of Rank's creative will, Becker was now able to set alongside the terror of extinction an ode to joy, the kingdom of death in balance with the kingdom of life" (68).

➤ Sharon Spencer publishes "The Music of the Womb: Nin's 'Feminine' Writing," a chapter in *Breaking the Sequence: Women's Experimental Fiction*. Spencer argues that Nin, as an outcome of her therapy with Rank, was one of the first women writers to promote "the need for a feminine theory and practice of literature" (165). Pointing to Nin's "womb-oriented writing," Spencer concludes that "the writing of the womb must be alive: that is, natural, spontaneous, flowing (to use one of Nin's favorite words). It must have warmth, color, vibrancy, and it must convey a sense of movement (often Nin's characters are stuck, immobile, or paralyzed), the momentum of growth. Woman's literature (a literature of flesh and blood) must create syntheses; it must reconnect what has been fragmented by excessive [Freudian] intellectual analysis" (ibid.).

2015

➤ Eli Zaretsky publishes *Political Freud: A History*, dismissing the efforts by Ferenczi and Rank in the mid-1920s to save psychoanalysis from Freud's therapeutic nihilism. "In analysis," Zaretsky writes, "the search for quick, affirmative, shortcuts came from Sandor Ferenczi and Otto Rank, who suggested an 'active therapy.' . . . Freud's goal of insight, Ferenczi and Rank explained, was 'entirely different from the healing factor'" (97). Justifying Freud's therapeutic nihilism, Zaretsky adds: "Freud didn't believe that patients came to analysts to get well; they came, rather, to satisfy powerful instinctual wishes that had been formed in infancy" (ibid.). It's difficult to find a more cynical attitude to psychotherapy. Zaretsky argues that the ideas of Ferenczi and Rank ended up advancing "the new post-Fordist, finance and information-based capitalism, whose imaginary centered on open, indeterminate, shifting networks, rhizomorphic contexts, and deterritorialized flows. The idea of a personal life interior to the individual was repudiated in favor of an emphasis on flexibility, sociality, and sensitivity to difference" (34). There is no evidence that either Ferenczi or Rank repudiated the "personal life interior to the individual." Exactly the opposite is true, as even a cursory reading of Ferenczi's *Clinical Diary* or Rank's *Will Therapy* would demonstrate. Zaretsky has chosen to reinforce Freud's Oedipal narrative and his "one-person" psychology, rather than accept the "two-person" or relational revolution begun by Ferenczi and Rank.

2016

➤ Elizabeth Barry et al. show in *Journal of Medical Humanities* how closely Samuel Beckett read Rank. *The Trauma of Birth*, which Beckett annotated extensively in his own hand, occupies "a central place in Beckett's texts" (130).

➤ In a brilliant précis of Rank's *Art and Artist*, James Gallant writes in *Fortnightly Review*: "Rank saw the passion for 'immortalization' at work everywhere in culture and civilization: collective ideologies and symbols, libraries and museums, embalming, monuments, historiography. Looking at the world from a Rankian perspective, one can see the will to transcend time and process in architecture and urban design, family and school reunions, antique collecting, diaries, revivals of 50s or 70s popular music, Elvis imitators, and genealogy studies" (n.p.).

➤ In *Psychoanalytic Review*, Daniel Sullivan publishes the first comprehensive study of Rank's psychology of emotions.

➤ Elisabeth Roudinesco publishes *Freud in His Time and Ours*, claiming— incorrectly—that "the Freudian clinic . . . nullified therapeutic nihilism, which consisted in categorizing psychic illnesses without ever listening to the patient" (217). The opposite is true. Roudinesco occludes the fact that Ferenczi and Rank, in the mid-1920s, fought against Freud's therapeutic nihilism and his refusal to listen to the "here-and-now" (Rank 1926:9) feelings of his patients, spending most of his time during the consulting hour interpreting the "then-and-there" (24n). To Freud, psychoanalysis was an objective scientific method for researching the Oedipal unconscious and making a living: "[P]sychoanalysis as a therapy may be worthless" he confessed to Ferenczi (1932:186) and other members of his inner circle, including Rank.

➤ Claude Barbré publishes "The Contrapuntal Play of Paradox: Likeness and Difference in the Theories of Rank," a chapter in *Psychoanalytic Perspectives on Identity and Difference: Navigating the Divide*. Writes Barbré: "Like Rollo May, Rank distinguished the analytic situation from the transference.... The analyst's personality and the emotional relationship with the analyst determine what will happen as much as the patient's past. Instead of uncovering the patient's past, the patient's ego is the focus. Creative will is liberated.... Accepting will means embracing self-creation—or, as Rank emphasized: 'The artist appoints himself or herself artist.'... The therapist participates in this recognition and renegotiation of the emerging self-acceptance" (199).

➤ In *Phenomenology of Pregnancy*, which explores the first-person subjective experience of pregnancy, Erik Bryngelsson publishes a chapter on "The Problem of Unity in Psychoanalysis: Birth Trauma and Separation." He concludes: "Freud claims that the biological birth has no real significance for the mental development of the individual. The psyche can only come into being through the Oedipus complex and its connections to male genitals.... [I]n contrast to Freud, [Rank] understands birth as a major event and as the separation through which the psyche comes into being" (13).

➤ Hugo Lagercrantz, professor of pediatrics at Stockholm's Karolinska Institute, publishes *Infant Brain Development*, reporting that the fetus mobilizes very high levels of catecholamines (stress hormones) during normal birth, thus confirming, through measurement, Rank's contention that there's a physiological—as well as a psychological—trauma of separation at birth. "When I showed the results to my colleagues in adult medicine," Lagercrantz writes, "they did not believe me. [But] the levels were even much higher than in adults during severe stress, like running a marathon or during child birth" (57–58).

➤ In *Between Self and Society: Inner Worlds and Outer Limits in the British Psychological Novel*, John Rodden draws on Rank to study British fiction since the mid-eighteenth century. As portrayed in British fiction, the inter-relationship between self and society, he concludes, alternates between individual and community, part and whole, particular and universal.

➤ Andre Walton publishes "Resolving the Paradox of Group Creativity" in *The Harvard Business Review* (online). "In *Art and Artist*," Walton writes, "Otto Rank suggests that people's desire to be creative stems from their need to feel immortal, symbolically at least, and to leave their indelible mark on future generations in the form of artworks. If Rank is to be believed, this drive to be unique may be the primary motivation for many of us to follow a path of creativity" (n.p.).

2017

➤ Edgar Schein, professor at the MIT Sloan School, founder of the academic study of organizational culture, and pioneer in leadership development, writes: "If we now . . . are arguing for an experientially based self-development and are accepting . . . of the importance of will in addition to brain and heart, perhaps it turns out that we are all Rankians" (quoted in Kramer 2017:344).

➤ Mark Griffiths publishes *The Challenge of Existential Social Work*, highlighting the legacy of Rank's existential thought for social workers worldwide.

➤ Judith Lebiez publishes "Matricide and the Trauma of Birth in Hofmannsthal's *Elektra*" in *Women in German Yearbook*, exploring "the links between birth trauma and the violence against women committed in the sexual, social, and symbolic fields" (28).

➤ Birgit Lang publishes "Fin-de-Siecle Investigations of the 'Creative Genius' in Psychiatry and Psychoanalysis," a chapter in *A History of the Case Study: Sexology, Psychoanalysis, Literature*. Concerning Rank's 685-page book on incest, she writes: "*The Incest Theme in Literature and Legend* (1912) has been called the 'most important single work of psychoanalytic criticism' in relation to literature. Already in his 1914 essay on the history of psychoanalysis, Freud acknowledged the importance of Rank's 'exhaustive work on the theme of incest,' which he saw 'easily tak[ing] the first place' in psychoanalytic studies focused on literature, trumping his own works" (79).

2018

➤ Susan Lanzoni publishes *Empathy: A History*, showing how Rank's advocacy of empathic understanding (*Einfühlung*) shaped the relationship therapy of Carl Rogers, Jessie Taft, and Virginia Robinson.

➤ Heather D. Humann publishes *Another Me: The Doppelganger in 21st Century Fiction, Television and Film*, refracting contemporary fiction, television, and film through the lens of Rank's *The Double*.

➤ Isaac F. Young, Daniel Sullivan, Sheridan Stewart, and Roman Palitsky publish "The Existential Approach to Place: Consequences for Emotional Experience" in *Journal of Environmental Psychology*. Rank, they write, "described a neurotic type who continually experiences alienation from the environment and, as a result, is prone to anxiety, as well as an adapted type who feels interconnected socially and with the environment, making them prone to guilt if they violate these bonds" (101).

➤ In "The Educator as Neurotic: A Rankean [sic] Analysis of Impotent Teachers in Film," published in *Free Associations*, Daniel Sullivan writes: "Otto Rank argued that, in the modern individualistic and child-focused era, the transmission of collective beliefs is no longer valued and the figure of the educator becomes obsolete. This analysis illuminates the significance of a common theme in films, namely the teacher who, though serviced with the task of training children, is himself impotent or childless. The protagonists of *Goodbye Mr. Chips* (1939), *The Browning Version* (1951), *Who's Afraid of Virginia Woolf?* (1966), and *Waterland* (1992) are variously portrayed as unable to produce their own offspring and trapped by an overly ruminative approach to life. Rank's analysis suggests that the educator protagonists in these films are incarnations of the modern neurotic personality, whom he described as a 'failed artist.' These impotent teachers also serve as symbols of the breakdown of cultural transmission in amnesic modernity" (n.p.).

2019

➢ Alison Stone publishes *Being Born: Birth and Philosophy*, with the aim of overcoming the forgetting of mothers and birth by Western philosophers such as Heidegger, who focuses only on death. Stone reverberates with the relational themes of *The Trauma of Birth*, taking from Rank "an insight into the lasting power in our lives of a kind of separation anxiety" (19).

2020

➢ Terry Koenig, Rick Spano, and John Thompson publish *Human Behavior Theory for Social Work Practice*, lauding Rank's prescience in advocating the values of human growth, diversity, and inclusion during the late 1920s. "It is noteworthy," they write, "that Rank, rejected and professionally oppressed by his former psychoanalytic community, was apparently only able to find an academic home with the Social Work faculty at the University of Pennsylvania" (111).

➢ Richard Pine publishes "Otto Rank and the Case of Lawrence Durrell," an article in *C. 20: An International Journal*, showing the influence of Rank's writings on the author of *The Alexandria Quartet*, one of the most celebrated novels of the 20th century. Pine writes that Durrell's close friends, Anaïs Nin and Henry Miller, "presented him with a copy of Otto Rank's *Art and Artist* which, together with *The Trauma of Birth* (which he already possessed), Durrell read assiduously and on which he made copious notes" (2).

➢ In a biography of the poet Sylvia Plath, Heather Clark (2020) writes that "The themes of rebirth and renewal are as central to her poems as depression, rage and destruction" (xxi). In her senior year at Smith College, Plath "hoped to read Otto Rank [on *The Double*] in German—'all fascinating stuff about the ego as symbolized in reflections (mirror and water), shadows, twins . . . dividing off and becoming an enemy, or omen of death . . . or a warning conscience.'" Clark adds: "This was the most serious scholarly work she had ever done. She hoped to write 'an adolescent story about doubles' after she finished her thesis—'every incident in my life begins to smack of the mirror image'" (341).

➢ Drawing on Rank, Eran Dorfman publishes *Double Trouble: The Doppelgänger from Romanticism to Postmodernism*. The double, writes Dorfman, "opens up the subject to multiplicity, since it reveals that the boundaries between I and world, I and other, I and me, are far from being clear" (3).

2021

➢ Kirk Schneider publishes "The Existential Unconscious: A Re-Visioning of Our Hidden Selves" on the *Psychology Today* website. Schneider writes: Rank's "existential unconscious unchains us from many classical conceptions of nonconscious processing, from the delimited investigations of the laboratory to the restrictive data sets, resonant as they may be in certain instances, of theorists such as Freud and Jung" (n.p.).

➤ Drawing on Rank's *Trauma of Birth*, Panagiotas Kostaras publishes a vivid account in *British Journal of Psychotherapy* of how "patients experiencing panic attacks describe their fear of death as a fear of nonexistence: they fear absolute nothingness, in which, nevertheless, perception and feelings remain intact" (637).

➤ Frank Tallis publishes *The Act of Living: What the Great Psychologists Can Teach Us About Surviving Discontent in an Age of Anxiety*. "Rank's willingness to empathize," writes Tallis, "to imagine what it is like to experience the symbiotic bliss of the womb, followed by expulsion, represents not only an impressive act of identification, but also an early example of the raised consciousness that mobilized for natural childbirth in the 1970s and ultimately made obstetrics a more humane profession" (52–53).

➤ Funded by the John Templeton Foundation, the newly created *International Society for the Science of Existential Psychology*, which promotes experimental research on ultimate human concerns, pays homage to Ernest Becker, Otto Rank, and Rollo May (among many other existentialists) on its website: https://www.issep.org/the-science-of-existential-psychology.

➤ Klaus Evertz, Ludwig Janus, and Rupert Linder publish an 817-page *Handbook of Prenatal and Perinatal Psychology: Integrating Research and Practice*. According to Evertz et al., "Rank stated that the strengthening of self-experience in the 'analytic situation' should enable the end of therapy to be associated with true independence and individuation with an enrichment of self-experience and a self-gain and not with forlornness and a loss of self as originally at birth" (4). Promoting the integration of all major schools of therapy, Evertz et al. add: "The field of psychotherapy, which had been earlier divided into individual schools and methods, is becoming increasingly integrated. Empirical research, neurophysiology, and psychotraumatology are gaining the attention they deserve. The areas of encounter and cooperation are developing in the various depth psychology approaches, such as body psychotherapy, depth-psychological psychotherapy, and psychoanalysis" (6).

2022

➤ Tim Lomas publishes "Making Waves in the Great Ocean: A Historical Perspective on the Emergence and Evolution of Wellbeing Scholarship" in *Journal of Positive Psychology*, identifying Rank as one of the pioneers of positive psychology.

➤ James Meyer and other curators at the National Gallery of Art in Washington, DC, organize an exhibition entitled *The Double: Identity and Difference in Art Since 1900*. As an adjunct to this exhibition, the National Gallery of Art co-publishes with Princeton University Press a 288-page book-catalog with the same title. Serving as one of the intellectual foundations for the exhibition, Rank's *The Double* (1925) included a film review. In the book-catalog, Tom Gunning recognizes Rank as the first psychoanalytic movie critic, "a bold move at a time when film was still viewed as a cheap fairground attraction. . . . Cinema, [Rank] speculated, might become the medium of the unconscious. . . . We could ask in turn whether the cinematic double became emblematic of the modern environment, in which we seem to be surrounded by endless photographic and electronic doppelgängers" (245).

➤ Agata Bielik-Robson, Professor of Jewish Studies at the University of Nottingham, publishes "Psychoanalysis as *Torat Hayim*: In Praise of Separation" in *European Judaism*. "If, as Otto Rank claims, 'the birth trauma is the ultimate biological basis of the psychical,' then the Jewish *torat hayim* [the teaching of life, i.e., 'choose life rather than death'] offers one of the most fundamental interpretations of what it means to be human. . . . Even if separation generates inevitable anxiety, it is a cost worth being paid for the ability to affirm one's singular existence" (66–67).

➤ In "Existential Empathy: The Challenge of 'Being' in Therapy and Counseling," Siebrecht Vanhooren reports in *Religions* that "therapists do not always feel comfortable with the existential concerns of their clients. Therapists seem to underestimate their clients' existential needs. . . . Existential empathy, or the capacity to resonate with the client's existential concerns and to communicate this empathy"—as did Otto Rank, Carl Rogers, and Rollo May—"could be enlarged in therapists in order to help clients find different avenues to be with their human condition" (1).

2023

➤ Robert Kugelmann publishes *The Soul in Soulless Psychology*, including a 20-page analysis of Rank's writings on the soul. The conclusions of experimental researchers in the field of "terror management theory," notes Kugelmann, "invoking the work of Otto Rank, point to the human awareness of personal mortality and the resultant anxiety as contributing to belief in the soul as a way of 'helping humans defy the finality of death.' . . . Along these lines Gadamer (1996) referred to the gift that the Titan, Prometheus, gave to struggling humanity: not the gift of fire but the gift of forgetfulness of mortality as enabling human flourishing. . . . There is another source for the soul, according to Preston, Gray and Wegner (2006), namely as a way 'to explain the unfathomable source of our own ability to do things merely by wanting them. The soul is a way of understanding the experience of conscious will.' . . . This inner source of action we observe in others as well. . . . To this, I would add that the experience of conscious will points to moments of transcendence of situational constraints, a connotation preserved in the illusion, if that is what it is, of the soul" (12).

➤ In *Humanistic Psychologist*, Robert Kramer publishes "Discovering the Existential Unconscious: Rollo May Encounters Otto Rank," the first comprehensive account of how Rank's writings on love and will, and life fear and death fear, influenced the development of existential therapy by Rollo May.

➤ Kirk Schneider publishes *Life Enhancing Anxiety: Key to a Sane World*, comparing psychoanalyst Robert Stolorow's *ontological unconscious* with Rank's *existential unconscious*. "In my understanding," writes Schneider, "these conceptions share similarities but also notable differences, such as Stolorow's emphasis on language as a hallmark of the ontological unconscious, whereas the existential unconscious may be seen as fundamentally pre-linguistic and embodied" (15n).

➤ Siebrecht Vanhooren publishes *Op de bodem: Existentiële thema's in psychotherapie en begeleiding* (On the bottom: Existential themes in psychotherapy and counseling), the first Dutch-language book that draws extensively on Rank. "According to Rank," writes Vanhooren, "the birth trauma, the split between the original mother-child whole, is the starting point of the desire to be able to feel at one with the whole again. Once the birth trauma has occurred, the person is stuck with being an identifiable, separate individual. Before birth, the fetus consists of a unity with the mother, said Rank. The meaning of the birth trauma is the breaking of this unity, being suddenly separated. From that point on, there's a yearning for ultimate re-connection. . . . Spiritual mystical experiences in which we strongly feel a union with what Rank calls '*das Ganze*,' or the whole, can also be understood in this way. . . . We do end up being thrown back—often to our regret and pain—on our individuality, but in an enriched way. The desire for fusion, according to Rank, refers to the spiritual idea that both before we are born and after we die, we completely merge and even disappear into that whole" (57–58).

➤ Naomi Klein applies Rank's ideas on the double in *Doppelganger: A Trip into the Mirror World* to explore the emergence of Artificial Intelligence—a "mirroring machine"—which Klein argues is an existential threat to authentic communication between human beings.

➤ John Bonaduce publishes "The Prenatal Origin of Myth, Religion, and Ritual" in *Journal for Prenatal and Perinatal Psychology and Health*. "It has been a century since Otto Rank boldly broke away from Freudian orthodoxy and declared that babies at birth are sentient and highly impressionable human beings," writes Bonaduce. "Since then, evidence for embryonic consciousness has been firmly established with data from neuroscience, biology, psychiatry, and medicine, always tending to earlier prenatal awareness models" (87).

➤ In November, the *First International Otto Rank Conference* is held online under the auspices of the Existential-Humanistic Institute (San Francisco), the Existential-Humanistic Institute (Pacific Northwest), the Existential-Humanistic Institute (Madrid), and K-U Leuven University (Belgium).

2024

➤ Daniel Sullivan, Alexis Goad, and Harrison J. Schmitt publish "Existential Psychology," a chapter in *The Routledge International Handbook of Existential Human Science*. "In North American therapeutic practice," they write, "*existential-humanistic psychology* emerged largely via the mediating influence of Rollo May. . . . This movement was substantively influenced by Otto Rank, who expanded the humanistic dimension of psychotherapy by incorporating insights from Nietzsche and other diverse sources. Existential-humanistic therapy is relatively distinctive in that it presents existentialism as a fundamental orientation that can be compatible with strategic use of more conventional therapeutic techniques (e.g., cognitive-behavioral)" (25; italics in the original).

➤ Laura Stephenson publishes *Cinema, Suffering and Psychoanalysis: The Mechanism of Self*. Drawing on *The Double*, she writes that Rank "claims that when the protagonist of the text is unable to accept his own guilt on a conscious level he relocates it from his own ego and places it onto another 'ego'" (64). Stephenson concludes: "Indeed, the double in cinema is a transient, otherworldly creature, sometimes aware of their own presence, other times not. . . . Rank interprets this meeting of past and present circumstances as uncanny, with the subject's attempts to ignore or forget the past only succeeding in cementing the past into the subject's present and future" (68–69).

➤ Ingrid Sara Ekenstierna completes a PhD dissertation at University of Queensland, Australia, entitled *The Part-Whole Relation: Otto Rank, David Bohm, and a Therapeutic Third*. She maps theoretical physicist David Bohm's philosophy of wholeness onto Rank's practice of psychotherapy. She shows strong congruences between the two and explores the *unio mystica* experience in the I-Thou relationship between therapist and client.

➤ In a chapter entitled, "Who Is Transferring What to Whom? Resistance to Lacan," published in *Negativity in Psychoanalysis: Theory and Clinic*, Ellie Ragland writes that "Rank has triumphed over Freud in America. Not only do psychiatrists use the short sessions Rank recommended, but psychotherapists do as well. In his writings about psychoanalysis and in his practice, Rank promoted ever shorter sessions and ever decreasing frequency" (18). Without knowing anything about Rank's influence on social work or his influence on Carl Rogers and Rollo May, Ragland alleges—incorrectly—that Rank did not listen empathically to his clients: "The patient's speech was not to be heeded. Rank assured mental health care workers that a cure should arise quickly because of their keen insight and vision" (ibid.). The opposite is true. Raglund asserts that Rank's therapy was "a clinical learning and unlearning experience that should be focused on *feelings*, not speech. Patient learning (and unlearning) occurs *quickly* as if the patient were coming out of a *birth trauma*" (ibid.; italics in the original). As a Lacanian, Raglund finds a focus on feelings in therapy objectionable, just as Freud did.

➤ Ludwig Janus publishes *The Enduring Effects of Prenatal Experiencing: Echoes from the Womb*. Pointing to Rank as the pioneer theorist of birth psychology and prenatal medicine, Janus provides the first English translation of Rank's case history, published in 1926 in Vol. 1 of *Technik der Psychoanalyse* (Technique of Psychoanalysis), of "a middle-aged woman with a dependence problem who had a difficult birth and who had then lost her mother when she was 12 years old" (64).

In press

➤ Will Wadlington will publish "Otto Rank's Original Contributions to Humanistic and Existential Psychology," a chapter in the *APA Handbook of Humanistic and Existential Psychology*, a two-volume work that provides a comprehensive overview by the American Psychological Association of the current state of humanistic and existential psychology worldwide and envisions its future direction.

German editions of Rank

➤ Over the last 25 years, German publisher Hans-Jürgen Wirth, founder of Psychosozial-Verlag in Giessen, Germany, has published six works by Rank: *Kunst und Künstler* (in 2000), which originally appeared only in English (as *Art and Artist* in 1932); three volumes of *Technik der Psychoanalyse* (in 2006), the last two of which were published in English as *Will Therapy* in 1936; *Das Trauma der Geburt* (in 2007); and *Grundzüge einer genetischen Psychologie* (in 2024). Wirth's German edition of the Freud-Rank letters was published in 2014.

Notes

Epigraphs

1 SOURCE: Rank, O. (1939). Hand-written note. Otto Rank Collection, Rare Book and Manuscript Library, Columbia University. Box 14.
2 SOURCE: p. 57 in Nin, A. (1973). On truth and reality. *Journal of the Otto Rank Association*, 8, 51–58.
3 SOURCE: p. 283 in Taft, J. (1933). *The dynamics of therapy in a controlled relationship*. New York: Macmillan.
4 SOURCE: p. 22 in Robinson, V. P. (1968). The influence of Rank in social work. *Journal of the Otto Rank Association*, 2, 5–50.
5 SOURCE: pp. 101–102 in Crosby, P. (1970). Letter to the Editors. *Journal of the Otto Rank Association*, 5, 101–102.

Chapter 1

1. See https://ccare.stanford.edu/about/related-organizations/.
2. See https://www.adultdevelopmentstudy.org/.
3. As of 2023, according to the Bureau of Labor Statistics, 751,900 social workers comprise the vast bulk of helping professionals in the United States. See https://www.bls.gov/ooh/community-and-social-service/social-workers.htm.
4. Today the University of Pennsylvania School of Social Work is called the University of Pennsylvania School of Social Policy and Practice; its leadership vision is "the passionate pursuit of social innovation, impact, and justice."
5. Ludwig Binswanger is usually credited with founding existential therapy. As a medical doctor, Binswanger was the first existential *psychiatrist*, but Rank, who was not a physician, was the first existential *therapist*. (For a highly readable account of key figures in the development of existential therapy, up to the present, see Cooper 2017.)
6. See https://www.issep.org/the-science-of-existential-psychology.

Chapter 2

1. The term "leadership development" was first used by Kurt Lewin in the 1940s. Creator of the field of experimental social psychology, Lewin also coined the term "group dynamics" (Goethals et al. 2004). Early on, Lewin (1926) wrote extensively about "the will," but neither Rank nor Lewin knew of the other's work in this area.
2. "I admire Rank's work on will therapy very much," Burns told me during a conversation we had in 2001 at the annual conference of the International Leadership Association. "It resonates closely with my own vision of 'transforming leadership' in order to create a more ethical, just society," said Burns (personal communication).
3. In 1994, the *Diagnostic and Statistical Manual* (DSM), the encyclopedia of mental disorders compiled by the American Psychiatric Association, officially dropped the word "neurosis."
4. For Rank, Taft, and Robinson, self-determination, a core value of the social work profession, is identical to self-leadership. "Social workers respect and promote the right of clients to self-determination and assist clients in their efforts to identify and clarify their goals," according to the Code of Ethics of the National Association of Social Workers. "Social workers may limit clients' right to self-determination [only] when, in the social workers' professional judgment, clients' actions or potential actions pose a serious, foreseeable, and imminent risk to themselves or others." See: https://www.socialworkers.org/About/Ethics/Code-of-Ethics/Code-of-Ethics-English/Social-Workers-Ethical-Responsibilities-to-Clients.
5. Here Rank reverses a position he had taken six years earlier, before he had crystallized his theory of the creative will. In an overreaction to the Freudian view of analysts as entirely passive, Rank (1926) went to the other extreme, advocating that analysts "must have the courage to completely withdraw the leadership [*Führung*] of the analysis from the patient" (20). However, within a short time, Rank re-thought and abandoned this view, and began promoting

the expression of self-leadership—i.e., creative willing—for *both* analyst and patient during the therapeutic hour.

6. See https://www.oxfordbibliographies.com/display/document/obo-9780195389678/obo-978 0195389678-0006.xml.

Chapter 3

1. In this book, I will linger on Rank's influence on Samuel Beckett, Martha Graham, Nella Larsen, Anaïs Nin, Betty Friedan, Henry Miller, Carl Whitaker, Jean-Lipman Blumen, D.W. Winnicott, Jacques Lacan, and Ernest Becker. For the others, I provide brief accounts in *Appendix B—Annotated Bibliography of Selected Writings on Rank*.

2. See https://www.nytimes.com/2023/12/28/books/review/denial-of-death-ernest-becker.html ?smid=tw-nytbooks&smtyp=cur.

3. See https://ihavenotv.com/flight-from-death.

4. See https://nebula.tv/videos/like-stories-of-old-redefining-the-antiwar-film.

5. See https://twobirdsfilm.com/films/allillusionsmustbebroken.

6. See https://lithub.com/how-do-we-live-with-the-knowledge-that-well-die.

7. It took over six decades for psychoanalysts to see the merits in Rank's arguments. "I believe that it is fair to say," writes Thomas Ogden (1994), "that contemporary psychoanalytic thinking is approaching a point where one can no longer simply speak of the analyst and the analysand as separate subjects who take one another for objects" (3). Some analysts still refuse to accept this view. Freud never did. In January 1927, Freud recounted to Ferenczi the two hours he had just spent with Einstein, who "understands as much about psychology as I do about physics, and so we had a very good conversation" (Freud & Ferenczi 2000:292).

8. "There is no such thing as a baby," psychoanalyst D.W. Winnicott (1964) famously wrote. "A baby cannot exist alone, but is essentially part of a relationship" (88). In *Bloomsbury/Freud: The Letters of James and Alix Strachey, 1924–1925*, Meisel and Kendrick (1985) show the influence of Rank's *The Trauma of Birth* on Winnicott, who was termed a *"Rankschüler"* (115)—a member of "Rank's school of thought"—by James Strachey, main editor of the *Standard Edition* of Freud's writings. I will return to Rank's influence on Winnicott in my Epilogue.

9. In October 2023, drawing on the latest discoveries in neuroscience and biology, Robert Sapolsky published *Determined: A Science of Life Without Free Will*. In the same month, drawing mostly on the same discoveries in neuroscience and biology, but making the opposite argument, Kevin Mitchell published *Free Agents: How Evolution Gave Us Free Will*. Which argument is correct? How should one choose between the two arguments? Is the choice "determined," as Sapolsky would have it, or "free," as Mitchell would have it? Echoing William James, Rank (1941a) writes in *Beyond Psychology*: "Even if human nature and man's behavior are absolutely determined, man's *belief* in his free will, ability to choose and individual responsibility would still be his 'psychology' and the real object of human psychology" (34; italics added).

10. Notable exceptions are Shedler (2010), Solms (2015; 2021), Leichsenring et al. (2023), Lilliengren (2023), and Richardson et al. (2023).

11. For a highly readable account of research on TMT, which touches on a vast array of topics, including human evolution, child development, religion, war, politics, and leadership, see Solomon et al. (2015).

12. The word "genocide" was coined in 1944 by Raphael Lemkin, a lawyer of Polish-Jewish origin, to describe the murder of millions of Jews by Hitler. For an account of recent genocides, see: https://news.un.org/en/tags/genocide.

13. Underlining is by Taft, who was quoting Rank. Taft's personal copy of the book is in the Otto Rank Collection, Columbia University Rare Book and Manuscript Library, Box 40.

14. Kierkegaard's book and Heidegger's book were in Rank's library at the time of his death (Rank 1941b). Heidegger published *Sein und Zeit* in 1927. Although Rank read Heidegger, he does not quote him; however, Rank (1932a) *does* quote Kierkegaard in *Art and Artist* (413) and in his diary of 1905, written when he was 21 years old (Taft 1958:37–38). That Rank read Kierkegaard and Heidegger, neither of whom Freud ever heard of, is emblematic of Rank's wide-ranging intellect.

Chapter 4

1. A copy of James's *The Varieties of Religious Experience* was in Rank's library at the time of his death (Rank 1941b).

2. See https://www.sipri.org/media/press-release/2023/world-military-expenditure-reaches-new-record-high-european-spending-surges.
3. For a video recording of Sagan, see https://www.youtube.com/watch?v=GO5FwsblpT8.
4. As I show in my Epilogue, for Rank, art and love offer a "creation-centered" rather than "dying-centered" mysticism for transcending death.
5. See https://geneva-academy.ch/galleries/today-s-armed-conflicts.

Chapter 5

1. Ira Progoff (1956) observes a similar stress on likeness in Jung's writings, which "began as an analysis of the cultural varieties of myths and symbols, but as [Jung] framed his theory of the archetypes he tended more and more to emphasize their underlying sameness rather than their historical differences" (235).
2. Permission to republish these quotes was kindly granted me by PEP. All the interviews can be seen here: https://www.youtube.com/watch?v=N8-VIi7tb44.
3. In 2022, drawing partly on the writings of Rank, the National Gallery of Art in Washington, DC held an exhibit on *The Double: Identity and Difference in Art Since 1900.* "This past July," writes Naomi Klein (2023b) in the *New York Times,* "Merriam-Webster announced on X, the platform formerly known as Twitter, that 'doppelgänger is currently one of our top lookups.'"
4. Rank's 1932 *Art and Artist* was in Ellison's library at the time of his death. See https://findingaids.loc.gov/exist_collections/ead3pdf/rbc/2016/rb016001.pdf. During the 1920s, psychoanalysis attracted a large number of Black intellectuals, who "deployed Freudianism to counter Victorian sexual repressiveness, expressed in the hygienic advocacy of Booker T. Washington and in the Puritanism of the Black church" (Zaretsky 2015:44).

Chapter 6

1. Rank's presentation copy is in Freud's library in London at 20 Maresfield Gardens, which is now one of the two Freud museums in the world. The other is located at *Berggasse 19,* Freud's apartment-office in Vienna.
2. I can find only two references to Rank on the website of the International Psychoanalytical Association: (a) "1914–1918, President: Karl Abraham; Secretary: Hanns Sachs; Succeeded by Acting Secretaries: Otto Rank, L. Levy, Sándor Radó." See https://www.ipa.world/en/en/IPA1/officers_past_and_current/ipa_officers_past_and_current.aspx. (b) "Over a period of several years in the nineteen-twenties, serious difficulties developed in the relationship of Rank to the other members of the Committee. He left the Committee and his place on it was taken in 1925 by Anna Freud." See https://www.ipa.world/IPA/en/IPA1/ipa_history/history_of_the_ipa.aspx.
3. For a recent example of *totgeschweigen,* the name Otto Rank is not mentioned in a 2022 article in *International Forum of Psychoanalysis* by Harold and Elsa Blum, entitled "Evolution of Freudian Psychoanalytic Thought in the Twentieth-Century USA: The Influence of the European Émigrés." However, Rank's closest collaborator, Sándor Ferenczi, at one time also *totgeschweigen,* is now fully accepted into mainstream psychoanalysis. Today, Ferenczi is heralded as the forerunner of relational psychoanalysis (Haynal 1993; Haynal 2002; Szekacs-Weisz & Keve 2012).
4. In 1929 and 1931 Rank published two books in German, *Technik der Psychoanalyse,* Vols. II and III, translated by Jessie Taft into English as *Will Therapy.* It's likely that Ferenczi read the German volumes (André Haynal, personal communication). In his *Clinical Diary,* written in 1932, Ferenczi draws on Rank's vocabulary of "will" and "life fear and death fear" to characterize his tormented relationship with Freud. In the literature of psychoanalysis, only Rank was using such language, so Ferenczi could not have gotten these ideas from anywhere other than Rank's just-published books, or perhaps from his conversations with Rank before their break. "Is the only possibility for my continued existence," wondered Ferenczi (1932), "the renunciation of the largest part of one's own self, in order to carry out the will of that higher power [Freud] to the end (as though it were my own)? . . . [I]s it worth it always to live the life (will) of another person—is such a life not almost death?" (212).

Chapter 7

1. In his first paper after publication of *The Trauma of Birth,* Freud (1924) expressed reluctance to "begin a criticism or an appreciation of Rank's view" (179) since he thought he could still influence Rank to correct himself, and return to the centrality of the Oedipus complex. But

two years later, seeing that Rank would not recant his "anti-Oedipal" views, Freud had decided to deliver a fatal blow.

2. The *Oxford Dictionary of Philosophy* defines *causa sui* as: "The (problematic) property possessed only by God, of being his own cause, i.e., independent of any other ground, yet containing within himself a sufficient explanation of his own being." See: https://www.oxfordreference.com/display/10.1093/oi/authority.20110803095555963.

Chapter 8

1. Recently, psychoanalyst Joel Whitebook (2017) published a biography of Freud, repeating what Rank said a century ago about the absence of the powerful mother in Freud's theories, yet he never cites Rank. Like almost all contemporary analysts, Whitebook is oblivious to Rank. The continuing neglect of Rank by modern analysts is exemplified by Whitebook's otherwise excellent biography.

2. As Ernest Jones "remarked in dismay, confidentially to Siegfried Bernfeld, 'Martha comes out of the letters excellently but Freud was very neurotic!' Jones could see that the state of being engaged had elicited an infantilism in Freud that must have been present all along" (Crews 2017:43).

Chapter 9

1. Ferenczi criticized transference only in the privacy of his *Clinical Diary*. In public, Ferenczi (1921) continued to insist that "the transference occurs spontaneously, the doctor needs only the skill not to disturb this process" (189).

2. Jacob Moreno, a psychiatrist and the founder of psychodrama, was the first to use the term "here-and-now" (Blatner 2005). It's possible that Rank borrowed the term from Moreno, a prominent theater director during the 1920s in Vienna who promoted spontaneity through the expression of creativity by his actors in the "here-and-now." At the *3rd World Congress of Existential Therapy: Living in the Here and Now*, Ernesto Spinelli (2023) observed: "Being in the here-and-how cannot be captured in prose because you are already then-and-there."

3. Throughout the 20th century, citations to Rank's writings far exceed citations to those of Ferenczi. For a comparison of their citations in English-language books, see: https://books.google.com/ngrams/graph?content=Otto+Rank%2CSandor+Ferenczi&year_start=1905&year_end=2019&corpus=en-2019&smoothing=3.

4. Rank drafted *The Trauma of Birth* in April 1923 and published it in December, the same month in which he and Ferenczi published *The Development of Psychoanalysis*. Rank's typist Editha Sterba recalls that he dictated the manuscript of *The Trauma of Birth* to her from "off the top of his head" (quoted in Lieberman 1985:201). But the large number of books and articles cited by Rank in his text suggests that he dictated only a preliminary draft to Sterba, perhaps just the short preface, and later went over the whole manuscript with great thoroughness, as he did with all his writings.

Chapter 10

1. By 2025, there will be an estimated one billion menopausal women in the world (Staszak 2023).

2. English professor Mark Edmunson (2023) maintains that "Freud championed female sexuality, and at the time at least, that meant he championed women" (98). But how could Freud champion female sexuality when it remained, according to psychoanalysts Cohler and Galatzer-Levy (2008), forever "unknown to Freud" (23)? For a philosophical exploration by a woman of why female sexuality remained forever "unknown to Freud," see Tuana (2004; 2006).

Chapter 11

1. After seeing his analyst for fifteen years, Woody Allen remarked: "I'll give it one more year and then I'll go to Lourdes'" (quoted in Burns & Burns-Lundgren 2015:29).

2. I thank Ruhama Veltfort, Rank's granddaughter, for allowing me to publish excerpts from these previously unpublished letters. E. James Lieberman provided me with transcripts.

3. See Hill & Norcross (2023) for the most recent evidence on the effectiveness of over two dozen psychotherapy skills and methods, all of which presuppose an authentic relationship between therapist and client: affirmation/validation; self-disclosure; immediacy; rupture repairs; questions; Socratic questions and guided discovery; empathic reflection; metaphors; interpretations; paradoxical interventions; advice, suggestions, and recommendations; between session homework; silence; dyadic synchrony; role induction; collaborative

assessment methods; strength-based methods; routine outcome monitoring; emotion regulation; chairwork; dream work; meditation, mindfulness, and acceptance; behavioral activation; and cognitive restructuring. https://global.oup.com/academic/product/psychotherapy-skills-and-methods-that-work-9780197611012?cc=hu&lang=en&#.

Chapter 12

1. Often pointing to "the beyond" in his writings, Rank used this term in *The Trauma of Birth* (1924:131); in *Art and Artist* (1932a:49n; 143; 144; 271; 292; 308; 339); and in *Beyond Psychology* (1941a:56; 58; 195). During her therapy with Rank, Anaïs Nin (1966) observed that Rank, unlike other analysts, "detours the obvious, and begins a vast expansion into the greater, the vaster, the beyond" (289). I return to "the beyond" in my Epilogue.

2. Historian of psychoanalysis André Haynal (2008) observes that Freud, even when he was suffering from the agonies of his oral cancer, distanced himself from the feelings registered in his own body. "The history of Freud's illness shows that he tried to avoid confrontation with [his body], and to treat it as unimportant. In his personal letters, the ill body remains *outside*— as another person, 'Konrad,' not he himself—and it is not taken into account," writes Haynal (2008:103; italics in the original) of Freud's cancer. After surgeries removed part of his jaw and upper palate, Freud was forced to insert a painful, ill-fitting prosthesis into his mouth. He asked Anna, who helped him remove the blood-soaked prosthesis at night before going to sleep and re-insert it, with an equal amount of blood spilled, in the morning, to treat the process with the objectivity of a surgeon, showing no feelings whatsoever. She complied for the next sixteen years, until his death in 1939. The expression of feelings was taboo (Jones 1957:101).

3. Rank's will therapy is a precursor of embodied approaches to therapy, such as meditation, somatic breathwork, and Gestalt therapy (Wadlington, in press). Paul Goodman, while constructing the theoretical basis for Gestalt therapy, leaned heavily on Rank, whose "formulation of the [here-and-now]," writes Goodman's biographer, "has the therapeutic moment in view more explicitly than any other" (Stoehr 1994:126).

Chapter 13

1. Jessie Taft (1958) attended this conference, the first time she heard Rank speak. "An acquaintance who had worked in Vienna with both Freud and Rank had told me of something new and different in Rank's theory as well as in his therapeutic technique that had aroused immediate interest, although I had known nothing of Rank previously except his name and a title, *The Myth of the Birth of the Hero*" (ix)

2. See my Epilogue for how Rank's pointing to the existential unconscious influenced D.W. Winnicott, Jacques Lacan, and Samuel Beckett.

3. A copy of Rudolf Otto's *Das Heilige* was in Rank's library at the time of his death (Rank 1941b).

4. In a footnote in *Art and Artist*, Rank (1932a), quoting archaeologist Heinrich Sitte, writes that Bach, in his *Chromatic Fantasia and Fugue*, "set his own family name to music . . . 'Out of the double cry of anguish: B [flat]–A–C–H [= B natural] . . . which comprises his whole human existence, in joy and sorrow, as if it were his portrait'" (79n).

Chapter 14

1. A copy of Whitehead's *Process and Reality* was in Rank's library at the time of his death (Rank 1941b).

2. The German edition of Buber's *Ich und Du* was in Rank's library at the time his death (Rank 1941b); he probably read it when it was published in 1923, the same year in which he wrote *The Trauma of Birth*.

3. As an example of extreme narcissism, Rank points to the psychopath, who rarely if ever experiences empathy or guilt-feeling. "This type, in spite of appearances, is actually *weak*-willed," unable to control harmful emotions (Rank 1996:254; italics in the original). In his therapy practice, Rank had little or no experience with psychopathy, so his ideas on it are undeveloped. "While it is true that people with [psychopathy] display a range of disconcerting tendencies— including low empathy and remorse, grandiosity, impulsivity, and sometimes aggressive or violent behavior—new findings show not only that people with psychopathy have varying degrees and types of this condition but that the condition and its precursors can be treated" (DeAngelis 2022:46).

Chapter 15

1. As noted earlier, one year before meeting Rogers, Rank (1935) had told a group of social workers: "The whole psychoanalytic approach is centered around the therapist. *Real therapy has to be centered around the client, his difficulties, his needs, his activities*" (262; italics in the original). Rank would almost certainly have used similar language with Rogers during their time together. But in *Will Therapy*, Rank (1936a) used the word "patient," not "client." Regardless of the term he used, Rank, the first nonmedical analyst, never saw patients (or clients) through the lens of physicians, who traditionally objectified patients, paying little or no attention to their feelings. According to Jessie Taft, "the absence of medical presupposition" (Rank 1936a:xi) was central to Rank's practice of relationship therapy.

2. Today, we would call this process *gaslighting* (Dorpat 1996), which Oxford University Press defines as: "The action of manipulating someone by psychological means into accepting a false depiction of reality or doubting their own sanity." Gaslighting was on the "Word of the Year—Shortlist" published in 2018 by OUP. See https://languages.oup.com/word-of-the-year/2018-shortlist/.

3. Researchers in person-centered therapy are now examining whether Rogers's three core conditions can be merged into a single condition: *positive regard*—which might be redefined as unconditional respect for the difference of the other person (Farber et al. 2022).

Chapter 16

1. Taft's personal copy of this book is in the Otto Rank Collection, Columbia University Rare Book and Manuscript Library, Box 40.

Chapter 18

1. Rank played a large role in Lacan's self-image. Literary critic Shuli Barzilai (1999) writes: "Lacan wanted all his life . . . simultaneously to occupy two positions: both that of beloved son and intellectual companion, held by Rank before his break with Freud, *and* that of independent, ambitious, even renegade, creator held by Rank thereafter" (29; italics in the original).

References

Abzug, R.H. (2021). *Psyche and soul in America: The spiritual odyssey of Rollo May*. New York: Oxford University Press.

Adams, P.L. (1987). The mother not the father. *Journal of the American Academy of Psychoanalysis, 15,* 465–480.

Ahad, B.S. (2010). *Freud upside down: African-American literature and psychoanalytic culture.* Champaign: University of Illinois Press.

Alic, M. (2001). Otto Rank. In Strickland, B. (Ed.). *The Gale encyclopedia of psychology* (2nd ed.). Detroit: Gale, 535–536.

Alyan, H. (2023, October 25). The Palestine double standard. *New York Times.* https://www.nytimes.com/2023/10/25/opinion/palestine-war-empathy.html.

American Psychoanalytic Association (2023). *Holmes Commission Final Report.* https://apsa.org/wp-content/uploads/2023/06/Holmes-Commission-Final-Report-2023-Report-rv6-19-23.pdf?ver.

Améry, J. (1999). *At the mind's limits: Contemplations by a survivor on Auschwitz and its realities.* Rosenfeld, S. & Rosenfeld, S.P. (Eds.). London: Granta.

Amundson, J. (1981). Will in the psychology of Otto Rank: A transpersonal perspective. *Journal of Transpersonal Psychology, 13,* 113–124.

Anzieu, D. (2021). New views on Freud's self-analysis and the discovery of psychoanalysis. Vanderwees, C. (Tr.). *American Imago, 78,* 463–484.

Arendt, H. (1973). *The origins of totalitarianism* (Rev. ed.). New York: Harcourt Brace & Company.

Arendt, H. (1978). *The life of the mind.* Thinking, Vol. 1. Willing, Vol. 2. McCarthy, M. (Ed.). New York: Harcourt Brace Jovanovich.

Arendt, H. (1998). *The human condition* (2nd ed.). Chicago, IL: University of Chicago Press.

Arlow, J.A. (2002). Transference as defense. *Journal of the American Psychoanalytic Association, 50,* 1139–1150.

Arnold, T. (1935). *Symbols of government*: New Haven, CT: Yale University Press.

Aron, L. (1996). *A meeting of minds: Mutuality in psychoanalysis.* Hillsdale, NJ: Analytic Press.

Bair, D. (1995). *Anaïs Nin: A biography.* New York: Penguin Books.

Balsam, R.H. (2012). *Women's bodies in psychoanalysis.* New York: Routledge.

Balsam, R.H. (2013). Freud, females, childbirth, and dissidence: Margarete Hilferding, Karen Horney and Otto Rank. *Psychoanalytic Review, 100,* 695–716.

Balsam, R.H. (2016). The war on women in psychoanalytic theory: Past to present. In Lament, C., King, R.A., Abrams, S., Brinich, P.M. & Knight R. (Eds.), *The war against women in psychoanalytic culture.* New Haven, CT: Yale University Press, 83–107.

Barbré, C. (1999). Reversing the crease: Nietzsche's influence on Otto Rank's concept of creative will and the birth of individuality. In Golomb, J., Santaniello, W. & Lehrer, R. (Eds.), *Nietzsche and depth psychology.* Albany, NY: State University of New York, 247–267.

Barbré, C. (2004). Otto Rank's psychology of will and soul and its spiritual implications for psychotherapeutic theory and practice. Unpublished PhD dissertation. Union Theological Seminary.

Barbré, C. (2012). Confusion of wills: Otto Rank's contribution to understanding children. *American Journal of Psychoanalysis, 72,* 409–417.

Barbré, C. (2016). The contrapuntal play of paradox: Likeness and difference in the theories of Otto Rank. In Willock, B., Bohm, C.C. & Curtis, R.C. (Eds.), *Psychoanalytic perspectives on identity and difference: Navigating the divide.* New York: Routledge, 192–201.

Barrett-Lennard, G.T. (1998). *Carl Rogers' helping system: Journey and substance*. Thousand Oaks, CA: Sage Publications.

Barry, E., Maude, U.F. & Alisbury, L. (2016). Introduction-Beckett, medicine and the brain. *Journal of Medical Humanities, 37*, 127–135.

Barzilai, S. (1999). *Lacan and the matter of origins*. Stanford, CA: Stanford University Press.

Becker, E. (1968). *The structure of evil: An essay on the unification of the science of man*. New York: Braziller.

Becker, E. (1973). *The denial of death*. With a foreword by Sam Keen. New York: Free Press (1997 paperback edition).

Becker, E. (1974). The spectrum of loneliness. In Liechty, D. (Ed.). (2005). *The Ernest Becker reader*. Seattle & London: Ernest Becker Foundation in association with the University of Washington Press, 231–234.

Becker, E. (1975). *Escape from evil*. New York: Free Press.

Becker, E. (1982). Growing up rugged: Fritz Perls and gestalt therapy. *ReVision, 5*, 6–14.

Beckett, S. (1994). *I can't go on, I'll go on: A Samuel Beckett reader*. Seaver, R.W. (Ed.). New York: Grove Atlantic.

Benatar, D. (2006). *Better never to have been: The harm of coming into existence*. New York: Oxford University Press.

Bennis, W. (1989). *On becoming a leader*. Reading, MA: Addison-Wesley Publishing.

Bergmann, M. (2004). *Understanding dissidence and controversy in the history of psychoanalysis*. New York: Other Press.

Bernstein, J. (2023, March 22). Not your daddy's Freud: A new generation of analysts and patients is embracing the father of psychoanalysis—in magazines and memes and many hours on the couch. *New York Times*.

Bettelheim, B. (1990). *Freud's Vienna and other essays*. New York: Alfred A. Knopf.

Bielik-Robson, A. (2022). Psychoanalysis as *Torat Hayim*: In praise of separation. *European Judaism, 55*, 55–70.

Billig, M. (2017). Banal nationalism and the imagining of politics. In Skey, M. & Antonsich, M. (Eds.). *Everyday nationhood: Theorising culture, identity and belonging after Banal Nationalism*. London: Palgrave Macmillan, 307–322.

Binswanger, L. (1942). *Ausgewählte Werke Band 2: Grundformen und Erkenntnis menschlichen Daseins*. Herzog, M. & Braun, H.J. (Eds.). Heidelberg: Roland Asanger Verlag, 1993.

Binswanger, L. (1963). *Being-in-the-world: Selected papers*. Needleman, J. (Tr.) New York: Basic Books.

Blackmore, D.L. (1992). "That unreasonable restless feeling": The homosexual subtexts of Nella Larsen's *Passing*. *African American Review, 26*, 475–484.

Blatner, A. (2005). Perspectives on Moreno, psychodrama, and creativity. *Journal of Creativity in Mental Health, 1*, 111–121.

Bloom, H. (1973). *The anxiety of influence: A theory of poetry*. New York: Oxford University Press.

Bloom, H. (1981). Freud and the poetic sublime: A catastrophe theory of creativity. In Meisel, P. (Ed.), *Freud: A collection of critical essays*. Englewood Cliffs, NJ: Prentice-Hall, 211–231.

Bloom, H. (1983). Reading Freud: Transference, taboo, and truth. In Cook, E., Hosek, C., Macpherson, J., Parker, P., & Patrick, J. (Eds.). *Centre and labyrinth: Essays in honour of Northrop Frye*. Toronto: University of Toronto Press, 309–329.

Bloom, H. (1986, March 23). Freud: The greatest modern writer. *New York Times Book Review*.

Bloom, H. (1991). The art of criticism: No.1. Interview by Antonio Weiss. *Paris Review, 118*, 178–232.

Bloom, P. (2016). *Against empathy: The case for rational compassion*. New York: Ecco.

Blum, H.P. (2022). The dawn of the Oedipus complex: A tale of two letters. In Weissberg, L. (Ed.). *Psychoanalysis, fatherhood, and the modern family*. New York: Palgrave Macmillan, 57–72.

Blum, H.P. & Blum, E.J. (2022). Evolution of Freudian psychoanalytic thought in the twentieth-century USA: The influence of the European émigrés. *International Forum of Psychoanalysis, 32*, 87–92.

Bohart, A.C. (2003). Person-centered psychotherapy and related experiential approaches. In Gurman, A.S. & Messer, S.B. (Eds.). *Essential psychotherapies: Theory and practice* (2nd ed.). New York: Guilford Press, 107–148.

Bohart, A. (2006). The active client. In Norcross, J.C., Beutler, L.E., & Levant, R.F. (Eds.). *Evidence-based practices in mental health: Debate and dialogue on the fundamental questions.* Washington DC: American Psychological Association, 218–226.

Bollas, C. (1987). *The shadow of the object: Psychoanalysis of the unthought known.* New York: Columbia University Press.

Bonaduce, J. (2023). The prenatal origin of myth, religion, and ritual. *Journal for Prenatal and Perinatal Psychology and Health 37*, 87–97.

Bradatan, C. (2023). *In praise of failure: Four lessons in humility.* Cambridge, MA: Harvard University Press.

Breger, L. (2000). *Freud: Darkness in the midst of vision.* New York: Wiley.

Bruce, J. (2023, May 26). Racism: The elephant in the consulting room. Webinar. International Psychoanalytical Association. https://www.ipa.world/en/en/IPA1/Webinars/Psychoanalysis_and_Racism_on_the_road_to_Cartagena.aspx.

Bryngelsson, E. (2016). The problem of unity in psychoanalysis: Birth trauma and separation. In Bornemark, J. & Smith, N. (Eds.). *Phenomenology of pregnancy.* Stockholm: Södertörn University Press, 225–250.

Buber, M. (1923). *I and thou.* Smith, R.G. (Tr.). Edinburgh: T.&T. Clark, 1937.

Burns, J.M. (1978). *Leadership.* New York: Harper & Row.

Burns, J.M. (2003). *Transforming leadership: A new pursuit of happiness.* New York: Atlantic Monthly Press.

Burns, T. & Burns-Lundgren, E. (2015). *Psychotherapy: A very short introduction.* New York: Oxford University Press.

Burston, D. (1996). *The wing of madness: The life and work of R.D. Laing.* Cambridge, MA: Harvard University Press, 1996.

Butler, J.A., Herzberg, G.E. & Miller, R.L. (Eds.) (2024). *Integral psychedelic therapy: The nonordinary art of psychospiritual healing.* New York: Routledge.

Carter, C.J. (2023, January 27). All the rage: The whiteness of psychoanalysis, and what it cannot dare to see. Online newsletter of Section IX, Psychoanalysis for Social Responsibility, Society of Psychoanalysis and Psychoanalytic Psychology, Division 39 of the American Psychological Association. https://psychoanalyticactivist.com/2023/01/27/all-the-rage-the-whiteness-of-psychoanalysis-and-what-it-cannot-dare-to-see/.

Cave, S. (2012). *Immortality: The quest to live forever and how it drives civilization.* New York: Crown Publishers.

Chalmers, D.J. (1995). Facing up to the problem of consciousness. *Journal of Consciousness Studies 2*, 200–219.

Chamberlain, L. (2000). *The secret artist: A close reading of Sigmund Freud.* New York: Seven Stories Press.

Chamberlain, M. (2022). *Misogyny in psychoanalysis.* Oxfordshire: Phoenix.

Charnock, R.N.E. (2011). Touching stories: Performances of intimacy in the diary of Anaïs Nin. Unpublished PhD dissertation. University of Sussex, U.K.

Chertok, L. & Stengers, I. (1992). *A critique of psychoanalytic reason: Hypnosis as a scientific problem from Lavoisier to Lacan.* Stanford, CA: Stanford University Press.

Child, I.L. (1991). Rankian psychology. In Craighead, W.E. & Nemeroff, C.B. (Eds.). *The Corsini encyclopedia of psychology and the behavioral sciences*, Vol. 4 (3rd ed.). New York: John Wiley & Sons, 1366–1367.

Clark, H. (2020). *Red comet: The short life and blazing art of Sylvia Plath.* New York: Alfred A. Knopf.

Clark, M. (1988). *Jacques Lacan: An annotated bibliography*, Vol. 1. New York: Garland.

Clark, R.W. (1980). *Freud: The man and the cause.* New York: Random House.

Cnaan, R.A., Dichter, M.E. & Draine, J. (2008). *A century of social work and social welfare at Penn.* Philadelphia: University of Pennsylvania Press.

Cohen, R. (2023, November 20). Between Israelis and Palestinians, a lethal psychological chasm grows. *New York Times.*

Cohler, B.J. & Galatzer-Levy, R. M. (2008). Freud, Anna, and the problem of female sexuality. *Psychoanalytic Inquiry, 28,* 3–26.

Coleridge, S.T. (1831). *The friend: A series of essays, to aid in the formation of fixed principles in politics, morals, and religion, with literary amusements interspersed.* Burlington: Chauncey Goodrich.

Columbia Library Columns (1984). Otto Rank century issue, *33,* 1–26.

Conroy, J.O. (2023, June 16). Inside the war tearing psychoanalysis apart: "The most hatred I've ever witnessed." *Guardian.*

Cooper, M. (2017). *Existential therapies* (2nd ed.). Thousand Oaks, CA: Sage Publications.

Cooper, M., O'Hara, M., Schmid, P. & Bohart, A. (Eds.) (2013). *The handbook of person-centred psychotherapy and counselling* (2nd ed.). New York: Palgrave Macmillan.

Coren, A. (2001). *Short-term psychotherapy: A psychodynamic approach.* London: Palgrave.

Crewe, S.E., Brown A.W., & Gourdine, R.M. (2008). Inabel Burns Lindsay: A social worker, educator, and administrator uncompromising in the pursuit of social justice for all. *Affilia: Feminist Inquiry in Social Work, 23,* 363–377.

Crews, F. (2017). *Freud: The making of an illusion.* New York: Metropolitan Books.

Crosby, P. (1970). Letter to the Editors. *Journal of the Otto Rank Association, 5,* 101–102.

Crosby, P. & Janus, L. (2017). Eine Analyse bei Otto Rank. *Forum der Psychoanalyse: Zeitschrift für psychodynamische Theorie und Praxis, 33,* 447–457.

Cummings, E.E. (1965). *A miscellany revised.* Firmage, G.J. (Ed.). New York: October House.

Cummings, E.E. (1991). *Complete poems 1904–1962.* Firmage, G.J. (Ed.). New York: Liveright.

Damasio, A. (1994). *Descartes' error: Emotion, reason, and the human brain.* New York: Avon Books.

Damasio, A. (2018). *The strange order of things: Life, feeling, and the making of cultures.* New York: Pantheon.

Davis, T.M. (1994). *Nella Larsen, novelist of the Harlem Renaissance: A Woman's life unveiled .* Baton Rouge: Louisiana State University Press.

DeAngelis, T. (2022, March). A broader view of psychopathy. *APA Monitor on Psychology, 53,* 46–51.

deCarvalho, R.J. (1999). Otto Rank, the Rankian circle in Philadelphia, and the origins of Carl Rogers' person-centered psychotherapy. *History of Psychology, 2,* 132–148.

Deegan, M.J. (1991). *Women in sociology: A bio-biographical sourcebook.* New York: Greenwood Press.

De Marchi, L. (1992). *Otto Rank: Pioniere misconosciuto.* Rome: Melasuna.

De Mille, A. (1991). *Martha: The life and work of Martha Graham: A biography.* New York: Random House.

Dewan, M.J. & Gupta, S. (1992). Congruence between Hindu philosophy and writings of Otto Rank. *Psychological Reports, 70,* 127–130.

Diprose, R. & Ziarek, E.P. (2018). *Arendt, natality and biopolitics: Toward democratic plurality and reproductive justice.* Edinburgh: Edinburgh University Press.

Dixon, N. (1999). *The organizational learning cycle: How we can learn collectively.* London: Gower.

H.D. (Hilda Doolittle) (1956). *Tribute to Freud.* New York: Pantheon.

Dominus, S. (2023, May 16). Does therapy really work? Let's unpack that. *New York Times Magazine.*

Dorfman, E. (2020). *Double trouble: The doppelgänger from romanticism to postmodernism.* New York: Routledge.

Dorpat, T.L. (1996). *Gaslighting, the double whammy, interrogation, and other methods of covert control in psychotherapy and analysis.* Northvale, NJ: Jason Aronson.

Du Bois, W.E.B. (1903a). *The souls of black folk.* New York: Dover, 1994.

Du Bois, W.E.B. (1903b). The talented tenth. In Washington, B.T. (Ed.). *The Negro problem: A series of articles by representative American Negroes of today.* New York: James Pott and Company, 31–75.

Dufresne, T. (2000). *Tales from the Freudian crypt: The death drive in text and context.* Stanford, CA: Stanford University Press.

Dufresne, T. (2007). *Against Freud: Critics talk back.* Stanford, CA: Stanford University Press.

Dupont, J. (Ed.) (2006). Otto Rank, l'accoucheur du sujet. *Le Coq-Héron, 187,* 1–79.

Dupont, J. (Ed.) (2012). Recognizing Otto Rank, an innovator. *American Journal of Psycho-analysis, 72,* 315–417.

Eccles, J. (1992). A divine design: Some questions on origins. In Margenau, H. & Varghese R.A. (Eds.). *Cosmos, bios, theos: Scientists reflect on science, God, and the origins of the universe, life, and homo sapiens.* La Salle, IL: Open Court, 160–164.

Economist. (2023, September 2–8). How paranoid nationalism corrupts.

Edmundson, M. (2023). *The age of guilt: The super-ego in the online world.* New Haven, CT: Yale University Press.

Ehrenreich, J.H. (1985). *The altruistic imagination: A history of social work and social policy in the United States.* Ithaca, NY: Cornell University Press.

Ekenstierna, I.S. (2024). *The part-whole relation: Otto Rank, David Bohm, and a therapeutic third.* Unpublished PhD dissertation. University of Queensland, Australia.

Ellingham, I. (2011). Carl Rogers's fateful wrong move in the development of Rogerian relational therapy: Retitling "relationship therapy" "non-directive therapy." *Person-Centered and Experiential Therapies, 10,* 181–197.

Ellis, H. (1923). *The dance of life.* Boston: Houghton Mifflin.

Elshtain, J.B. (2015, February 3). Identity, the state and sacrifice. *Library of Social Science Newsletter.* Online only. https://www.libraryofsocialscience.com/newsletter/posts/2015/2015-02-03-Elshtain.html

Evans, R. (1975). *Carl Rogers: The man and his ideas.* New York: E.P. Dutton.

Evertz, K., Janus, L. & Linder, R. (Eds.) (2021). *Handbook of prenatal and perinatal psychology: Integrating research and practice.* Cham: Springer Nature.

Fallend, K. (2012). *Caroline Newton, Jessie Taft, Virginia Robinson: Spurensuche in der Geschichte der Psychoanalyse und Sozialarbeit.* Vienna: Erhard Löcker.

Falzeder, E. (1998). Family tree matters. *Journal of Analytical Psychology, 43,* 127–154.

Falzeder, E. (2015). *Psychoanalytic filiations: Mapping the psychoanalytic movement.* London: Karnac.

Falzeder, E. (2016). Freud the analyst and therapist. In Kollreuter, A. (Ed.). *What is this Professor Freud like? A diary of an analysis with historical comments.* London: Karnac, 87–102.

Farber, B.A., Suzuki, J.Y., & Ort, D. (2022). What is positive regard, and why is it important? In Farber, B.A., Suzuki, J.Y., & Ort, D. *Understanding and enhancing positive regard in psychotherapy: Carl Rogers and beyond.* Washington, DC: American Psychological Association, 13–37.

Ferenczi, S. (1921). The further development of the "active technique" in psychoanalysis. In Borossa, J. (Ed.). *Sándor Ferenczi: Selected writings.* London: Penguin Books, 187–204, 1988.

Ferenczi, S. (1932). *The clinical diary of Sándor Ferenczi.* Dupont, J. (Ed.). Balint, M. & Jackson, N.Z. (Trs.). Cambridge, MA: Harvard University Press, 1988.

Ferenczi, S. & Rank, O. (1924). *The development of psychoanalysis.* Newton, C. (Tr.). New York: Dover, 1956.

Finkelstein, H. (1996). *Salvador Dalí's art and writing, 1927–1942: The metamorphoses of Narcissus.* Cambridge, UK: Cambridge University Press.

Fisher, M. (2022, February 24). Putin's case for war, annotated. *New York Times*.

Fortune, C. (1993). The case of "RN": Sandor Ferenczi's radical experiment in psychoanalysis. In Aron, L., & Harris, A. (Eds.). *The legacy of Sándor Ferenczi*. New York: Analytic Press, 101–120.

Fox, M. (1995). Otto Rank on the artistic journey as a spiritual journey, the spiritual journey as an artistic journey. In Fox, M. *Wrestling with the prophets: Essays on creation spirituality and everyday life*. San Francisco: HarperCollins, 199–242.

Fox, M. (2002). *Creativity: Where the divine and the human meet*. New York: Jeremy Tarcher/Putnam.

Fox, M. (2014). Psychotherapy and the "unio mystica": Meister Eckhart meets Otto Rank. In Fox, M. *Meister Eckhart: A mystic-warrior for our times*. San Francisco: New World Library, 139–156.

Franko, M. (2012). *Martha Graham in love and war: The life in the work*. New York: Oxford University Press.

Frederiksen-Goldsen, K.I., Lindhorst, T., Kemp, S.P. & Walters, K.L. (2009). "My ever dear": Social work's "lesbian" foremothers—a call for scholarship. *Affilia: Feminist Inquiry in Social Work, 24*, 325–336.

Freud, A. (1954). The widening scope of indications for psychoanalysis. *The writings of Anna Freud*, Vol. 4. New York: International Universities Press, 356–376, 1968.

Freud, A. (1966). *The ego and the mechanisms of defense*. New York: International Universities Press.

Freud, E. L. (Ed.) (1960). *Letters of Sigmund Freud*. Stern, T. & Stern, J. (Trs.). New York: Basic Books.

Freud, M. (1958). *Sigmund Freud: Man and father*. New York: Vanguard.

Freud, S. (1905). Three essays on the theory of sexuality. In Strachey, J. (Ed. and Tr.). *The standard edition of the complete psychological works of Sigmund Freud*, Vol. 7. London: Hogarth, 125–245, 1953.

Freud, S. (1912). Recommendations to physicians practicing psychoanalysis. In Strachey, J. (Ed. and Tr.). *The standard edition of the complete psychological works of Sigmund Freud*, Vol. 12. London: Hogarth, 109–120, 1958.

Freud, S. (1914). On narcissism: An introduction. In Strachey, J. (Ed. and Tr.). *The standard edition of the complete psychological works of Sigmund Freud*, Vol. 14. London: Hogarth, 73–102, 1958.

Freud, S. (1915). The unconscious. In Strachey, J. (Ed. and Tr.). *The standard edition of the complete psychological works of Sigmund Freud*, Vol. 14. London: Hogarth, 159–215, 1958.

Freud, S. (1916). Some character types met within psychoanalytic work. In Strachey, J. (Ed. and Tr.). *The standard edition of the complete psychological works of Sigmund Freud*, Vol. 14. London: Hogarth, 303–333, 1958.

Freud S. (1916–1917). *Introductory lectures on psycho-analysis*. In Strachey, J. (Ed. and Tr.). *The standard edition of the complete psychological works of Sigmund Freud*, Vols. 15–16. London: Hogarth, 13–463, 1963.

Freud S. (1920). *Beyond the pleasure principle*. In Strachey, J. (Ed. and Tr.). *The standard edition of the complete psychological works of Sigmund Freud*, Vol. 18. London: Hogarth, 3–66, 1958.

Freud S. (1921). *Group psychology and the analysis of the ego*. In Strachey, J. (Ed. and Tr.). *The standard edition of the complete psychological works of Sigmund Freud*, Vol. 18. London: Hogarth, 67–143, 1958.

Freud, S. (1923a). *The ego and the id*. In Strachey, J. (Ed. and Tr.). *The standard edition of the complete psychological works of Sigmund Freud*, Vol. 19. London: Hogarth, 3–59, 1961.

Freud, S. (1923b). Two encyclopaedia articles. In Strachey, J. (Ed. and Tr.). *The standard edition of the complete psychological works of Sigmund Freud*, Vol. 18. London: Hogarth, 235–262, 1961.

Freud, S. (1924). The dissolution of the Oedipus complex. In Strachey, J. (Ed. and Tr.). *The standard edition of the complete psychological works of Sigmund Freud*, Vol. 19. London: Hogarth, 173–179, 1961.

Freud, S. (1925). Some psychic consequences of the anatomical difference between the sexes. In Strachey, J. (Ed. and Tr.). *The standard edition of the complete psychological works of Sigmund Freud*, Vol. 19. London: Hogarth, 243–260, 1961.

Freud, S. (1926a). Inhibitions, symptoms and anxiety. In Strachey, J. (Ed. and Tr.). *The standard edition of the complete psychological works of Sigmund Freud*, Vol. 20. London: Hogarth, 77–178, 1964.

Freud, S. (1926b). The question of lay analysis. In Strachey, J. (Ed. and Tr.). *The standard edition of the complete psychological works of Sigmund Freud*, Vol. 20. London: Hogarth, 177–258, 1964.

Freud, S. (1927). The future of an illusion. In Strachey, J. (Ed. and Tr.). *The standard edition of the complete psychological works of Sigmund Freud*, Vol. 21. London: Hogarth, 3–56, 1964.

Freud, S. (1930). Civilization and its discontents. In Strachey, J. (Ed. and Tr.). *The standard edition of the complete psychological works of Sigmund Freud*, Vol. 21. London: Hogarth, 59–145, 1964.

Freud, S. (1933). New introductory lectures on psychoanalysis. In Strachey, J. (Ed. and Tr.). *The standard edition of the complete psychological works of Sigmund Freud*, Vol. 22. London: Hogarth, 3–182, 1964.

Freud, S. (1937). Analysis terminable and interminable. In Strachey, J. (Ed. and Tr.). *The standard edition of the complete psychological works of Sigmund Freud*, Vol. 23. London: Hogarth, 211–254, 1974.

Freud, S. (1939). Moses and monotheism. In Strachey, J. (Ed. and Tr.). *The standard edition of the complete psychological works of Sigmund Freud*, Vol. 23. London: Hogarth, 3–140, 1974.

Freud, S. (1940). An outline of psycho-analysis. In Strachey, J. (Ed. and Tr.). *The standard edition of the complete psychological works of Sigmund Freud*, Vol. 23. London: Hogarth, 141–207, 1974.

Freud, S. (1992). *The diary of Sigmund Freud, 1929–1939: A record of the final decade*. Molnar, M. (Ed.). New York: Charles Scribner's Sons.

Freud, S. & Eitingon, M. (2004). *Briefwechsel 1906–1939, Band II*. Schröter, M. (Ed.). Tübingen: edition diskord.

Freud, S. & Ferenczi, S. (1993). *The correspondence of Sigmund Freud and Sándor Ferenczi: Vol. 1, 1908–1914*. Brabant, E., Falzeder E. & Giampieri-Deutsch, P. (Eds.). Hoffer, P.T. (Tr.). Cambridge, MA: Harvard University Press.

Freud, S. & Ferenczi, S. (2000). *The correspondence of Sigmund Freud and Sándor Ferenczi: Vol. 3, 1920–1933*. Falzeder E. & Brabant, E. (Eds.). Hoffer, P.T. (Tr.). Cambridge, MA: Harvard University Press.

Freund, P. (Ed.) (1959). *The myth of the birth of the hero and other writings by Otto Rank*. New York: Vintage Books.

Frie, R. (2021, December 9). Dark shadows: Erich Fromm, social psychoanalysis and systemic racism. Lecture. International University of Psychoanalysis, Berlin. https://www.ipu-berlin.de/en/the-significance-of-erich-fromms-thinking-for-psychoanalytic-practice/.

Friedan, B. (1963). *The feminine mystique*. New York: Dell.

Friedan, B. (2013). *The feminine mystique: A Norton critical edition*. Fermaglich, K., & Fine, L.(Eds.). New York: W.W. Norton.

Friedman, M. (1967). *To deny our nothingness: Contemporary images of man*. New York: Delacorte.

Fromm, E. (1959). *Sigmund Freud's mission: An analysis of his personality and influence*. New York: Harper & Brothers Publishers.

Furman, R. (2002). Jessie Taft and the functional school: The impact of our history. *Canadian Social Work, 4*, 7–13.

Gallant, J. (2016). Otto Rank: Variations on a theme. *Fortnightly Review.* https://fortnightlyreview.co.uk/2016/11/otto-rank/.

Garai, J.E. (1977). The will and empathy in art therapy. *Journal of the Otto Rank Association, 12,* 32–53.

Gates, H.L. & Oliver, T.H. (Eds.) (1999). Du Bois, W.E. *The souls of black folk: A Norton critical edition.* New York: W.W. Norton.

Gay, P. (1988). *Freud: A life for our times.* New York: W.W. Norton.

Geismar, M. (1973). Evading art and society. *Chicago Review 24,* 85–92.

Gendlin, E. T. (1988). Obituary: Carl Rogers (1902–1987). *American Psychologist, 43,* 127–128.

Gentile, J. (2018). Trump, Freud and the puzzle of femininity. *Los Angeles Review of Books.* https://thephilosophicalsalon.com/trump-freud-and-the-puzzle-of-femininity.

Goethals, G.R., Sorenson, G.J., & Burns, J.M. (2004). *Encyclopedia of leadership.* (Vols. 1–4). Thousand Oaks, CA: Sage Publications.

Goldenberg, I., Stanton, M. & Goldenberg, H. (2017). *Family therapy: An overview.* Boston: Cengage.

Goldsmith, J.A. & Laks, B. (2019). *Battle in the mind fields.* Chicago, IL: University of Chicago Press.

Goldwert, M. (1985). Otto Rank and man's urge to immortality. *Journal of the History of the Behavioral Sciences, 21,* 169–177.

Gómez-Márquez J. (2021). What is life? *Molecular Biology Reports, 48,* 6223–6230.

Govrin, A. (2016). *Conservative and radical perspectives on psychoanalytic knowledge: The fascinated and the disenchanted.* New York: Routledge.

Graham, J.S. (1960). Otto Rank and Martin Buber: The healing potentialities of dialogue. Unpublished MA thesis. Cornell University.

Graybeal, C. (2001). Strengths-based social work assessments: Transforming the dominant paradigm. *Families in Society: The Journal of Contemporary Social Services, 82,* 233–242.

Grayling, A.C. (2000, February 26). The last word on nationalism. *Guardian.*

Green, A. (2023). *On the destruction and death drives.* Levine, H.B.(Ed.). Jaron, S. (Tr.). Oxfordshire: Phoenix.

Greening, T. (1995). Commentary by the editor. Special issue: Carl Rogers—the man and his ideas. *Journal of Humanistic Psychology, 35,* 4–6.

Griffiths, M. (2017). *The challenge of existential social work.* New York: Red Globe Press.

Groddeck, G. (2001). Rank in Freud's school. Rudnytsky, P.L. (Tr.). *American Imago, 58,* 841–845.

Grof, S. (1985). *Beyond the brain: Birth, death, and transcendence in psychotherapy.* Albany: State University of New York Press.

Grosskurth, P. (1991). *The secret ring: Freud's inner circle and the politics of psychoanalysis.* Reading, MA: Addison-Wesley.

Guralnik, O. (2023, May 16). I'm a couples therapist. Something new is happening in relationships. *New York Times Magazine.*

Haggbloom, S.J., Warnick, R., Warnick, J.E., Jones, V.K., Yarbrough, G.L., Russell, T.M., Borecky, C.M., McGahhey R., Powell, J.L., Beavers, J. & Monte, E. (2002). The 100 most eminent psychologists of the 20th century. *Review of General Psychology, 6,* 139–152.

Hall W. (2022). Why was early therapeutic research on psychedelic drugs abandoned? *Psychological Medicine, 52,* 26–31.

Halliwell, M. (1999). *Romantic science and the experience of self: Transatlantic crosscurrents from William James to Oliver Sacks.* Aldershot: Ashgate.

Hampden-Turner, C. (1982). *Maps of the mind.* New York: Macmillan.

Hankiss, E. (2001). *Fears and symbols: An introduction to the study of Western civilization.* Budapest and New York: Central European University Press.

Hardarson, T., Van Landuyt, L. & Jones, G. (2012). The blastocyst. *Human Reproduction, 27*, i72–i91.

Harrison I.B. (1979). On Freud's view of the infant-mother relationship and of the oceanic feeling—some subjective influences. *Journal of the American Psychoanalytic Association, 27*, 399–421.

Haynal, A. (1993). Ferenczi and the origins of the psychoanalytic technique. In Aron, L. & Harris, A. (Eds.). *The legacy of Sándor Ferenczi.* Hillsdale, NJ: Analytic Press, 53–74.

Haynal, A. (2002). *Disappearing and reviving: Sándor Ferenczi in the history of psychoanalysis.* London: Karnac.

Haynal A. (2008). Freud, his illness, and ourselves. *American Journal of Psychoanalysis, 68*, 103–116.

Haynes, K.S. (2014). Social workers as leaders. *Social Work Today.* Online only. https://www.socialworktoday.com/archive/exc_040714.shtml.

Hedges, C. (2002). *War is a force that gives us meaning.* New York: PublicAffairs.

Heidenreich, T., Noyon, A., Worrell, M., & Menzies, R. (2021). Existential approaches and cognitive behavior therapy: Challenges and potential. *International Journal of Cognitive Therapy, 14*, 209–234.

Heisenberg, W. (1958). *Physics and philosophy.* New York: Harper & Brothers.

Heller, J.B. (1973). Freud's father and mother. In Ruitenbeck, H.M. (Ed.). *Freud as we knew him.* Detroit: Wayne State University Press, 334–340.

Helson, R. & Pals, J.L. (2000). Creative potential, creative achievement, and personal growth. *Journal of Personality, 68*, 1–27.

Hill, C.E. & Norcross, J.C. (Eds.) (2023). *Psychotherapy skills and methods that work.* New York: Oxford University Press. Online edition. https://doi.org/10.1093/oso/9780197611012.001.0001.

Hinshelwood, R.D. (2023). *The mystery of emotions: Seeking a theory of what we feel.* Bicester: Phoenix.

Hoffman, I.Z. (2006). The myths of free association and the potentials of the analytic relationship. *International Journal of Psychoanalysis, 87*, 43–61.

Hoffman, L. (2017). *Un homme manqué*: Freud's engagement with Alfred Adler's masculine protest: Commentary on Balsam. *Journal of the American Psychoanalytic Association, 65*, 99–108.

Homans, P. (1989). *The ability to mourn: Disillusionment and the social origins of psychoanalysis.* Chicago, IL: University of Chicago Press.

Horney, K. (1924). On the genesis of the castration complex in women. *International Journal of Psychoanalysis, 5*, 50–65.

Hudson, L. (1992, July). Illicit inspiration. *Times* [London] *Literary Supplement*, 7.

Humann, H.D. (2018). *Another me: The doppelganger in 21st century fiction, television and film.* Jefferson: McFarland & Company.

Hutchinson, G.B. (2006). *In search of Nella Larsen: A biography of the color line.* Cambridge, MA: Harvard University Press.

Hyman, S.E. (1962). *The tangled bank: Darwin, Marx, Frazer and Freud as imaginative writers.* New York: Atheneum.

International Society for the Science of Existential Psychology. Website. https://www.issep.org/the-science-of-existential-psychology.

Isono, M. (2011). *Otto Rank: The creator of a relation-based psychology of the self: Toward a theory of affects.* Unpublished PhD dissertation. Institute for Contemporary Psychoanalysis, Los Angeles, CA.

Isono, M. (2012). An exploration in the will psychology of Otto Rank: Human intentionality and individuality. *American Journal of Psychoanalysis, 72*, 397–408.

James, W. (1902). *The varieties of religious experience: A study in human nature.* New York: Modern Library, 1929.

Janus, L. (Ed.). (1998). Die Wiederentdeckung Otto Ranks für die Psychoanalyse. *psychosozial*, *73*, 1–168.

Janus, L. (2024). *The enduring effects of prenatal experiencing: Echoes from the womb*. Dowling, T. (Tr.). New Castle upon Tyne: Cambridge Scholars Publishing.

Jason, P.K. (1978). Doubles/Don Juans: Anaïs Nin and Otto Rank. *Mosaic: An Interdisciplinary Critical Journal*, *11*, 81–94.

Johnson, R.E. (1975). *In quest of a new psychology: Toward a redefinition of humanism*. New York: Human Science Press.

John-Steiner, V. (1989). From life to diary to art in the work of Anaïs Nin. In Wallace, D.B. & Gruber, H.E. (Eds.). *Creative people at work: Twelve cognitive studies*. New York: Oxford University Press, 209–226.

Johnston, W.M. (1983). *The Austrian mind: An intellectual and social history 1848–1938*. Berkeley: University of California Press.

Jones, E. (1953). *The life and work of Sigmund Freud (Vol. 1). The formative years and the great discoveries, 1856–1900*. New York: Basic Books.

Jones, E. (1955). *The life and work of Sigmund Freud (Vol. 2). The years of maturity, 1901–1919*. New York: Basic Books.

Jones, E. (1957). *The life and work of Sigmund Freud (Vol. 3). The last phase, 1919–1939*. New York: Basic Books.

Jones, J. (1960). Otto Rank: A forgotten heresy. *Commentary*, *30*, 219–229.

Jong, E. (1993). *The devil at large: Erica Jong on Henry Miller*. New York: Turtle Bay Books.

Josselson, R. (2008). *Irvin D. Yalom: On psychotherapy and the human condition*. New York: Jorge Pinto Books.

Kahn, M. (1997). *Between therapist and client: The new relationship* (2nd ed.). New York: W.H. Freeman and Company.

Kainer, R.G.K. & Kainer, S. (2003). The anxiety of influence in the creation of theory. In Roland, A., Ulanov, B. & Barbré, C. (Eds.). *Creative dissent: Psychoanalysis in evolution*. Westport, CT: Praeger, 3–10.

Kamin, R. (2002). *Otto Rank's critique of psychoanalysis in light of philosophical hermeneutics*. Unpublished PhD dissertation. California School of Professional Psychology at Alameda.

Karpf, F. (1953). *The psychology and psychotherapy of Otto Rank: An historical and comparative introduction*. New York: Philosophical Library.

Katsafanas, P. (2018). Nietzsche's account of self-conscious agency. *Philosophical Explorations: An International Journal for the Philosophy of Mind and Action*, *21*, 122–137.

Kaufman, S.B. (2020). *Transcend: The new science of self-actualization*. New York: Tarcher-Perigee.

Keen, S. (2006). *The future of evil*. New York: Becker Press.

Kellerman, B. (2024). *Leadership from bad to worse: What happens when bad festers*. New York: Oxford University Press.

Kierkegaard, S. (1843). *Repetition: An essay in experimental psychology*. Lowrie, W. (Tr.). Princeton, NJ: Princeton University Press, 1946.

Kindersley, D. (2012). *The psychology book*. London: DK Publishers.

Kirschenbaum, H. (1979). *On becoming Carl Rogers*. New York: Delacorte.

Kirschenbaum, H. (2007). *The life and work of Carl Rogers*. Ross-on-Wye: PCCS Books.

Kirschenbaum, H. & Henderson, V.L. (Eds.) (1989a). *Carl Rogers: Dialogues*. Boston: Houghton Mifflin.

Kirschenbaum, H. & Henderson, V.L. (Eds.) (1989b). *The Carl Rogers reader*. Boston: Houghton Mifflin.

Kirschenbaum, H. & Jourdan, A. (2005). The current status of Carl Rogers and the person-centered approach. *Psychotherapy: Theory, Research, Practice, Training*, *42*, 37–51.

Klein, D.B. (1985). *Jewish origins of the psychoanalytic movement*. Chicago, IL: University of Chicago Press. (Originally published 1981 by Praeger.)

Klein, G. (1992). *The atheist and the holy city: Encounters and reflections.* Cambridge, MA: MIT Press.

Klein, N. (2023a). *Doppelganger: A trip into the mirror world.* New York: Farrar, Straus and Giroux.

Klein, N. (2023b, September 13). To know yourself, consider your Doppelganger. *New York Times.*

Knowlson, J. (1996). *Damned to fame: The life of Samuel Beckett.* London: Bloomsbury.

Koenig, T, Spano, R. & Thompson, J. (2020). *Human behavior theory for social work practice.* Thousand Oaks, CA: Sage Publications.

Kollreuter, A. (Ed.). (2016). *What is this Professor Freud like? A diary of an analysis with historical comments.* London: Karnac.

Kostaras, P. (2021). The maternal uterus as the primary object and its role in anxiety. *British Journal of Psychotherapy, 37,* 637–654.

Kramer, R. (1997). Otto Rank and "the cause." In Dufresne, T. (Ed.). *Freud under analysis: Essays in honor of Paul Roazen.* Northvale, NJ: Jason Aronson, 221–247.

Kramer, R. (2012). Otto Rank on emotional intelligence, unlearning and self-leadership. *American Journal of Psychoanalysis, 72,* 326–351.

Kramer, R. (2017). Review of E. Schein, *Humble consulting: How to provide real help faster* (Berrett-Koehler, 2016). In *Academy of Management Learning & Education, 16,* 342–345.

Kramer, R. (2023). Discovering the existential unconscious: Rollo May encounters Otto Rank. *Humanistic Psychologist, 51,* 15–35.

Krim, M. (1999). Otto Rank: Unacknowledged genius. *Contemporary Psychoanalysis, 35,* 166–170.

Kristeva, J. (2001). *Hannah Arendt: Life is a narrative.* Collins, F. (Tr.). Toronto: Toronto University Press.

Kuchuck, S. (2021). *The relational revolution in psychoanalysis and psychotherapy.* London: Confer Books.

Kugelmann, R. (2023). *The soul in soulless psychology.* Cambridge, UK: Cambridge University Press.

Lacan, J. (1977). *Écrits: A selection.* Sheridan, A. (Tr.). New York: W.W. Norton.

Lacan, J. (1981). *The four fundamental concepts of psycho-analysis.* Sheridan A. (Tr.). New York: W.W. Norton.

Lacan, J. (1985). *Feminine sexuality: Jacques Lacan and the école freudienne.* Mitchell, J. & Rose, J. (Eds.). Rose, J. (Tr.). New York: W.W. Norton.

Lacan, J. (1989). Science and the truth. Fink, B. (Tr.). *Newsletter of the Freudian Field.* Spring/Fall, *3,* 4–22.

Lacan, J. (2014). *Anxiety: The seminar of Jacques Lacan, Book X.* Miller, J.-A. (Ed.). Price, A.R. (Tr.). Cambridge, UK: Polity Press.

Lagercrantz, H. (2016). *Infant brain development: Formation of the mind and the emergence of consciousness.* Cham: Springer International Publishing.

Lament, C., King, R.A., Abrams, S., Brinich, P.M. & Knight R. (2016). The war against women in psychoanalytic culture. *Psychoanalytic Studies of the Child, 69,* 35–152.

Landy, R.J. (2008). *The couch and the stage: Integrating words and action in psychotherapy.* Lanham, MD: Jason Aronson.

Lang A., Ott P., Del Giudice R., Schabus M. (2020). Memory traces formed in utero: Newborns' autonomic and neuronal responses to prenatal stimuli and the maternal voice. *Brain Sciences, 10,* 837.

Lang, B. (2017, September 21). Fin-de-siècle investigations of the "creative genius" in psychiatry and psychoanalysis. In *A history of the case study: Sexology, psychoanalysis, literature.* Manchester Scholarship Online. https://www.manchesterhive.com/display/9781526106117/9781526106117.00006.xml.

Langman, L. (1961). The estrangement from being: An existential analysis of Otto Rank's psychology. *Journal of Existential Psychiatry, 1,* 455–477.

Langstroth, L. (1955). *Structure of the ego: An anatomic and physiologic interpretation of the psyche, based on the psychology of Otto Rank.* Stanford, CA: Stanford University Press.

Lanzoni, S. (2018). *Empathy: A history.* New Haven, CT: Yale University Press.

Larsen, N. (1928). *Quicksand.* In Zahar, R. (Ed.). *Harlem renaissance: Five novels of the 1920s.* New York: Library of America, 297–432, 2011.

Lavin, S. (2004). *Form follows libido: Architecture and Richard Neutra in a psychoanalytic culture.* Cambridge, MA: MIT Press.

Lawrence, D.H. (1920). *Women in love.* New York: Viking, 1960.

Lawrence, D.H. (1921). *Fantasia of the unconscious* and *Psychoanalysis and the unconscious.* New York: Penguin Books, 1977.

Lawrence, D.H. (1932). *Apocalypse.* New York: Viking.

Leader, Z. (1991). *Writer's block.* Baltimore: Johns Hopkins University Press.

Lebiez, J. (2017). Matricide and the trauma of birth in Hofmannsthal's *Elektra.* In Maierhofer, W. & Smith, C. (Eds.). *Women in German yearbook,* Vol. 33. Lincoln: University of Nebraska Press, 28–51.

Leichsenring, F., Abbass, A., Heim, N., Keefe, J.R., Kisely, S., Luyten, P., Rabung, S., & Steinert, C. (2023). The status of psychodynamic psychotherapy as an empirically supported treatment for common mental disorders—An umbrella review based on updated criteria. *World Psychiatry, 22,* 286–304.

Leitner, M. (1997). Too Rankian for the Freudians, or too Freudian for the Rankians: Otto Rank's contributions to psychoanalysis in the 1920s. *Journal of the American Academy of Psychoanalysis, 25,* 37–70.

Leitner, M. (1998). *Freud, Rank und die Folgen: ein Schlüsselkonflikt für die Psychoanalyse.* Vienna: Turia + Kant.

Levenson, H. (2010). *Brief dynamic therapy.* Washington, DC: American Psychological Association.

Lewin, K. (1926). *Vorsatz, Wille und Bedürfnis. Psychologische Forschung, 7,* 330–385.

Lewis, J.S. (1991). Carl Rogers and the person-centered approach: Social work applications now and for the future. In Greene, R.R. (Ed.). *Human Behavior Theory and Social Work Practice* (2nd ed.). London and New York: Routledge, 166–172.

Lieberman, E.J. (1979). The Rank-Wilbur correspondence. *Journal of the Otto Rank Association, 14,* 7–24.

Lieberman, E.J. (1985). *Acts of will: The life and work of Otto Rank.* New York: Free Press.

Lieberman, E.J. (2012). Rankian will. *American Journal of Psychoanalysis, 72,* 320–325.

Lieberman, E.J. & Kramer, R. (Eds.) (2012). *The Letters of Sigmund Freud and Otto Rank: Inside Psychoanalysis.* Richter, G.C. (Tr.). Baltimore: Johns Hopkins University Press.

Liechty, D. (Ed.). (2005). *The Ernest Becker reader.* Seattle: Ernest Becker Foundation in association with the University of Washington Press.

Lifton, R.J. (1983). *The broken connection: On death and the continuity of life.* New York: Basic Books.

Lilliengren, P. (2023). A comprehensive overview of randomized controlled trials of psychodynamic psychotherapies. *Psychoanalytic Psychotherapy, 37,* 117–140.

Lipman-Blumen, J. (1996). *The connective edge: Leading in an interdependent world.* San Francisco: Jossey-Bass.

Lipman-Blumen, J. (2005, January/February). The allure of toxic leaders: Why followers rarely escape their clutches. *Ivey Business Journal,* 1–8.

Lipman-Blumen, J. (2006). *The allure of toxic leaders: Why we follow destructive bosses and corrupt politicians—and how we can survive them.* New York: Oxford University Press.

Lipman-Blumen, J. (2007). Toxic leaders and the fundamental vulnerability of being alive. In Shamir, B. Pillai, R., Bligh, M.C., & Uhl-Bien, M. (Eds.). *Follower-centered perspectives on leadership: A tribute to the memory of James R. Meindl.* Greenwich: Information Age Publishing, 1–17.

Lomas, T. (2022). Making waves in the great ocean: A historical perspective on the emergence and evolution of wellbeing scholarship. *Journal of Positive Psychology, 17*, 1–14.

Loy, D. (1996). *Lack and transcendence: The problem of death and life in psychotherapy, existentialism, and Buddhism*. New Jersey: Humanities Press.

Lugrin, Y. (2012). The Rank-Ferenczi relationship, as seen from France. *American Journal of Psychoanalysis, 72*, 352–381.

MacKinnon, D.W. (1975). IPAR's contribution to the conceptualization and the study of creativity. In Taylor, I.A. & Getzels, J.W. (Eds.). *Perspectives in creativity*. Chicago: Aldine Publishing Company, 60–89.

Magnone, L. (2024). Beata "Tola" Rank: Out from the footnote. In Naszkowska, K. (Ed.). *Early women psychoanalysts: History, biography, and contemporary relevance*. New York: Routledge, 57–76.

Mahony, P.J. (1984). *Cries of the wolf man*. New York: International Universities Press.

Mahony, P.J. (1987). *Freud as a writer*. New Haven, CT: Yale University Press.

Makari, G. (2008). *Revolution in mind: The creation of psychoanalysis*. New York: Harper-Collins.

Manz, C.C. (1986). Self-leadership: Toward an expanded theory of self-influence processes in organizations. *Academy of Management Review, 11*, 585–600.

Manz, C.C. (2015). Taking the self-leadership high road: Smooth surface or potholes ahead? *Academy of Management Perspectives, 29*, 132–151.

Manz, C.C. & Sims H.P. (1991). Super leadership: Beyond the myth of heroic leadership. *Organizational Dynamics, 19*, 18–35.

Marinelli, L. & Mayer, A. (2003). *Dreaming by the book: Freud's The Interpretation of Dreams and the history of the psychoanalytic movement*. Fairfield, S. (Tr.). New York: Other Press.

Marmor, J. (1979). Short-term dynamic psychotherapy. *American Journal of Psychiatry, 136*, 149–155.

Martin, J. (2014). Ernest Becker at Simon Fraser University (1969–1974). *Journal of Humanistic Psychology, 54*, 66–112.

Masson, J.M. (Ed. &Tr.) (1985). *The complete letters of Sigmund Freud to Wilhelm Fliess 1887–1904*. Cambridge, MA: Harvard University Press.

Matson, F.W. (1964). *The broken image: Man, science and society*. New York: Braziller.

May, R. (1953). *Man's search for himself*. New York: W.W. Norton.

May, R. (1969). *Love and will*. New York: W.W. Norton.

May, R. (1972). *Power and innocence*. New York: W.W. Norton.

May, R. (1975). *The courage to create*. New York: W.W. Norton.

May, R. (1977). *The meaning of anxiety* (Rev. ed.). New York: W.W. Norton. (Original work published 1950.)

May, R. (1983). *The discovery of being: Writings in existential psychology*. New York: W.W. Norton.

May, R. (1985). *My quest for beauty*. San Francisco: Saybrook.

May, R. (1989). *The art of counseling* (Rev. ed.). New York: Gardner Press. (Original work published 1939.)

May, R. (1991). *The cry for myth*. New York: W.W. Norton.

May, R. (1996). Foreword. In Kramer, R. (Ed.). *A psychology of difference: The American lectures*. Princeton, NJ: Princeton University Press, xi–xii.

May, U. (2018). *Freud at work: On the history of psychoanalytic theory and practice, with an analysis of Freud's patient record books*. Abingdon: Routledge.

McGlynn, J. (2023, September 22). Russia is preparing the next generation to die for their country. *Moscow Times*. https://www.themoscowtimes.com/2023/09/22/russia-is-preparing-the-next-generation-to-die-for-their-country-a82536.

McGuire, W. (Ed.) (1974). *The Freud/Jung letters: The correspondence between Sigmund Freud and C.G. Jung*. Manheim, R. & Hull, R.F.C. (Trs.). Princeton, NJ: Princeton University Press.

McKitterick, B. (2015). *Self-leadership in social work: Reflections from practice.* Bristol: Policy Press.

McNeil, D.R. (2010). *Sex and race in the black Atlantic: Mulatto devils and multiracial messiahs.* New York: Routledge.

Meisel, O. & Kendrik, W. (Eds.). (1985). *Bloomsbury/Freud: The letters of James and Alix Strachey, 1924–1925.* New York: Basic Books.

Menaker, E. (1982). *Otto Rank: A rediscovered legacy.* New York: Columbia University Press.

Menaker, E. (1984). The ethical and the empathic in the thinking of Otto Rank. *American Imago, 41,* 343–351.

Menaker, E. (1995a). *The freedom to inquire: Self psychological perspectives on women's issues, masochism, and the therapeutic relationship.* Northvale, NJ: Jason Aronson.

Menaker, E. (1995b). *Misplaced loyalties.* New Brunswick, NJ: Transaction Publishers.

Menaker, E. (1996). *Separation, will, and creativity: The wisdom of Otto Rank.* Northvale, NJ: Jason Aronson.

Menand, L. (2012). Freud, anxiety and the cold war. In Burnham, J. (Ed.). *After Freud left: A century of psychoanalysis in America.* Chicago, IL: University of Chicago Press, 189–207.

Menand, L. (2021). *The free world: Art and thought in the cold war.* New York: Farrar, Straus and Giroux.

Merkur, D. (2010). Otto Rank's *Will Therapy.* In Merkur, D. (Ed.). *Contemporary psychoanalytic studies: Explorations of the psychoanalytic mystics,* Vol. 11. Amsterdam-New York: Rodopi, 53–70.

Mertens, R. (2012, May–June). Jessie Taft (1882–1960): A matriarch of modern social work. *University of Chicago Magazine,* 60–63.

Meyer, J. (Ed.) (2022). *The double: Identity and difference in art since 1900.* Washington, DC: National Gallery of Art in association with Princeton University Press.

Mitchell, K. (2023). *Free agents: How evolution gave us free will.* Princeton, NJ: Princeton University Press.

Mitchell, S.A. (1988). *Relational concepts in psychoanalysis: An integration.* Cambridge, MA: Harvard University Press.

Mitzen, J. (2006). Ontological security in world politics: State identity and the security dilemma. *European Journal of International Relations, 12,* 341–370.

Mizen, C.S. & Hook, J. (2020). Relational and affective neuroscience: a quiet revolution in psychiatric and psychotherapeutic practice. *BJPsych Advances, 26,* 356–366.

Moorjani, A. (2004). Beckett and psychoanalysis. In Oppenheim, L. (Ed.). *Palgrave advances in Samuel Beckett studies.* New York: Palgrave Macmillan, 172–193.

Morgan, G. (2006). *Images of organization* (2nd ed.). Thousand Oaks, CA: Sage Publication.

Morson, G.S. (2023, June 22). Death and the hedgehog. *New York Review of Books, 70,* 40–42.

Moskowitz, M. (2014). Quoted in "Black Psychoanalysts Speak." https://www.youtube.com/watch?v=N8-VIi7tb44.

Müller, B. (2003). The influence of Otto Rank's concept of creative will on gestalt therapy. In Lobb, M.S. & Amendt-Lyon, N. (Eds.). *Creative license: The art of gestalt therapy.* Vienna: Springer, 129–140.

Munroe, R.L. (1955). *Schools of psychoanalytic thought.* New York: Dryden Press.

Musser, G. (2023). *Putting ourselves back in the equation: Why physicists are studying human consciousness and AI to unravel the mysteries of the universe.* New York: Farrar, Straus and Giroux.

Neill, J.R. & Kinskern, D.P. (1982). *From psyche to system: The evolving therapy of Carl Whitaker.* New York: Guilford Press.

Neufeld, G. & Maté G. (2014). *Hold on to your kids: Why parents need to matter more than peers.* New York: Ballantine Books.

Nietzsche, F. (1887). *On the genealogy of morals.* Kaufman, W. & Hollingdale, R.J. (Trs.). *Ecco Homo* (1908). New York: Vintage Books [combined edition], 1967.

Nin, A. (1966). *The Diary of Anaïs Nin, Volume 1: 1931–34.* Stuhlmann, G. (Ed.). New York: Swallow Press and Harcourt, Brace and World.

Nin, A. (1967). *The Diary of Anaïs Nin, Volume 2: 1934–39.* Stuhlmann, G. (Ed.). New York: Swallow Press and Harcourt, Brace and World.

Nin, A. (1968). Review of *Art and Artist. Journal of the Otto Rank Association, 3,* 94–97.

Nin, A. (1973). On truth and reality. *Journal of the Otto Rank Association, 8,* 51–58.

Nin, A. (1976). *In favor of the sensitive man and other essays.* New York: Harcourt Brace Jovanovich.

Norcross, J.C. & Lambert, M.J. (2019). Evidence-based psychotherapy relationships: The third task force. In Norcross, J.C. & Lambert, M.J. (Eds.). *Psychotherapy relationships that work,* Vol. 1. New York: Oxford University Press, 1–23.

Norcross, J.C. & Cooper, M. (2021). *Personalizing psychotherapy: Assessing and accommodating patient preferences.* Washington, DC: American Psychological Association.

Novey, R. (1983). Otto Rank: Beginnings, endings, and current experience. *Journal of the American Psychoanalytic Association, 31,* 985–1002.

Nussbaum, M.C. (2001). *Upheavals of thought: The intelligence of emotions.* Cambridge, UK: Cambridge University Press.

Obaid, F.P. (2012). Sigmund Freud and Otto Rank: Debates and confrontations about anxiety and birth. *International Journal of Psychoanalysis, 93,* 693–715.

O'Dowd, W.T. (1986). Otto Rank and time-limited psychotherapy. *Psychotherapy, 23,* 140–149.

Ogden, T. (1994). The analytic third: Working with intersubjective clinical facts. *Psychoanalytic Quarterly, 75,* 3–19.

O'Hara, M. (2015). About Carl Rogers. Website. http://carlrrogers.org/aboutCarlRogers.html.

Okamoto, A., Dattilio, F.M., Dobson, K.S., & Kazantzis, N. (2019). The therapeutic relationship in cognitive–behavioral therapy: Essential features and common challenges. *Practice Innovations, 4,* 112–123.

O'Mahony, S. (2023). *The guru, the bagman & the sceptic: A story of science, sex & psychoanalysis.* London: Head Zeus.

Orange, D. (1995). *Emotional understanding: Studies in psychoanalytic epistemology.* New York: Guilford Press.

Orban P. (1988). Validating Otto Rank's work. *Anaïs, 6,* 110–125.

Otto, R. (1924). *The idea of the holy: An inquiry into the non-rational factor in the idea of the divine and its relation to the rational,* 2nd ed. Harvey, J.W. (Tr.). London: Oxford University Press, 1957.

Pascal, B. (1670). *The pensées.* Cohen, J.M. (Tr.). New York: Penguin, 1961.

Paskauskas, R.A. (Ed.) (1993). *The complete correspondence of Sigmund Freud and Ernest Jones, 1908–1939.* Cambridge, MA: Harvard University Press.

Pavloski, L. & Darga, S.T. (2002). *Twentieth-century literary criticism,* Vol. 115. Detroit: Gale, 220–353.

Perls, F., Hefferline, R. & Goodman, P. (1951). *Gestalt therapy.* New York: Delta.

Pine, R. (2020). Otto Rank and the case of Lawrence Durrell. *C. 20: An International Journal,* Issue No. 5, 1–13.

Plamper, J. (2015). *The history of emotions: An introduction.* Tribe, K. (Tr.). New York: Oxford University Press.

Plant, R.J. (2016). Betty Friedan. In Marso, L.J. (Ed.). *Fifty-one key feminist thinkers.* Abingdon: Routledge, 72–77.

Polster, E. (1968). A contemporary psychotherapy. In Pursglove, P.D. (Ed.). *Recognitions in gestalt therapy.* New York: Funk & Wagnalls, 3–19.

Pollan, M. (2018). *How to change your mind: What the new science of psychedelics teaches us about consciousness, dying, addiction, depression, and transcendence.* New York: Penguin/Random House.

Progoff, I. (1956). *The death and rebirth of psychology: An integrative evaluation of Freud, Adler, Jung and Rank and the impact of their culminating insights on modern man.* New York: Julian Press.

Rabinowitz, P., Good, G. & Cozad, L. (1989). Rollo May: A man of meaning and myth. *Journal of Counseling and Development, 67,* 436–441.

Rachman, A.W. (2018). *Elizabeth Severn: The "evil genius" of psychoanalysis.* New York: Routledge.

Ragland, E. (2024). Who is transferring what to whom? Resistance to Lacan. In Rousselle, D. & Murphy, M.G. (Eds.). *Negativity in psychoanalysis: Theory and clinic.* New York: Routledge, 3–60.

Rank, B. [Tola] (1923, May). Zur Rolle der Frau in der Entwicklung der menschlichen Geselschaft. Lecture given at the Vienna Psychoanalytic Society.

Rank, O. (1904). *Tagebücher.* Otto Rank Collection. Columbia University Rare Book and Manuscript Library. Box 8.

Rank, O. (1907). *The artist.* Salomon, E. & Lieberman, E.J. (Trs.). *Journal of the Otto Rank Association, 15,* 5–63. Revised 1925 edition.

Rank, O. (1910). *A dream that interprets itself.* Kramer, R. (Ed.). Richter, G.C. (Tr.). Oxfordshire: Karnac, 2024.

Rank, O. (1912). *The incest theme in literature and legend: Fundamentals of a psychology of literary creation.* Introduction by Rudnytsky, P.L. Richter, G.C. (Tr.). Baltimore: Johns Hopkins University Press, 1992.

Rank, O. (1922a). *The myth of the birth of the hero: A psychological exploration of myth.* Expanded and updated edition. Introduction by Segal, R. Richter, G.C. & Lieberman E.J. (Trs.). Baltimore: Johns Hopkins University Press, 2004. First edition published 1909.

Rank, O. (1922b). *The Don Juan legend.* Introduction by Winter, D.G. (Tr.). Princeton, NJ: Princeton University Press, 1975.

Rank, O. (1924). *The trauma of birth.* New York: Dover, 1993.

Rank, O. (1925). *The double: A psychoanalytic study.* Introduction by Tucker, H. (Tr.). Chapel Hill: University of North Carolina Press, 1971. First edition published 1914.

Rank, O. (1926). *Technik der Psychoanalyse, Band I: Die Analytische Situation.* Janus, L. & Wirth, H.-J. (Eds.). Giessen: Psychosozial-Verlag, 2006.

Rank, O. (1927). *Grundzüge einer genetischen Psychologie auf Grund der Psychoanalyse der Ichstruktur, I. Teil.* Leipzig & Vienna: Franz Deuticke.

Rank, O. (1928). *Grundzüge einer genetischen Psychologie auf Grund der Psychoanalyse der Ichstruktur, II. Teil.* Leipzig & Vienna: Franz Deuticke.

Rank, O. (1930). *Psychology and the soul: A study of the origin, conceptual evolution and nature of the soul.* Introduction by Lieberman, E.J. Richter, G.C. & Lieberman, E.J. (Trs). Baltimore: Johns Hopkins University Press, 1998.

Rank, O. (1932a). *Art and artist: Creative urge and personality development.* Atkinson, C.F. (Tr.). New York: Alfred A. Knopf.

Rank, O. (1932b). *Modern education.* Moxon, M. (Tr.). New York: Alfred A. Knopf.

Rank, O. (1934). Transcript of two letters to Anaïs Nin. Courtesy of E. James Lieberman.

Rank, O. (1935). Active and passive therapy. In Rank, O. *A psychology of difference: The American lectures.* Kramer, R. (Ed.). Foreword by May, R. Princeton, NJ: Princeton University Press, 260–262, 1996.

Rank, O. (1936a). *Will therapy: An analysis of the therapeutic process in terms of relationship.* Taft, J. (Tr.). New York: Alfred A. Knopf [translation of *Technik der Psychoanalyse, Band II: Die analytische Reaktion in ihren konstruktiven Elementen.* Leipzig & Vienna: Franz Deuticke, 1929 and *Technik der Psychoanalyse, Band III: Die Analyse des Analytikers und seiner Rolle in der Gesamtsituation.* Leipzig & Vienna: Franz Deuticke, 1931].

Rank, O. (1936b). *Truth and reality: A life history of the human will*. Taft, J. (Tr.). New York: Alfred A. Knopf [translation of *Wahrheit und Wirklichkeit: Entwurf einer Philosophie des Seelischen*. Leipzig & Vienna: Franz Deuticke, 1929].

Rank, O. (1938, December 11). Inscription in Rank's copy of Shakespeare's *Sonnets*, gifted to Jessie Taft. Otto Rank Collection, Rare Book and Manuscript Library, Columbia University. Box 40.

Rank, O. (1939). Handwritten note. Otto Rank Collection, Rare Book and Manuscript Library, Columbia University. Box 14.

Rank, O. (1941a). *Beyond psychology*. New York: Dover, 1958.

Rank, O. (1941b). In the matter of the estate of Otto Rank. Otto Rank Collection, Rare Book and Manuscript Library. Columbia University. Box 40.

Rank, O. (1981). Literary autobiography. *Journal of the Otto Rank Association, 16*, 3–38.

Rank, O. (1989). Sons and daughters: Incest, psychoanalysis, and family conflicts in Anglo-Saxon literature. Stuhlmann, G. (Tr.). *Anais, 7*, 59–68.

Rank, O. (1996). *A psychology of difference: The American lectures*. Kramer, R. (Ed.). Foreword by May, R. Princeton, NJ: Princeton University Press.

Rank-Veltfort, H. (2002). Rank-Minzer (Munzer), Beata (1886–1961). In De Mijolla, A. (Ed.). *International Dictionary of Psychoanalysis*. New York: Macmillan, 1443–1444.

Raphael-Leff, J. (2016). "Two-in-one body": Unconscious representations and ethical dimensions of inter-corporeality in childbirth. In Bornemark, J. & Smith, N. (Eds.). *Phenomenology of pregnancy*. Stockholm: Södertörn University Press, 157–198.

Raskin, N.J. (1948). The development of nondirective therapy. *Journal of Consulting Psychology, 12*, 92–110.

Raskin, N.J., Rogers, C.R. & Witty, M.C. (2019). Client-centered therapy. In Wedding, D. & Corsini, R.J. (Eds.). *Current psychotherapies* (11th ed.). Boston: Cengage, 101–156.

Reuland, J. (2015). The social worker's license: Reconstructing social selves in the work of Jessie Taft and Charlotte Perkins Gilman. *Modernism/modernity, 22*, 1–22.

Richardson, H., Ernst, J., Drill, R., Gill, A., Hunnicutt, P., Silver, Z., Coger, M., & Beinashowitz, J. (2023). In the patient's own words: A qualitative study of what patients find helpful in psychodynamic psychotherapy. *Journal of Mental Health Training, Education and Practice, 18*, 325–337.

Ricoeur, P. (1970). *Freud and philosophy: An essay on interpretation*. Savage, D. (Tr.). New Haven, CT: Yale University Press.

Rieff, P. (1959). *Freud: The mind of the moralist*. New York: Viking.

Rieff, P. (1966). *The triumph of the therapeutic*. New York: Harper & Row.

Roazen, P. (1974). *Freud and his followers*. New York: Alfred A. Knopf.

Roazen, P. (1990). Tola Rank. *Journal of American Academy of Psychoanalysis, 18*, 247–259.

Roazen, P. (1993). *Meeting Freud's family*. Amherst: University of Massachusetts Press.

Roazen, P. (1995). *How Freud worked: First-hand accounts of patients*. Northvale, NJ: Jason Aronson.

Roazen, P. (1999). Introduction. In Agassi, J.B. (Ed.). *Martin Buber on psychology and psychotherapy: Essays, letters, and dialogue*. Syracuse, NY: Syracuse University Press, xix–xxvi.

Roazen, P. (2001). *The historiography of psychoanalysis*. New Brunswick, NJ: Transaction Publishers.

Roazen, P. (2002). *The trauma of Freud: Controversies in psychoanalysis*. New Brunswick, NJ: Transaction Publishers.

Roazen, P. & Swerdloff, B. (Eds.) (1995). *Heresy: Sándor Radó and the psychoanalytic movement*. Northvale, NJ: Jason Aronson.

Robinson, V.P. (1930). *A changing psychology in social work*. Chapel Hill: University of North Carolina Press.

Robinson, V.P. (1968). The influence of Rank in social work. *Journal of the Otto Rank Association, 2*, 5–50.

Rodden, J. (2016). *Between self and society: Inner worlds and outer limits in the British psychological novel*. Austin: University of Texas Press.

Rogers, C.R. (1939). *The clinical treatment of the problem child*. Boston: Houghton Mifflin.

Rogers, C.R. (1951). *Client-centered therapy: Its current practice, implication, theory*. Boston: Houghton Mifflin.

Rogers, C.R. (1959). A theory of therapy, personality, and interpersonal relationships as developed in the client-centered framework. In Koch, S. (Ed.). *Psychology: A study of a science*, Vol. 3. New York: McGraw-Hill, 184–256.

Rogers, C.R. (1961). *On becoming a person*. Boston: Houghton Mifflin.

Rogers, C.R. (1967a). The interpersonal relationship: The core of guidance. In Rogers, C.R. & Stevens, B. (Eds.). *Person to person: The problem of being human*. New York: Pocket Books, 85–101.

Rogers, C.R. (1967b). Autobiography. In Boring, E.G. & Lindzey, G. (Eds.). *A history of psychology in autobiography*, Vol. 5. New York: Appleton, 343–384.

Rogers, C.R. (1973). Letter to Virgina Robinson, October 15, 1972. *Journal of the Otto Rank Association*, 8, 95.

Rogers, C.R. (1978). Do we need "a" reality? *Dawnpoint*, 1, 6–9.

Rogers, C.R. (1980). *A way of being*. Boston: Houghton Mifflin.

Rogers, C.R. (1983). *Conversations with Carl Rogers* [Videotape]. Produced by the Encinitas Center for Family and Personal Development.

Rogers, C.R. (1986). Client-centered therapy. In Kutash, I.L. & Wolf, A. (Eds.). *Psychotherapist's casebook*. San Francisco: Jossey-Bass, 197–208.

Rogers, C.R. (1995). What understanding and acceptance mean to me. *Journal of Humanistic Psychology*, 35, 7–22.

Rogers, C.R. & Russell, D.E. (2002). *Carl Rogers: The quiet revolutionary: An oral history*. Roseville, CA: Penmarin Books.

Rogers, R. (1970). *A psychoanalytic study of the double in literature*. Detroit: Wayne State University Press.

Roland, A., Ulanov, B. & Barbré, C. (Eds.) (2003). *Creative dissent: Psychoanalysis in evolution*. Westport, CT: Praeger.

Romm, S. (1983). *The unwelcome intruder: Freud's struggle with cancer*. New York: Praeger.

Rose, J. (2023, September 21). The analyst. *New York Review of Books*, 70, 49–51.

Roudinesco, E. (2016). *Freud in his time and ours*. Cambridge, MA: Harvard University Press.

Rudnytsky, P.L. (1991). *The psychoanalytic vocation: Rank, Winnicott, and the legacy of Freud*. New Haven, CT: Yale University Press.

Rudnytsky, P.L. (2002). *Reading psychoanalysis: Freud, Rank, Ferenczi, Groddeck*. Ithaca, NY: Cornell University Press.

Sachs, H. (1944). *Freud: Master and friend*. Cambridge, MA: Harvard University Press.

Safran, J.D. & Kriss, A. (2014). Psychoanalytic psychotherapies. In Wedding, D. & Corsini, R.J. (Eds.). *Current psychotherapies* (10th ed.). Boston: Brooks/Cole Cengage, 19–54.

Safran, J.D., Kriss, A. & Foley, V.K. (2019). Psychodynamic psychotherapies. In Wedding, D. & Corsini, R.J. (Eds.). *Current psychotherapies* (11th ed.). Boston: Cengage, 21–57.

Safran, J.D. & Muran, J.C. (2000). *Negotiating the therapeutic alliance: A relational treatment guide*. New York: Guilford Press.

Sakanaka, M. (2015). The person-centered approach in Japan as demonstrated in a publication review (1951–2008). In Mikuni, M. (Ed.). *The person-centered approach in Japan: Blending a Western approach with Japanese culture*. Ross-on-Wye: PCCS Books, 157–181.

Salamon, S.I. (2019). Insight and responsibility: A psychodynamic-existential approach to psychotherapy. *Humanistic Psychologist*, 47, 52–75.

Sanders, P. (Ed.) (2012). *The tribes of the person-centered nation: An introduction to the schools of therapy related to the person-centered approach* (2nd ed.). Ross-on-Wye: PCCS Books.

Santayana, G. (1922). *Soliloquies in England and later soliloquies*. New York: Scribner.

Sapolsky, R. (2023). *Determined: A science of life without free will.* New York: Penguin/Random House.

Sass, L. (1992). *Madness and modernism: Insanity in the light of modern art, literature, and thought.* New York: Basic Books.

Schein, E.H. (2009). *Helping: How to offer, give, and receive help.* San Francisco: Jossey-Bass.

Schmitt, A. (1980). Will therapy of Otto Rank. In Herink, R. (Ed.). *The psychotherapy handbook.* New York: New American Library, 701–703.

Schneider, K.J. (2021, November 25). The existential unconscious: A re-visioning of our hidden selves. *Psychology Today* website. https://www.psychologytoday.com/us/blog/awakening-awe/202111/the-existential-unconscious-re-visioning-our-hidden-selves.

Schneider, K.J. (2023). *Life enhancing anxiety: Key to a sane world.* Colorado Springs: University Professors Press.

Schneider, K.J. & May, R. (1995). *The psychology of existence. An integrative clinical perspective.* New York: McGraw-Hill.

Schorske, C. (2023, May 21). I had to quit therapy to finally be ready for it. *New York Times Magazine,* 52.

Schrödinger, E. (1944). *What is life? The physical aspect of the living cell.* London: Cambridge University Press.

Schur, M. (1972). *Freud: Living and dying.* London: Hogarth Press and the Institute of Psychoanalysis.

Schwartz, A. (1973). The Trauma of Birth and Rank's departure from Freud. *Review of Existential Psychology and Psychiatry, 12,* 75–92.

Seidenman, E.W. (1978). In therapy with Otto Rank 1936–38. *Journal of the Otto Rank Association, 13,* 51–64.

Seif, N.G. (1980). *Otto Rank: On human evil.* Unpublished PhD dissertation. Yeshiva University.

Seif, N.G. (1984). Otto Rank: On the nature of the hero. *American Imago, 41,* 373–384.

Segal, R. (2011). Mysticism and psychoanalysis. *Religious Studies Review, 37,* 1–18.

Searles, H.F. (1975). The patient as therapist to his analyst. In Giovacchini, P. (Ed.). *Tactics and techniques in psychoanalytic therapy,* Vol. 2. New York: Jason Aronson, 95–151.

Sehgal, P. (2023, August 14). How the writer and critic Jacqueline Rose puts the world on the couch. *New Yorker,* 12–18.

Severn, E. (2017). *The discovery of the self: A study in psychological cure.* Rudnytsky, P.L. (Ed.). New York: Routledge.

Shahar, G. & Schiller, M. (2016). A conqueror by stealth: Introduction to the special issue on humanism, existentialism, and psychotherapy integration. *Journal of Psychotherapy Integration, 26,* 1–4.

Shedler, J. (2010). The efficacy of psychodynamic psychotherapy. *American Psychologist, 65,* 98–109.

Sheets-Johnstone, M. (2008). *The roots of morality.* University Park: Pennsylvania State University Press.

Shuman, M.L. (2007). *"A woman's face, or worse": Otto Rank and the modernist identity.* Unpublished PhD dissertation. University of South Florida.

Sievers, B. (1994). *Work, death, and life itself: Essays on management and organization.* Berlin: Walter de Gruyter.

Sloterdijk, P. (1998). *Sphären I: Blasen. Mikrosphärologie.* Frankfurt am Main: Suhrkamp Verlag. See also: Sloterdijk, P. (2011). *Spheres: Bubbles Volume I: Microspherology.* Los Angeles: Semiotexte(e).

Smith, E.W.L. (2012). *The psychology of artists and the arts.* Jefferson, NC: McFarland & Company.

Smith, H. (1992). *Forgotten truth: the common vision of the world's religions.* San Francisco: HarperOne.

Smith, J.C. (1990). *The neurotic foundations of social order: Psychoanalytic roots of patriarchy.* New York: New York University Press.

Smith, K.K., & Berg, D.N. (1987). *Paradoxes of group life: Understanding conflict, paralysis, and movement in group dynamics.* San Francisco: Jossey-Bass.

Smith, R. (2010). It's nothing: Beckett and anxiety. In Caselli, D. (Ed.). *Beckett and nothing: Trying to understand Beckett.* Manchester and New York: Manchester University Press, 192–212.

Sollod, R.N. (1978). Carl Rogers and the origins of client-centered therapy. *Professional Psychology, 9*, 93–104.

Solms, M. (2015). *The feeling brain: selected papers on neuropsychoanalysis.* London: Karnac.

Solms, M. (2021). *The hidden spring: A journey to the source of consciousness.* New York: W.W. Norton.

Solomon, S., Greenberg, J. & Pyszczynski, T. (2015). *The worm at the core: On the role of death in life.* New York: Random House.

Spector, J.J. (1973). *The aesthetics of Freud: A study in psychoanalysis and art.* New York: Praeger.

Spencer, S. (1982). Delivering the woman artist from the silence of the womb: Otto Rank's influence on Anaïs Nin. *Psychoanalytic Review, 69*, 111–129.

Spencer, S. (1997). Beyond therapy: The enduring love of Anaïs Nin for Otto Rank. In Nalbantian, S. (Ed.). *Anaïs Nin: Literary perspectives.* New York: Palgrave Macmillan, 97–111.

Spencer, S. (2014). The music of the womb: Anaïs Nin's "feminine writing." In Friedman, E.G. & Fuchs, M. (Eds.). *Breaking the sequence: Women's experimental fiction.* Princeton, NJ: Princeton University Press, 161–173.

Spinelli, E. (2023, May 5). Keynote speech. *3rd World Congress of Existential Therapy: Living in the Here and Now.* Athens, Greece.

Spiro, Jack D. (1979). *Man and cosmos: The educational theories of Otto Rank.* Unpublished PhD dissertation. University of Virginia.

Spitz, E.H. (1991). *Image and insight: Essays in psychoanalysis and the arts.* New York: Columbia University Press.

Sprengnether, M. (1990). *The spectral mother: Freud, feminism, and psychoanalysis.* Ithaca, NY: Cornell University Press.

Stapp, H.P. (2017). *Quantum theory and free will: How mental intentions translate into bodily actions.* New York: Springer.

Staszak, K. (2023, November 3). Breaking the taboo of menopause at the workplace. https://worldcrunch.com/culture-society/menopause-at-work.

Stein, E.S. (2010). Otto Rank: Pioneering ideas for social work theory and practice. *Psychoanalytic Social Work, 17*, 116–131.

Stepansky, P.E. (Ed.) (1988). *The memoirs of Margaret S. Mahler.* New York: Free Press.

Stephenson, L. (2024). *Cinema, suffering and psychoanalysis: The mechanism of self.* New York: Bloomsbury.

Sterba, R.F. (1982). *Reminiscences of a Viennese psychoanalyst.* Detroit: Wayne State University Press.

Stevens, R. (1983). *Freud and psychoanalysis: An exposition and appraisal.* Milton Keynes: Open University.

Stoehr, T. (1994). *Here now next: Paul Goodman and the origins of gestalt therapy.* San Francisco: Jossey-Bass.

Stolorow, R. & Atwood, G. (1979). *Faces in a cloud: Subjectivity in personality theory.* New York: Jason Aronson.

Stone, A. (2019). *Being born: Birth and philosophy.* New York: Oxford University Press.

Storr, A. (1989). *Freud: A very short introduction.* New York: Oxford University Press.

Stuhlmann, G. (Ed.) (1979). *Henry Miller: Letters to Anaïs Nin.* London: Sheldon Press.

Suler, J. (1993). *Contemporary psychoanalysis and eastern thought.* Albany: State University of New York Press.

Sullivan, D. (2016). Person-environment mergence and separation: Otto Rank's psychology of emotion, personality, and culture. *Psychoanalytic Review, 103,* 743–770.

Sullivan, D. (2018). The educator as neurotic: A Rankean [sic] analysis of impotent teachers in film. *Free Associations, 73,* 41–63.

Sullivan, D., Goad, A. & Schmitt, H.J. (2024). Existential psychology. In Wardle, H., Rapport, N. & Piette, A. (Eds.). *The Routledge international handbook of existential human science.* London: Routledge, 23–35.

Sulloway, F. (1979). *Freud: Biologist of the mind.* New York: Basic Books.

Sullum, J. (2000, July). Curing the therapeutic state: Thomas Szasz interviewed by Jacob Sullum: Thomas Szasz on the medicalization of American life. *Reason.* https://reason.com/archives/2000/07/01/curing-the-therapeutic-state-t/.

Sward, K. (1980). Self-actualization and women: Rank and Freud contrasted. *Journal of Humanistic Psychology, 20,* 5–26.

Szekacs-Weisz, J. & Keve, T. (Eds.) (2012). *Ferenczi and his world: Rekindling the spirit of the Budapest school.* London: Routledge.

Taft, J. (1933). *The dynamics of therapy in a controlled relationship.* New York: Macmillan. 1962.

Taft, J. (1946) (Ed.). *The role of the baby in the placement process.* Philadelphia: University of Pennsylvania School of Social Work.

Taft, J. (1958). *Otto Rank: A biographical study based on notebooks, letters, collected writings, therapeutic achievements and personal associations.* New York: Julian Press.

Taft, J. (1968). Rank's contribution to education. *Journal of the Otto Rank Association, 3,* 75–89.

Tallis, F. (2021). *The act of living: What the great psychologists can teach us about surviving discontent in an age of anxiety.* London: Picador.

Tamir, Y. (2019). *Why nationalism.* Princeton, NJ: Princeton University Press.

Tate, C. (1996). Freud and his "Negro": Psychoanalysis as ally and enemy of African Americans. *Journal for the Psychoanalysis of Culture & Society, 1,* 53–62.

Taylor, M.C. (1987). *Altarity.* Chicago, IL: University of Chicago Press.

Thorne, B. (1992). *Carl Rogers.* Thousand Oaks, CA: Sage Publications.

Thorne, B. & Sanders, P. (2013). *Carl Rogers.* Thousand Oaks, CA: Sage Publications.

Tillich, P. (1952). *The courage to be.* New Haven, CT: Yale University Press.

Tookey, H. (2003). *Anaïs Nin, fictionality and femininity: Playing a thousand roles.* New York: Oxford University Press.

Tropman, J.E. (2020). *Supervision, management, and leadership: An introduction to building community benefit organizations.* New York: Oxford University Press.

Tuana, N. (2004). Coming to understand: Orgasm and the epistemology of ignorance. *Hypatia, 19,* 194–232.

Tuana, N. (2006). The speculum of ignorance. *Hypatia, 21,* 1–19.

Tucker, H. (1971). Introduction. *The double: A psychoanalytic study* [by Otto Rank]. Chapel Hill: University of North Carolina Press, xiii–xxii.

Ulfig, N., Setzer M., & Bohl J. (2003). Ontogeny of the human amygdala. *Annals of the New York Academy of Sciences, 985,* 22–33.

Vanhooren, S. (2022). Existential empathy: The challenge of 'being' in therapy and counseling. *Religions, 13,* 1–11.

Vanhooren, S. (2023). *Op de bodem: Existentiële thema's in psychotherapie en begeleiding.* Kapellen: Pelckmans.

Vanhooren, S., Grosemans, A., & Breynaert, J. (2022). Focusing, the felt sense, and meaning in life. *Person-Centered & Experiential Psychotherapies, 21,* 250–268.

Vidal, G. (1993). *United States: Essays 1952–1992.* New York: Random House.

Volosinov, V.N. (1987). *Freudianism: A critical sketch.* Bruss, N.H. (Ed.). Titunik, I.R. (Tr.). Bloomington: Indiana University Press.

Wadlington, W. (1983). *Otto Rank's art of psychotherapy*. Unpublished PhD dissertation. Penn State University.

Wadlington, W. (2001). Otto Rank's art. *Humanistic Psychologist, 29,* 280–311.

Wadlington, W. (2005). The *Birth of Tragedy* and the *Trauma of Birth*. *Humanistic Psychologist, 33,* 175–186.

Wadlington, W. (2011). Otto Rank 1884–1939. In Runco, M.A. & Pritzker, S.R. (Eds.). *Encyclopedia of creativity* (2nd ed.), Vol. 2. New York: Springer, 279–285.

Wadlington, W. (2012). The art of living in Otto Rank's will therapy. *American Journal of Psychoanalysis, 72,* 382–396.

Wadlington, W. (in press). Otto Rank's original contributions to humanistic and existential psychology. In Hoffman, L. (Ed.), Vallejos, L. X., Hocoy D., Tummala-Narra, P. & DeRobertis, E.M. (Assoc. Eds.). *APA handbook of humanistic and existential psychology: Vol. 1. History, research, philosophy, and theory.* Washington, DC: American Psychological Association.

Wall, J.N. (1976). Suffering and charity. *Journal of the Otto Rank Association, 11,* 29–32.

Wallerstein, R.S. (2002). Psychoanalytic therapy research: Its coming of age. *Psychoanalytic Inquiry, 23,* 375–404.

Walton, A. (2016, January 25). Resolving the paradox of group creativity. *Harvard Business Review.* Online only. https://hbr.org/2016/01/resolving-the-paradox-of-group-creativity?autocomplete=true.

Wampold B.E. (2001). *The great psychotherapy debate: Model, methods, and findings.* Mahwah, NJ: Erlbaum.

Wampold, B.E., & Imel, Z.E. (2015). *The great psychotherapy debate: The evidence for what makes psychotherapy work* (2nd ed.). New York: Routledge/Taylor & Francis Group.

Wardle, H., Rapport, N. & Piette, A. (Eds.) (2024). *The Routledge international handbook of existential human science.* London: Routledge.

Watt, S. (1986). O'Neill and Otto Rank: Doubles, "death instincts," and The *Trauma of Birth. Contemporary Drama, 20,* 211–230.

Webber, A.J. (1996). *The Doppelgänger: Double visions in German literature.* Oxford: Clarendon Press.

Wedding, D. & Corsini, R.J. (2019). *Current psychotherapies* (11th ed.). Boston: Cengage.

Weinstein, F. (2001). *Freud, psychoanalysis, social theory: The unfilled promise.* Albany: State University of New York.

Werbart A. & Lagerlöf, S. (2022). How much time does psychoanalysis take? The duration of psychoanalytic treatments from Freud's cases to the Swedish clinical practice of today. *International Journal of Psychoanalysis, 103,* 786–805.

Westerink, H. (2009). *A dark trace: Sigmund Freud on the sense of guilt.* Leuven: Leuven University Press.

Whitebook, J. (2017). *Freud: An intellectual biography.* Cambridge, UK: Cambridge University Press.

Whitehead, A.N. (1929). *Process and reality: An essay in cosmology.* Griffin, D.R. & Sherburne, D.W. (Eds.). New York: Free Press, 1978.

Wilson, C. (1972). *New pathways in psychology: Maslow and the post-Freudian revolution.* London: Littlehampton Book Series Ltd.

Winnicott, D.W. (1949). Birth memories, birth trauma, and anxiety. In *Through paediatrics to psycho-analysis: Collected papers.* New York: Basic Books, 174–193.

Winnicott, D.W. (1964). *The child, the family, and the outside world.* London: Pelican Books.

Winnicott, D.W. (1986). *Home is where we start from: Essays by a psychoanalyst.* Winnicott, C. (Ed.). New York: W.W. Norton.

Winnicott, D.W. (1989). *Psycho-analytic explorations.* Cambridge, MA: Harvard University Press.

Wirth, H.-J. (2007). Schismatic processes in the psychoanalytic movement and their impact on the formation of theories. *International Forum of Psychoanalysis, 16,* 4–11.

Wittels, F. (1924). *Sigmund Freud*. London: George Allen & Unwin.

Wittenberger, G., & Tögel, C. (Eds.) (1999–2001). *Die Rundbriefe des "Geheimen Komitees"* (Vols. 1–4). Tübingen: edition discord.

Wittgenstein, L. (1921). *Tractatus logico-philosophicus*. Pears, D.F. & McGuinness, B.F. (Trs.). New York: Humanities Press, New York, 1961.

Wolfe, H. (2023, May 14). IPA news: From the officers. International Psychoanalytical Association website. https://www.ipa.world/en/en/IPA1/board_of_representatives/From_the_Officers.aspx.

Wolitzky, D.L. & Eagle, M.N. (1992). Psychoanalytic theories of psychotherapy. In Freedheim, D.K. (Ed.). *History of psychotherapy: A century of change*. Washington, DC: American Psychological Association, 39–96.

Yaden, D.B., Giorgi, S., Jordan, M., Buffone, A., Eichstaedt, J.C., Schwartz, H.A., Ungar, L., & Bloom, P. (2024). Characterizing empathy and compassion using computational linguistic analysis. *Emotion, 24*, 106–115.

Yalom, I. (1980). *Existential psychotherapy*. New York: Basic Books.

Yalom, I. & Elkin, G. (1974). *Every day gets a little closer: A twice-told therapy*. New York. Basic Books.

Yamada, A.M., Rozas, L.M.W., & Cross-Denny, B. (2015). Intersectionality and social work. https://oxfordre.com/socialwork/display/10.1093/acrefore/9780199975839.001.0001/acrefore-9780199975839-e-961.

Yerushalmi, Y.H. (1991). *Freud's Moses: Judaism terminable and interminable*. New Haven, CT: Yale University Press.

Young, I.F., Sullivan, D., Stewart, S. & Palitsky, R. (2018). The existential approach to place: Consequences for emotional experience. *Journal of Environmental Psychology, 60*, 100–109.

Young-Bruehl, E. (1988). *Anna Freud: A biography*. New York: Summit Books.

Zahidi, S. (Ed.) (2023). *World economic forum global gender gap*. Cologny/Geneva: Switzerland.

Zaretsky, E. (2004). *Secrets of the soul: A social and cultural history of psychoanalysis*. New York: Alfred A. Knopf.

Zaretsky, E. (2015). *Political Freud: A history*. New York: Columbia University Press.

Zilcha-Mano, S., Fisher, H., Dolev-Amit, T., Keefe, J.R. & Barber, J.P. (2023). Interpretation. In Hill, C.E. & Norcross, J.C. (Eds.). *Psychotherapy skills and methods that work*. New York: Oxford University Press, 165-198. https://doi.org/10.1093/oso/9780197611012.001.0001.

Zottl, A. (1980). *Erziehung zum Über-Menschen: Individualität, Kreativität und Wille bei Otto Rank*. Paderborn: Egger-Verlag.

Zottl, A. (1982). *Otto Rank: Das Lebenswerk eines Dissidenten der Psychoanalyse*. Munich: Kindler.

Author's Note

Some material in this book was adapted from previous publications:

1. Robert Kramer, "The Birth of Client-Centered Therapy: Carl Rogers, Otto Rank, and 'The Beyond.'" *Journal of Humanistic Psychology*, Vol. 35, No. 4, pp. 54–110. Copyright ©1995 by Sage Publications. Reprinted by permission of Sage Publications.
2. Robert Kramer, "Chronology of Rank's Life (1884–1939)" and "Introduction". Used with permission of Princeton University Press, from Otto Rank, *A Psychology of Difference: The American Lectures*, 1996; permission conveyed through Copyright Clearance Center, Inc.
3. Robert Kramer, "Rank on Emotional Intelligence, Unlearning and Self-Leadership." *American Journal of Psychoanalysis*, 2012, Vol. 72, pp. 326–371. Used with permission of Giselle Galdi, Editor-in-Chief.
4. Robert Kramer, "'I Am Boiling with Rage': Why Did Freud Banish Rank?" *Psychoanalyse im Widerspruch*, 2015. Vol. 53, pp. 31–43. Used with permission of Parfen Laszig, Editor-in-Chief.
5. Robert Kramer, *The Birth of Relationship Therapy: Carl Rogers Meets Otto Rank*, 2nd revised ed., 2022. Psychosozial-Verlag. Copyright © Robert Kramer.
6. Robert Kramer, "Discovering the Existential Unconscious: Rollo May Encounters Otto Rank." *Humanistic Psychologist*, Vol. 51, No. 1, pp. 15–35. Reproduced with permission from American Psychological Association. No further reproduction or distribution is permitted.

Index

For the benefit of digital users, indexed terms that span two pages (e.g., 52–53) may, on occasion, appear on only one of those pages.

"above-I" (*Über-Ich*). *See* super-ego
Abzug, Robert, 197–198, 240
actualizing tendency. *See also* creative will; self-actualization
  Rogers on, 4, 207
Adams, Paul L., 250
agape, 192
  Becker on, 41, 243
  eros and, 41, 192, 221, 243, 247
  Freud and, 221
  nature of, 192, 221
  Rank on, 221, 229
  Rogers and, 192
Ahad, Badia Sahar, 58–59, 61, 264–265
Alic, Margaret, 258–259
Amundsen, Jon, 246–247
"Analysis Terminable and Interminable" (Freud), 118, 124–126, 140–141, 149. *See also* interminable analysis
Angst, 9, 110, 163, 218. *See also* anxiety; existential despair; *Urangst*
  nature of, 38, 110
anxiety, 12, 86, *163f*. *See also* castration anxiety and castration theory; existential anxiety; primal fear/primal anxiety
  The Denial of Death (Becker) and, xxii, 49, 165, 211, 218
  origin and causes of, 86, 233, 246–247. *See also* birth trauma
  The Trauma of Birth and, 70, 75, 81, 86, 110, 113, 242–243, 246–247
Arendt, Hannah, 112, 232
  on birth/natality, 112, 216, 231–232
  critique of psychoanalysis, 112
  Heidegger and, 112
  The Human Condition, 112, 231–232
  on politics, 112, 232
Aron, Lewis, 255–256
art, xv, 59, 152–153
  feelings and, 155–156
  love and, 182–183, 212–214, 224

Art and Artist: Creative Urge and Personality Development (Rank), xii, 25, 39, 60–61, 171, 182–183, 213
  Becker and, xii, 49
  on sexuality, 35, 151, 222
  on therapy, 144, 212
artiste manqué (failed artist), 10
  woman as, 20, 22
artistic personality, creative, 60
attachment and detachment in analysis, 130. *See also* separation–individuation: from therapist
Atwood, George, 245
authenticity, 30, 115, 145, 190–191
authentic relationship, 113–114, 142. *See also specific topics*

Balsam, Rosemary S., 123–124, 127, 267
Barbré, Claude, 257, 261, 268–269
Barry, Elizabeth, 268–269
Barzilai, Shuli, 257, 281 n.1
Becker, Ernest, xii, xxii, 9, 28, *29f*, 41, 49, 178, 211, 220, 226, 231, 251–252, 267–268. *See also Denial of Death*
  Art and Artist (Rank) and, xii, 49
  Escape from Evil, xxii, 35, 40–41, 43–44, 50, 197–198, 243–244
  heroes, heroism, and, 28, 43–44, 88, 251
  life force and, 49, 156, 220
  on loneliness and ontological motives of human condition, 41, 243
  on nation-states, 41, 46–47
  on psychoanalysis, 161–162
  on quest for immortality, 28, 40–41, 43–44, 49, 251–252, 263–267
  on Rank, xxii, 28, 50, 147, 211
  on sex, 223
  on *Todestrieb* (death drive), 40–41
  on toxic leaders, 50–51
Beckett, Samuel, 226, 233–234, 255–256, 261, 268–269
Berg, David, 250

Bergmann, Martin A., 261
Beyond, the, xxii, 148, 204, *213f*, 218–219, 224,
    280 n.1. *See also* existential
    unconscious; "other world"
  Lacan on, 222–223
  "negotiating" with the problem of, 148, 169,
    206, 210, 230
  surrender, dissolution, and, 213–214
beyond psychology, xv, xxi, xxii, 7, 148, 207,
    225
Bielik-Robson, Agata, 272–273
birth
  Hannah Arendt on, 112, 216, 231–232
  as triumph, 225
birth memories, 227–229
birth trauma, 87, 111, 227–229, *228f*, 232. *See
    also* primal trauma; *Trauma of Birth*
  anxieties and fears related to, 70–71
  Beckett and, 233–234
  conceptions and characterizations of, xiii, 9,
    70, 272–273
  culture, mythology, and, 111
  difference and, 110
  Freud and, 89
  Lacan on, 267–268
  nature of, 70–71, 110, 157, 165, 273–274
  as "original wound," xiii, xv, 110, 227–228
  physiological, *228f*, 228–229
  R.D. Laing and, 255–256
  separation trauma at birth, 110, 157, 165,
    229, 234, 268–269
  therapy and, 70, 264–265, 274–275
  Winnicott on, 223, 228
  women and, 23
Blacks, 6, 57–58, 61–62. *See also* race
  Black analysts, 53–57
  Rank and, 58
Bonaduce, John, 273–274
Breger, Louis, 258
brief therapy, xvii, 130, 258–259, 264–265. *See
    also* time-limited therapy
Bryngelsson, Erik, 268–269
Buber, Martin, 120, 181, 212, 257, 280 n.2. *See
    also* I–Thou relationship
Burns, James MacGregor, 18, 276 n.2
  on leadership, 13–15, 276 n.2
Burston, Daniel, 255–256

castration anxiety and castration theory, 73, 98,
    110, 246–247. *See also* Oedipus
    complex
  separation from mother and, 86
causa sui, 171, 279 n.2

Freud's *causa sui* project, 88, 221, 224
Cave, Stephen, 265–267
Chamberlain, Lesley, 101, 258
charismatic leaders, 15, 43, 51
Child, Irvin L., 251–252
child as leader, 24
Civilization and Its Discontents (Freud), 19–20,
    22–23, 37–38, 167
Clark, Heather, 271
client-centered therapy. *See*
    person-centered/client-centered
    therapy
Cnaan, Ram, 263–264
cognitive-behavioral therapy (CBT), 2
Coleridge, Samuel Taylor, 217
collectivism, 40. *See also* nationalism;
    nation-states
community and individuality, 6, 178
compassion and empathy, 5. *See also* empathy;
    indifference
confrontation, 177, 197
congruence, 190–191. *See also* authenticity
consciousness, 153, 165, 230
  double, 57
  Freud and, 224
  of living, 163–165, 168, 218
    difference and, 176, 225
    nature of, 163, 168, 218
    pain and terror of (mere), 164
Coren, Alex, 258–259
cosmic emotion, 207. *See also* creative will
cosmic forces, 207
  cosmic primal force, 156, 160, 201, 207, 253.
    See also will
cosmic love, 139
cosmic process, 166. *See also* mystical union
  identity with the, xiv, 213
cosmology, xiv
counter-transference, 103, 120–121, 202–204.
    See also self-disclosure of therapist
  racism and, 62–63
counter-will, 122, 247–248. *See also* daimonic;
    resistance; will conflict between
    therapist and patient
  creative will and, 131–132, 174–175, 199
  Freud on, 145, 174, 202
  integration of will and, 247–248, 258,
    263–264
  nature of, 142, 199, 267–268
  terminology and related terms, 122,
    131–132, 142, 145, 155, 175, 199, 202
  in therapy, 107, 122, 145, 174, 175, 199, 202,
    205, 247–248

"courage to be," 173
creative artistic personality, 60
creative potential, 1, 17–18
creative will, 17–18, 22, 155, 162. *See also* life
    force
  Anaïs Nin and, 26, 123, 137–138, 251
  counter-will and, 131–132, 174–175, 199
  energizing and releasing, xxi, 4–5
  vs. guilt-feeling, 171
  life force and, xx, 13, 17–18, 49, 87, 105–106,
    155, 157, 201
  Martha Graham on, 157
  nature of, xx, 4, 157
  Rank's first use of the term, 22
  Rogers and, 4, 191
  self-leadership and, 13, 16, 24–26
  terminology and related terms, xx, 4, 169,
    207
  therapeutic relationship and, xx, 5, 202
  women's, xxi, 22, 25–26, 234. *See also*
    women: will of
creativity, xv, 23, 25, 201
  difference and, 17–18, 226
  guilt-feeling and, 169–170, 171–173, 175
  immortality and, 25, 247, 265, 268–269
  nature of, 60–61
Creativity: Where the Divine and the Human
    Meet (Fox), xiii
Crewe, Sandra E., 62
Crosby, Phoebe, 133–134, 147, 203–204
culture, 111
Cummings, E.E., 224–225

daimonic, the, 197, *198f*, 199, 204. *See also*
    counter-will
  creative power and, 142, 201–202
  and the demonic, 199, 202
  nature of, 197
  Rogers and, 147–148, 197, 199, 202, 205
  Rollo May and, 142, 147–148, 197–199, 202
  terminology and related terms, 142, 197, 199
  therapy and, 197, 199, 201–202, 205
  vs. *Todestrieb* (death drive), 199, 202
Dalí, Salvador, 255–256
Darga, Scott T., 259–260
"David and Goliath" battle between Rank and
    Freud, 68, *69f*, 76–77, 89
David and Goliath dream, Freud's, 250–251
"David and Goliath" letter (Freud), 74–76
death, 111. *See also Denial of Death*;
    "dying-centered" mysticism
  Heidegger and, 112–113

transcending, 28, 41, 43, 49, 155–156, 226.
    See also immortality
death drive. *See Todestrieb*
death fear (*Todesangst*), 48, 51, 58, 110, 175,
    190, 219. *See also* death: transcending;
    extinction; immortality; mortality:
    denial of
  cannot be eradicated, 166
  vs. life fear (*Lebensangst*), xxi–xxi–xxii, 9,
    169
  nature of, xxi, 211
  and politics, 41, 45, 50–51, 255–256
  terminology, 38
  and "the other," 35–36, 40, 49–50, 166
  vs. *Todestrieb* (death drive) as cause of
    aggression, 12, 38, 40–41, 43, 50, 162
  unlived/unused life and, 9, 169
  Urangst and, 12, 162, 211
  Will Therapy and, 12, 38
deCarvalho, Roy J., 257
de Marchi, Luigi, 252–253
democratic leaders, 16, 23
demonic, the, 201–202
  and the daimonic, 199, 202
  Todestrieb (death drive) and, 38, 199
Denial of Death, The (Becker), 43–44, 156, 168,
    220
  on anxiety and terror, xxii, 49, 165, 211, 218
  awards and tributes to, 27–28
  on causes of suffering, 251–252
  Freud and, 68, 88, 211
  on meaning and existential matters, 225–226
  Rank and, xii, xxii, 9, 28, 68, 88, 147, 166,
    211, 242–243
  on therapy, 211
dependency on analyst. *See also* interminable
    analysis
  transference and, 192, 203, 212
"depth-psychology," 224
destiny/fate, 218–219. *See also* determinism
  making vs. being, 219
  Nietzsche on, 176
  self-determination and, 9, 168, 176, 201
detachment. *See also* separation–individuation
  from ancient primal mother, 71
  from therapist, 130, 212
determinism. *See also* destiny/fate
  vs. free will/freedom, 33, 168, 171
  Freud and, 33, 153–154
Development of Psychoanalysis, The (Ferenczi
    & Rank), 108–109
Dewan, Mantosh J., 252–253

difference, xix–xix, 163, 224–225. *See also* fear:
of difference; likeness; psychology of
difference; *specific topics*
  acceptance and appreciation of, 205
  affirmation of the other's, 6, 203
  empathy and, 6
  existential meaning of, 51
  giving up. *See* merger; surrender
  love and, 210–211
  nature of, 160, 226
  separateness, separation, and, 78, 160, 174,
    191, 194, 205
  and suffering, 9, 174
differentiation (of self from non-self), 145, 174,
    176, 182, 211, 222. *See also*
    separation–individuation
  of client from therapist, 140, 204–205
"Discovering the Existential Unconscious:
    Rollo May Encounters Otto Rank"
    (Kramer), 273–274
diversity, 136
  vs. interdependence, 15
Doppelgänger (the double), 57–58, 273–274
Dorfman, Eran, 271
Double, The (Rank), 57–58, 65, 246–247,
    257–259, 271–273
  difference and, xix–xix–xx, 57
  W.E.B. Du Bois and, 57–58
  writers and writings influenced by, 58, 242,
    263–264
"Double as Immortal Self, The" (Rank), 57
double consciousness, 57
dreams, 135. *See also* Freud, Sigmund: dreams
    of; interpretation of dreams
  of immortality, 44–45, 48, 50
  Rank's, 83
"Dream That Interprets Itself, A" (Rank), 65
Du Bois, W.E.B., 57–58
Dufresne, Todd, 258
Dupont, Judith, 98, 262, 265–267
Durrell, Lawrence, 271
"dying-centered" mysticism, 40–41, 45, 50,
    231–232
"dying-centered" politics, 46, 232

Eagle, Morris N., 252–253
Ego and the Id, The (Freud), 19, 72, 74
ego death. *See* "other," death fear and; self:
    dissolution of
egoism, 182. *See also* narcissism
  love abolishes, 181, 210
Ekenstierna, Ingrid Sara, 274–275

emotional coldness of therapists, 32, 109, 120,
    129. *See also* indifference; surgeon
emotions/feelings, 13, 153, 156, 161–162, 207.
    See also intellectual knowledge
  accepting all, 161
  art, creativity, and, 155–156
  difference and, 225
  Freud and, 157
  Freud on, 1, 116–118, 153, 161
  listening to, 8, 13, 155, 192–193
  negative psychoanalytic attitudes toward,
    115–117, 161–162
  Nietzsche on rationality, intellect, and,
    154–155
  Rank on, 115, 160–161
  Samuel Beckett on, 234
  separating vs. uniting, 161–162
  sexuality and, 116–117
  and the soul, 32
  terminology, 115
  will and, 155, 157, 225
empathic identification, 107, 213
empathic listening, 5–6, 8, 32, 192–193. *See
    also* listening
empathy, 1, 210, 215, 229. *See also under*
    mutuality
  compassion and, 5
  existential, 227, 272–273
  interpretation and, 1, 30, 32
  listening with, 6
  microcosmic and macrocosmic levels of, 213
  nature of, 6
  Rank and, 6, 8, 30, 32, 205, 212–214,
    228–229, 271–272
  Rogers and, 4–6, 192–193, 194–195,
    202–203, 205, 207
  spirituality and, 214
  for "the other," 50, 213, 229
Empathy: A History (Lanzoni), 6, 107
empowerment. *See* self-empowerment
end phase of therapy, 70, 106–107, 111, 130,
    200, 203–204. *See also* interminable
    analysis; separation phase of
    relationship therapy; time-limited
    therapy
  and the daimonic, 199, 201–202
  "destroying" the therapist, 204–205
  goals of, 106–107, 111
  intrauterine kicking and, 200–202
  Phoebe Crosby on, 134, 203–204
  purpose of scheduling the, 202
  self-determination and, 111, 201–202

end phase of therapy (*Continued*)
  self-leadership emerging during, 106, 204.
    See also self-leadership: therapy and
eros, 192
  agape and, 41, 192, 221, 243, 247
Es (the It), 153, 155, 229
ethical development, 22, 75, 80
ethics, 156. *See also* super-ego
  emotions and, 156
  leadership, followership, and, 13–14
  men, fathers, and, 19, 25–26, 78–79
  Oedipus complex and, 78–79
  women and, 19–20, 80–81, 124
Evertz, Klaus, 271–272
evil, 36, 43. *See also* demonic
  nation-states and, 39–40, 46
  the quest for immortality and, 39–41, 43–44,
    46
existence. *See also* nonexistence vs. existence
  mystery of, xiii–xiv, 52, 169, 215, 223–224,
    230, 232, 259–260
existential anxiety, 45, 111, 233, 242–243. *See
    also Angst*; death fear; life fear; *Urangst*
existential despair, 110, 165, 211, 242–243. *See
    also Angst*; loneliness; Nothingness
  Rollo May on, 164–165, 214–215, 218
existential guilt, 15, 171, 174. *See also* guilt
  Kierkegaard on, 172, 218–219
  Rank on, 52, 160, 175, 185, 220–221, 257,
    260
  will and, 160, 174, 185, 257, 260
existential-humanistic psychology, 11, 13,
    273–275
  Rank as first analyst to integrate, 11
existentialism, 216–219. *See also* Kierkegaard,
    Søren; nonexistence vs. existence
existential empathy, 227, 272–273
existential-humanistic therapy, 2, 273–275
existential therapy, xiv, 8, 10, 110, 254–255,
    276 n.5. *See also* May, Rollo
existential unconscious, 259–261, 271–274
  nature of, 164, 233, 259–261, 273–274
  ontological unconscious and, 273–274
  philosophers on, 217
  Rank on, 164, 233
  use of the term, 164
extinction, fear of, 43, 49

Fallend, Karl, 265–267
Falzeder, Ernst, 61–62, 119, 256–257
family therapy, 30–31
fate. *See* destiny/fate

father. *See also* Oedipus complex;
    super-ego/"above-I"
  Freud on the, 19, 78, 80–81, 86, 95, 98, 154
  Rank on the, 20, 76, 80–81, 83, 87, 98
  relative power of mother and, 20, 64, 67, 77,
    80–81, 83. *See also under*
    super-ego/"above-I"
father–daughter relationship, 123, 126
father's will, 19
  vs. mother's will, 77, 80–81, 83, 89, 154
  Oedipus complex and, 25–26, 80, 90
  super-ego, ethics, and, 19, 25–26, 78, 154.
    See also super-ego/"above-I"
fear. *See also* anxiety; primal fear/primal
    anxiety; *Urangst*; *specific fears*
  of difference, xxi, 35–36. *See also* difference
  "fear and trembling," 110, 218
female sexuality. *See also* penis envy
  Freud on, 124–127, 279 n.2
Feminine Mystique, The (Friedan), 127–129
femininity, Freud on, 124
  repudiation of femininity, 22, 25–26, 98, 118,
    124–126, 150, 153
feminism, xiii, 136–137. *See also Feminine
    Mystique*; life fear: women and
  Rank and, 250, 251–252, 254–255
Ferenczi, Sándor, C6P33nn.3–4, 98, *102f*, 108,
    115, 175
  on analyst insensitivity as obstacle to
    healing, 116
  on analyst's empathy and caring, 104–105
  The Clinical Diary of Sándor Ferenczi,
    102–103, 116, 211, 250–251
  criticism of psychoanalytic treatment, 117,
    130, 179
    interminable analysis and, 102–103, 130,
      179
  The Development of Psychoanalysis, 108–109
  Elizabeth Severn and, 131–132
  on Freud, 98–99, 103, 179
    criticism of Freud as clinician, 94, 96, 103,
      109, 117, 179, 211
  Freud's analysis of, 95–96, 120
  Freud's correspondence with, 81, 84–85, 88,
    95–97
  on Freud's lack of insight, 94, 124
  on Freud's personality and pathology, 94–97
  Freud's relationship with, xviii, 76, 83–84,
    94–96, 103, 109, 120, 250–251, 278 n.4
  prospect of analyzing Freud, 95–97, 140–141
  Rank's relationship with, 76, 84–85, 94,
    250–251

Ferenczi's turning against Rank, xviii, 67,
    76, 83, 85, 109, 248, 250–251
  Secret Committee and, 67, 76, 109, 115
  on therapeutic relationship, 203, 210–211
  The Trauma of Birth (Rank) and, xviii, 71, 76
  use of Rank's vocabulary, 250–251, 278 n.4
  on women, 94–95
Finkelstein, Haim, 255–256
Fox, Matthew, xii–xvi, 254–255, 259–260,
    267–268
Franko, Mark, 265–267
free will vs. determinism. *See under*
    destiny/fate; determinism
Freud, Amalia (mother), 90, 96
  death, 126–127
  Ferenczi and, 94–97, 179
  Freud's cancer and, 70, 93, 97, 141
  Freud's relationship with, 88, 91, *92f*, 93–94
    enmeshment, 90–93, 95–96, 99, 101,
      140–141, 179, 227
    Freud's lack of insight into and reluctance
      to analyze, 90, 93–94, 97, 101, 140–141,
      227
    and Freud's views on female psychology,
      90, 94–95, 98, 124, 126–127
    and Freud's views on technique, 101
    negative feelings toward Amalia, 90–92,
      95, 97, 124, 141, 227
  personality, 90–91, 93
  photographs of, 91–92, *92f*
  Rank and, 93–95, 97–98, 124, 179
  sexuality and, 94–95, 98
  as *Urmutter* of psychoanalysis, 88, 90, 99,
    179
Freud, Anna, *125f*
  Esther Menaker and, 129
  Freud and, 68, 80, 123, *125f*, 126, 157
  Freud's analysis of, 118
  on Rank, 68
  on "real relationship," 121
  on relationship therapy, 121
Freud, Jakob (father), 91, 95
Freud, Martha Bernays (wife), 99–101, *100f*
Freud, Martin (son), 91
Freud, Oliver (son), 91
Freud, Sigmund, 19–20. *See also specific topics*
  on analyst's emotional experience, 1
  anti-Americanism, 141
  assumptions about human nature, 25–26
  cancer, 70, 75, 91, 93, 96, 120, 141, 258–259,
    280 n.2
    and Amalia Freud (mother), 70, 93, 97,
      141

prosthesis, 91, 280 n.2
  "psychic root" of, 97
  surgeries, 71–72, 74–75, 91, 93, 97, 280 n.2
character, 78, 101
as clinician, 120
  attitudes toward patients, 61–62, 103,
    117–118, 120, 150, 268
  effectiveness, 118
  "lured transference" to get love from
    patients, 211
  technique, 120
death of, xix, 221
  Rank and the, 87, 221
determinism and, 33, 153–154
dreams of, 72–73, 250–251
  David and Goliath dream, 250–251
  Rank's interpretation of, 65, 72–75, 84,
    250–251
on homogeneity of human nature, 53
language and, 98
  metaphors, 98–99
on mother–infant relationship, 87
on mother–son relationship, 103, 121,
    140–141
personality, xviii, 78, 83, 101, 120, 127, 144
  "small boy," 91–93, 98, 103, 179
photographs of, *37f*, 91–92, *92f*, *125f*
and the pre-Oedipal mother, 83, 141, 154,
    251. *See also under* Freud, Amalia;
    Trauma of Birth
psychopathology, 68, 94–95, 179–180, 220,
    279 n.2. *See also under* Ferenczi, Sándor
  infantilism, 91–92, 95, 99–101, 141, 220,
    279 n.2
  narcissistic rage, xviii, xix, 81, 95
race and, 62. *See also* "negroes"
on Rank, 66. *See also under* Freud–Rank
    conflict
  negative characterizations, xviii, 87, 101
  positive characterizations, 65–66, 76, 83
Rank's characterizations of, 68, 83, 88, 124
  "[no] more insight than a small boy"
    (Rank), xviii, 86, 93–94, 101, 124
Rank's writings and, 76
science and, xvii–xviii, 24–26, 29–30, 33, 127
self-analysis of
  and the creation of psychoanalysis, 127
  limitations of the, 90, 99, 127
  and Oedipus complex, 25–26, 73, 76, 78,
    90
sexuality, 94–95
on technique, 32, 119–120

Freud, Sigmund (*Continued*)
  therapeutic nihilism, 103–104, 108–109, 117, 221, 268–269
  unacknowledged intellectual debts, 88
  United States and, 141
  vasectomy/self-castration, 72
  on will, 25. *See also under* counter-will; women: will of
  will and, 19
  women and, 25–26, 77, 94, 251. *See also under* women
  women friends, 80
  women's power and, 19–20, 22
  women's sexuality and, 80, 94–95, 98
  writings of. *See also specific writings*
    Rank's editing and proofreading, 86
    as revealing Freud's unconscious, 98–99
Freudians
  in social work, 26
    criticism of Rank, 24
  vendetta against Rank, xix, 68
Freud–Rank conflict, xviii–xix, 68, 77, 81–83, 86
  "David and Goliath" battle, 68, 69f, 76–77, 89
  final parting, 67–68, 86–87
  Freud's criticisms of Rank, xviii, 33, 81
  Freud's "treacherous assassination" of Rank, xviii, 84–87, 95
  Rank's criticisms of Freud, 29–30, 68
Freud–Rank relationship, xvii–xix, 66, 73. *See also* "David and Goliath" battle between Rank and Freud
  Freud's reactions to Rank, xviii–xix
  letters, 83
    Freud's "David and Goliath" letter, 74–76
  mutual analysis, 84
  Rank as "heir" of Freud, xvii–xviii, 66, 68
  Rank's feelings toward Freud, 83–84
Freund, Philip, 241
Friedan, Betty, 127–129, 128f
fusion. *See* merger; Oneness/wholeness

Gallant, James, 268–269
Garai, Josef E., 244
Gay, Peter, 67, 90, 250–251
Geismar, Maxwell, 242–243
gender differences, 35, 52. *See also specific topics*
genocide, 36, 40
Gestalt therapy, 253–254
God, 210
  father and, 19, 80

Rollo May on, 214–215
  transference and the analyst as, 211–212
Goldwert, Marvin, 248–249
Goodman, Paul, 253–254
Graham, Martha, 157–159, 158f, 169–170
Griffiths, Mark, 25, 270
Groddeck, Georg, 258–259
Grof, Stanislav, 248–249
Grosskurth, Phyllis, 251–252
group psychology. *See under* immortality
guilt, 160, 167–169, 171. *See also* existential guilt
  Becker on, 41, 211
  consciousness of, 171
  difference and, 52, 160
  real vs. imaginary, 169–170
  therapy and, 172–173, 204, 211
guilt-feeling. *See also* existential guilt
  creativity and, 169–170, 171–173, 175
  Freud's, 75, 220
  nature of, 160, 168–169, 171–172
  separation–individuation and, 168, 172
  will and, 52, 167–168, 169–173, 175, 185
Gunning, Tom, 272–273
Gupta, Sanjay, 252–253

Halliwell, Martin, 257
Hampden-Turner, Charles, 247
Hankiss, Elemér, 258–259
Haynal, André, 250–251, 280 n.2
Heidegger, Martin
  death and, 112–113
  Hannah Arendt and, 112
  Rank and, 277 n.14
Helson, Ravenna, 258
"here-and-now," 1, 105, 279 n.2. *See also* present moment
heroes and heroism, 43, 88. *See also* leadership; *Myth of the Birth of the Hero*
  Becker and, 28, 43–44, 88, 251
  immortality and, 41–43, 251
  mysticism, religion, and, 40–41, 44, 167
  war and, 28, 41, 44
Hoffman, Irwin Z., 262
Homans, Peter, 251
homosexuality, 135
  Jessie Taft and, 135–136
  Rank and, 135–136
  Sigmund and Anna Freud and, 118, 123
humanistic psychology, 109. *See also* existential-humanistic psychology
Humann, Heather D., 270–271
human nature

Freud's theory of, 25–26, 52, 152–154
Rank's theory of, 146–147, 150, 152–153
Rogers on, 146, 188, 197, 199

id (*das Es*/"the It"). *See also* structural theory
  Freud on feelings and, 118, 153
  will and, 74, 153, 155, 229
ideologies and immortality, 39–41, 263–264
immortality, 44, 68, 153, 265. *See also* mortality
  artists and, 25, 152, 171
  and belief in the soul, 32–33
  creativity and, 25, 247, 265, 268–269
  and the double, 57
  dreams of, 44–45, 48, 50
  group/collective, 40, 42–45, 153. *See also*
    nation-states: immortality and
  heroism and, 41–43, 251
  ideologies and, 39–41, 263–264
  nationalism and, 39, 42
  nation-states and, 39–41, 42–46, 48, 50–51,
    153, 231–232
  quest for, 25, 39–40, 43–44, 248–249, 262,
    265–267, 268–269
    Becker on, 28, 40–41, 43–44, 251–252,
      263–267
    and evil, 39–41, 43–44, 46
    and fear of death, 247, 251–252. *See also*
      death fear
    and group psychology, 40, 42–44
  species, 152
  war and, 41, 44, 46
  women as threat to man's, 88
Incest Theme in Literature and Legend, The
  (Rank), 65, 270
independence. *See* dependency on analyst;
  self-determination; will
indeterminism, principle of, 33. *See also*
  quantum physics
indifference (*Indifferenz*/"neutrality"). *See also*
  emotional coldness of therapists;
  neutrality; surgeon; transference
  Ferenczi's criticism of, 116, 175, 252–253
  Freud and, 116, 119–120, 180
  meanings and translations of the term, 119,
    252–253
  and transference, 180, 192
individuality. *See also* difference
  and community, 6, 178
  Hannah Arendt on, 112, 231–232
  will and, 152

individuation. *See* separation–individuation
infantilizing patients, 104, 179, 204
inferiority vs. superiority and difference, 163
Inhibitions, Symptoms and Anxiety (Freud)
  critique of Rank, xviii, 85–87, 93, 95,
    246–247. *See also* Freud–Rank conflict:
    Freud's "treacherous assassination" of
    Rank
  Ferenczi and, 95
  Rank and the publication of, 86, 95
insight, 116–117
  Freud on, 1, 94, 97
  Rank and, 180–181, 259–260, 268
  resistance to, 97, 104
  Rogers and, 4, 149
intellectual knowledge (vs. emotional
  experience), 32, 164, 180, 189, 190
interminable analysis, 140. *See also* "Analysis
  Terminable and Interminable"
  Ferenczi on, 102–103, 130, 179
  Freud and, 127, 130, 140–141, 161, 179, 220
  Rank and, 140–141, 175, 179, 212
  transference and, 102–103, 179, 192, 212
internalization. *See also* super-ego/"above-I"
  first internalized object, 71–72, 80–81, 86–87
  of mother, 70–71, 80–81, 87
International Psychoanalytical Association
  (IPA), 56–57
interpretation, 144, 149, 178, 180. *See also*
  insight
  empathy and, 1, 30, 32
  limits of, 1, 32, 177–178, 180–181, 194,
    201–202
  pitfalls of, 30, 32, 103–104, 142, 177, 191
  Rank on, 1, 30, 32, 104, 174, 177–178,
    180–181, 194, 201–202
  relationship and, 1, 30, 149
  resisting analyst's interpretations, 38, 80, 122,
    144, 145, 150, 174–175, 179, 199, 202
  of transference, 38, 103–105, 149, 180
interpretation of dreams, 65
  Rank's interpretation of Freud's dreams, 65,
    72–75, 84, 250–251
Interpretation of Dreams, The (Freud), 78, 98
  Rank and, 65, 73
intersectional identities, 57
Isono, Masayo, 265
I–Thou relationship, 178, 181, 200, 212, 257.
    See also Buber, Martin
  Freud and, 118–120
  vs. I–It relationship, 118–120
  Rank and, 181, 183, 257

Janus, Ludwig, 256–257, 274–275
Jason, Philip K., 244–245
Johnson, Richard, 243–244
John-Steiner, Vera, 251
Jones, Ernest, xviii, xxii, 93–94
  distortions and fabrications, xxii, 87, 243,
    254–255
  on Freud, 101, 279 n.2
  Freud biography, xxii
  on Rank, 87, 93–94, 243, 254–255
  vs. Rank, 81–82, 85, 108–109
Josselson, Ruthellen, 263–264

Kainer, Rochelle, 260
Kainer, Selig, 260
Kamin, Robert Joel, 259–260
Karpf, Fay, 179, 240
Kaufman, Scott Barry, 231
Kendrick, Walter, 248–249
Kierkegaard, Søren, xxi, 110, 218, 219f, 277
  n.14
Kindersley, Dorling, 265–267
Klein, Dennis, 248–249
Klein, Naomi, 273–274
Knowlson, James, 255–256
Koenig, Terry, 271
Kostaras, Panagiotas, 271–272
Krim, Murray, 257
Kugelmann, Robert, 33, 273–274

Lacan, Jacques, 222–223, 267–268
  on creation, 224
  Freud and, 98, 141
  Rank and, 256–257, 274–275, 281 n.1
Lagercrantz, Hugo, 229, 268–269
Laing, R.D., 255–256
Landy, Robert J., 263–264
Lang, Birgit, 270
Langstroth, Lovell, 240
Lanzoni, Susan, 6, 107, 270–271
Larsen, Nella, 59–61, 60f
Lavin, Sylvia, 261
Lawrence, D.H., 215, 226
  Nietzsche and, 215
  Rank on, 215
Leader, Zachary, 251–252
leaders
  charismatic, 15, 43, 51
  toxic, 43, 45, 50–51, 232, 261–262
leadership
  as art form, 14
  heroes and, 13, 43. See also Myth of the Birth
    of the Hero

James MacGregor Burns on, 13–15
  practicing, 14
  as a relationship, 13
leadership development, 13
  will therapy and, 16
learning. See unlearning
Lebensangst. See life fear
Lebiez, Judith, 270
Leitner, Marina, 256–257
Levenson, Hanna, 264–265
Lewisohn, Ludwig, 265–267
libido. See also sex drive
  Freud on, 116, 124
Lieberman, E. James, xxii, 40, 57–58, 73, 82, 98,
    147, 248–249
life fear (Lebensangst), 110, 219. See also Angst
  and autonomy, 51
  cannot be eradicated, 166
  charismatic leaders and, 15
  vs. death fear (Todesangst), xxi–xxii, 9, 12,
    169
  nature of, xxi, 15, 211, 216, 218
  Rogers and, 190
  Urangst and, 12, 162, 211
  will and, 162
  women and, 22, 77, 128
life force, xx, 26, 207. See also cosmic forces;
    creative will
  Becker and, 49, 156, 220
  creative will and, xx, 13, 17–18, 49, 87,
    105–106, 155, 157, 201
  Freud and, 22, 220
  nature of, 150–151, 157
  neurotics and, 162
  Rollo May and, 197
  self-leadership and, 10, 13, 162
  will and, 32, 142, 150–151, 162
  women and, 22, 87
life/living. See also consciousness: of living
  nature of, 151, 167
  unlived/unused life and failing to live, 9, 169,
    171
Lifton, Robert J., 247–248
likeness, 37
  difference and
    creativity and, 52
    integrating, 194, 203, 207
    simultaneous experience of, 203, 207
    tension between, 52, 57–58, 174, 178–179,
      198–199, 243
  psychoanalysis and, 53, 55, 112, 202
Lipman-Blumen, Jean, 15, 45, 50–51, 255–256,
    261–262

listening, 32
    active, 4–5
    empathic, 5–6, 8, 32, 192–193
    to feelings, 8, 13, 155, 192–193
    Rogers and, 4–6, 192–193
Lomas, Tim, 272–273
loneliness, 41–42, 111, 243
    birth trauma and, 110–111
    difference and, 9, 41, 52, 110, 174, 243
lost unity, searching for and restoring, 214
love, 133, 181. *See also agape; eros*
    abolishes egoism, 181, 210
    art and, 182–183, 212–214, 224
    cosmic, 139
    darker side of, 105, 204, 210
    difference, Oneness, and, 213–215
    empathy and, 148, 192, 210
    Freud and, 120, 178–179, 211
    I–Thou relationship and, 178, 181, 210, 235
    mutual, 182–183, 203, 221, 229
    nature of, 181, 210
    of patient for therapist, 102–103. *See also*
        transference love
    and therapist's need for love, 120, 202,
        204, 211
    in relationship therapy, 105–106, 133–134,
        143, 183, 203, 212
    Rogers and, 192, 202
    separation and, 203–204
    types of, 210–211
love and will, 106, 162, 165, 168, 176, 178,
        179–180
    integration of, 140, 146
    Rollo May and, 10
Love and Will (May), 77, 214–215, 221, 242.
        See also daimonic: Rollo May and
Loy, David, 255–256

MacKinnon, Donald, 243–244
macrocosm. *See* microcosm (of individual
        psyche) and macrocosm
Mahony, Patrick J., 248
Makari, George, 263–264
Malraux, André, 226
Marinelli, Lydia, 260
Marmor, Judd, 245
Martin, Jack, 49, 267–268
masculine ideology, 121–122
    Rank on, xvi, xxi, 16, 23, 121
    women's liberation from, xxi, 23
Maslow, Abraham, 10–11
Maté, Gabor, 267–268
Matson, Floyd W., 241

May, Rollo, 173, 240, 243–244, 251
    on birth trauma, 9
    and the daimonic, 142, 147–148, 197–199,
        202
    on existential despair, 164–165, 214–215,
        218
    Irvin Yalom and, 12, 77
    Love and Will, 77, 214–215, 221, 242. *See
        also* daimonic: Rollo May and
    overview, 10–11
    Power and Innocence, 197–199
    on Rank, 10–11, 146, 240, 244, 248–249,
        251–252, 254–256
    Rank's influence on, 10
    Rogers and, 146–148, 199
    self-leadership and, 10
    as therapist, 10
    on transference, 192
Mayer, Andreas, 260
Meisel, Perry, 248–249
Menaker, Bill, 127–129
Menaker, Esther, 229
    Anna Freud and, 129
    Misplaced Loyalties, 129, 254–255
    Otto Rank: A Rediscovered Legacy, 36, 247
    Rank and, xix, 36, 68, 88, 129, 144, 248,
        254–255, 256–257
    *Separation, Will and Creativity: The Wisdom
        of Otto Rank*, 255–257
    women, feminism, and, 36, 127
merger, 213–214, 273–274. *See also*
        Oneness/wholeness
    desire for, 41, 107, 166, 176, 210, 254–255
    with therapist, 70, 107, 145
Merkur, Dan, 230, 264–265
Meyer, James, 272–273
microcosm (of individual psyche) and
        macrocosm (of universe), 182–183,
        208, 226
    Carl Rogers and, 207–208, 214
    The Denial of Death and, 166, 168
    difference and, 225
    empathy and, 213–214
    and negotiating with "the Beyond," 230
    Rank on connection between, xiv, 134,
        156–157
    separation, union, and, 166–167, 214–215
"midwife," therapist as, 111, 185, 190, 208
Miller, Henry
    Anaïs Nin and, 142–144, *143f*, 199
    Rank and, 142–144, 199
Miller, Jacques-Alain, 267–268
Milton, John, 245–246

Moorjani, Angela, 233–234, 261
Morgan, Gareth, 262
mortality. *See also* immortality
    denial of, 36, 43, 88. *See also Denial of Death*
    relational, 113
mother–child relationship, xviii, 87. *See also Urmutter; specific topics*
    clinging to mother, 81
    vs. father–child relationship. *See under* father; father's will
    internalization of mother, 70–71, 80–81, 87
    man's denial of his mother-origin and mortality, 36, 88
"mother love" (from therapist in relationship therapy), 105–106, 143
Müller, Bertram, 260
Munroe, Ruth, 240
Muran, Christopher J., 258
mutuality
    mutual empathic relationship, xv–xvi, 182, 207, 212, 229
    mutual empathy, 5–6, 183, 205, 210, 214–215
    mutual love, 182–183, 203, 221, 229
    mutual recognition, 210, 229
    of therapeutic relationship, 18, 31, 105, 114, 202–203, 212
mystery of existence, xiii–xiv, 52, 169, 215, 223–224, 230, 232, 259–260
mystical union (*unio mystica*), xiv, xv, 208, 212, 214, 267–268
    Freud and, 227
    Rogers and, 207–208, 214
    Rollo May on, 214–215, 242
    therapeutic relationship and, 229
mysticism, 264–265. *See also* Beyond; "dying-centered" mysticism; spirituality; transcendence
    creation-centered, 231–232
    etymology of the term, 230
    Lacan and, 222–223
    life-enhancing, 232
    nature of, 230
    in politics, 41–42, 231
    Rogers and, 206–207
    universality of, 230–232
    Wittgenstein's, 230
Myth of the Birth of the Hero, The (Rank), 14–15, 43, 65, 138
mythologies. *See* heroes and heroism

narcissism, 178–179, 182, 280 n.3. *See also* egoism
natality, Hannah Arendt on, 112, 232

National Gallery of Art exhibition on *The Double*, 272–273, 278 n.3
national ideologies. *See under* immortality
nationalism, 42–43, 46–48
nation-states, 232. *See under* immortality; Russian invasion of Ukraine
    Becker on, 41, 46–47
    dying in the name of, 41, 231
    evil and, 39–40, 46
    Hannah Arendt on, 112, 232
    heroism and, 41–43, 46–47
    as "home-like," 48, 50, 111
    immortality and, 39–41, 42–46, 48, 50, 153, 231–232
    nature of, 46–48
    and the womb, 111–112
"negroes," Freud calling his patients, 61–62, 126
Neufeld, Gordon, 267–268
neurosis
    nature of and causes of, xiv, 10, 70, 162–163, 165, 174, 201
    as self-willed, 162
    use of the term, 16
Neutra, Richard, 261
neutrality, 174, 192. *See also* indifference
    terminology and meanings of the term, 119, 252–253
Nietzsche, Friedrich, 154, *177f*, 215
    contrasted with Rank, 167, 257
    on fate, 176
    Freud and, 88
    on rationality, intellect, and feeling, 154–155
    will and, 77, 154, 167, 195, 257
Nin, Anaïs
    creative will and, 26, 123, 137–138, 251
    Henry Miller and, 142–144, *143f*, 199
    lovers, 139–140, 142
    on Rank, xiii, 16, 26, 58, 115, 123, 137–138, 161, 187, 226, 227, 280 n.1
    on Rank's death, 140
    Rank's letters to, 139, 223
    Rank's relationship with, 58, 137–140, 161
    therapy with Rank, 137–139, 142, 187, 247, 251, 267–268
    women, womanhood, and, 26, 123, 137–138, 140, 251, 267–268
    writings, 137, 139–140, 260, 267–268
        The Diary of Anaïs Nin, 137–138, 187
9/11 terrorist attacks, 48
nonbeing, existential awareness of, 233
nonexistence vs. existence, 52–53, 227
Nothingness, 168, 216, 220, 226, 233
    birth and, 112, 164, 222–224

death and, 48, 164
denying our, 41, 226
difference and, 215, 224–225
fear of, 38, 48
Pascal on, 217
and the unconscious, 164
Novey, Rita, 247–248

Obaid, Francisco, 265–267
observer and observed, 29. See also quantum
    physics
oceanic feeling, 227–228. See also mystical
    union; Oneness/wholeness
O'Dowd, William T., 249
Oedipus complex, 25–26. See also castration
    anxiety and castration theory
    birth trauma and, 70–71
    Freudian diagnosis and, 25–26
    Freud on, xvii–xviii, 19, 25–26, 39, 71, 78
    Freud's self-analysis and, 25–26, 73, 76, 78,
        90
    vs. the pre-Oedipal, xviii, 70–71, 76
    Rank's disagreements with Freudian view of,
        xviii, 26–27, 39, 68, 71, 76
    super-ego and, 19, 25–26, 72–73, 79, 86, 154
    transference and, 26, 30
    The Trauma of Birth and, xviii, 71, 76, 80–81
    women, femininity, and, 19, 25–26
Oneness/wholeness, xiv, 183, 190, 207, 214. See
    also merger; mystical union; surrender
    birth and the loss of, 111, 157, 165
    empathy and, 229
    existential guilt and, 174
    healing and, 9, 165, 182, 190, 208
    separation, union, and, 9, 157, 165, 174, 176,
        207–208
    and the womb, 165, 229
    yearning for, 41, 111, 157, 165
Orban, Peter, 250–251
"other, the," 160, 168, 171. See also separateness
    acceptance vs. nonacceptance of, 231
    aggression toward, 35–36, 40, 49
    death fear and, 35–36, 40, 49–50, 166
    difference and, 6, 36, 41, 211, 214, 231
    empathy for, 50, 213, 229. See also empathy
    love and, 183, 210
    Oneness and, 214, 229
    will and, 211
"other world," 213–214. See also Beyond
    Rank on, 206, 210, 212
    Rogers on "other-worldly" realm, 7, 148,
        206–207, 214
"Otto Rank and 'The Cause'" (Kramer), 256

Pals, Jennifer L., 258
part–whole problem, 179, 182, 274–275
    solutions to, 165–166, 182, 212
Pascal, Blaise, 218
paternal domination, 20–21
patriarchy, xiii, xv, xvi, 23, 35, 251
    and creative will, 22
    Freud's, xiii, xiv, 22–23, 35, 68, 123, 245–246,
        248–249. See also under Freud,
        Sigmund
    in psychoanalysis, 68, 123
Pavloski, Linda, 259–260
Peck, Wilda, 132–133
penis envy, 59, 80, 124–126
person-centered/client-centered therapy, xvii,
    xx, 8. See also Rogers, Carl
    birth of, 189–190
    central message of, 4
    core conditions of, 4, 190–193, 194–195, 281
        n.3. See also empathy
    Rank and, 7–8, 146, 150, 194, 205
    Rogers on, 190–191
    terminology and related terms, 7–8
    transference in, 192, 211
    in various countries, 8
Pine, Richard, 271
Plath, Sylvia, 271
Plowden, Mary, 142
polarities in relationship therapy, 5, 145, 182,
    205
politics, 44. See also under immortality
    death fear (Todesangst) and, 41, 45, 50–51,
        255–256
    Hannah Arendt on, 112, 232
    mysticism in, 41–42, 231
Pollan, Michael, 252–253
Polster, Erving, 242
power, 19. See also will; women: power
    power over vs. power with, 26
    of social work clients, 26
powerlessness, 23, 197
    women and, 20, 22–23, 51, 197
prenatal psychology and womb experience,
    111–112, 227, 229, 267–268
    Ludwig Janus on, 256–257, 274–275
    Rank on, xiv, 70, 111, 165, 214, 273–275
pre-Oedipal mother. See also Trauma of Birth
    Freud and, 83, 141, 154, 251
    Rank and, 83
"pre-Oedipal," origin of the term, xviii, 81
pre-Oedipal phase, 94, 96. See also Trauma of
    Birth
    Freud and, 84–85, 88, 94

pre-Oedipal phase (*Continued*)
vs. Oedipus complex, xviii, 70–71, 76
Rank's theory of, 81–85, 88, 91–92, 130
present moment, 103, 105, 177–178, 211. *See also* "here-and-now"
primal fear/primal anxiety, 12, 71, 81, 110, 216. *See also Urangst*
primal life force. *See* cosmic forces; life force
primal repression, 20, 71, 81, 140–141
primal trauma, 140–141, 228. *See also* birth trauma; primal fear/primal anxiety
Progoff, Ira, 241
projective identification, 108, 133, 175, 204
psychoanalytic cancel culture, 68
psychoanalytic treatment. *See also specific topics*
"classical psychoanalysis," 175
harmful effects, 32, 102, 161, 175. *See also* interminable analysis
interminable analysis, 102–103, 127, 130, 140–141, 161, 175, 179, 212, 220
length of, 130. *See also* brief therapy; interminable analysis; time-limited therapy
transference and, 192
primary obstacle to healing in, 116
Rank's criticisms of, 120, 150
terminology, 175
therapeutic factors in. *See also specific topics*
Ferenczi and Rank on, 104–105, 108–109
Rank on, 104
Psychology and the Soul (Rank), 28, 32–33
Freud's critique of, 33
motives for writing, 39
psychology of difference, 23, 222. *See also* difference
vs. Freud's psychology of likeness, 52–53, 62, 112, 137, 152
intersectional identities and, 57
Rank on, xix–xx, 52–53, 222
Rogers and, 191, 205
social work and, xx, 57, 62, 136–137
The Trauma of Birth and, 110, 225
Psychology of Difference, A (Rank), 7–8, 10, 52, 255–256

quantum physics, xvi, 28–30, 32–33

race, 6, 52–53. *See also* Blacks
Freud and, 62, 126. *See also* "negroes"
psychology of likeness and, 202
racism, 6, 36, 58
in psychoanalysis, 53–57, 62–63

Ragland, Ellie, 274–275
Rank, Beata "Tola" (wife), 80, *108f*, 115
as analyst, 20–21
Freud and, 82, 93, 139
on Rank, 82, 115
Rank on, 80
Rank's relationship with, 21, 32, 65, 107–108, 139
women and, 20–21, 80, 154
Rank, Helene (daughter), 107, *108f*, 139
Rank, Otto
alter-ego ("Huck"), 57
character and integrity, 65, 83–84, 98
characterizations of, xiii–xvii, 10, 27–28, 66–67, 107, 149, 225, 234, 241, 243, 254–255, 258–260. *See also* "David and Goliath" battle between Rank and Freud; Freud, Sigmund: on Rank
Anaïs Nin's, 187, 226
criticisms of, 131. *See also* Freud, Sigmund: on Rank
death, xix, 221, 234
feelings, 115
forced to either recant or fight back, 82–83. *See also under Trauma of Birth*
in historical context, 10–11
interdisciplinary thought, 28
letter of apology to Secret Committee, 82–83
personality, xv, 16, 82–83, 107, 115, 131, 138
photographs of, *3f*, *54f*, *64f*, *186f*
pioneering work of, 11, 13. *See also Trauma of Birth*: as groundbreaking
positions held by, 66–67
prominent figures influenced by, 27
psychopathology, 84
alleged "psychosis," 68, 87
mood swings, 87
as therapist, 137–138
invoice and fee, *132f*
technique, 187
therapeutic failures, 131
writings of, 64–65, 147, 208. *See also specific writings*
epigraphs in the, xx–xxi
"real relationship," 181, 211. *See also* I–Thou relationship; therapeutic relationship
Anna Freud on, 121
vs. transference, 26, 30, 104–105, 109, 120–121, 144, 149, 180, 192, 210–212, 242
reductionism, Freud's, 116, 151
relational mortality, 113
relational psychoanalysis, 8, 77

relationship(s), 2. *See also* I–Thou relationship;
  romantic relationships; therapeutic
  relationship
 healing effects of, 1–4
 Rank's definition of, 1, 114
 Rogers on, 4–5, 196
 willingness to be oneself within, 1
relationship therapy, 1, 29–30, 32, 187. *See also*
  time-limited therapy; will therapy;
  specific topics
 aims of, 133, 162
 beginning phase of, 105
 empathy in, 8, 105, 107
 Freudian criticism of, 121, 140
 love in, 105–106, 133–134, 143, 183, 203, 212
 overview and nature of, 8, 110, 133, 135, 145,
  205, 229
 vs. psychoanalysis, 31, 121, 149
 Rank's invention of, 107–108, 150
 Rogers and, 8, 149, 188, 196
 terminology and related terms, 8, 145, 150
 therapeutic factors in, 26, 145. *See also*
  authentic relationship
 will therapy and, 145, 150, 187
religion, xiv, 19, 210
 Rank on, xiv, 153, 167, 216
repression. *See* primal repression
resistance, 104
 counter-will/daimonic and, 122, 131–132,
  145, 175, 179, 199, 202. *See also*
  counter-will
 Freud on, 38, 140, 144–145, 150, 174–175,
  179, 202
 to insight, 97, 104
 positive will and, 120, 140, 175, 264–265
 Rank on, 175–176
 resisting analyst's interpretations, 38, 80, 122,
  144, 145, 150, 174–175, 179, 199, 202
 Todestrieb (death drive) as cause of, 38, 80,
  122, 150, 199
Roazen, Paul, 101, 129, 251–252, 254–255, 257
 on Rank and Freud, 243, 257–259
Robinson, Virginia, xx, 16–17, 106, 135–136,
  137*f*, 149, 160
Rodden, John, 268–269
Rogers, Carl, 148*f*, 149, 205–206, 216. *See also*
  person-centered/client-centered
  therapy
 on actualizing tendency, 4, 207
 anger and, 202
 characterizations of, 7, 146, 191
 and the daimonic, 147–148, 197, 199, 202,
  205

empathy and, 4–6, 192–193, 194–195,
  202–203, 205, 207
 essential contribution, 6
 insight and, 4, 149
 language and metaphors, 7
 legacy, xvii, 2–6, 7–8
 limitations, 202
 on listening, 4–5
 "overall hypothesis," 196–197
 personality, 191, 202–203
 professional evolution, 4–5
 psychology of difference and, 191, 205
 on Rank, 2, 185, 188
 Rank compared with, 188, 190–191, 197
 Rank's influence on, 2–4, 7–8, 146, 185–188,
  189–190, 234
 Rank's weekend with, 149–150, 152–153,
  185–187, 189–190
 relationship therapy and, 8, 149, 188, 196
 Rollo May and, 146–148, 199
 on self, 209, 211
 self-empowerment of clients, 4
 on separateness, 6, 191, 193–194
 on spirituality, 7, 148, 205–208, 214–215
 on therapist as "midwife," 190, 208
 transcendence and, 148, 205–208
 on transference, 192, 211
 will and, 4, 191
 writings, 4
  Counseling and Psychotherapy, 2, 190
Rogers, Robert, 242
romantic relationships, transference and
  projective identification in, 108
Roudinesco, Elisabeth, 268–269
Rudnytsky, Peter, 251–252, 259–260
Russian invasion of Ukraine, 45–46

Safran, Jeremy, 258
Schein, Edgar, 17, 270
Schmitt, Abraham, 245–246
Schneider, Kirk J., 254–255, 271–274
Schopenhauer, Arthur, 152–154
Schwartz, Albert, 242–243
science
 Freud and, xvii, 24–26, 29–30, 33, 127
 limitations, 151, 215–217
 psychoanalysis as "scientific," 259–260
 Rank and, 24, 29–30, 32, 216–217, 259–260
Secret Committee, 85, 139, 251–252
 Ferenczi and, 67, 76, 109, 115
 Freud's power in, 66–67
 Freud's support for Rank in, 66–67, 82, 85
 overview and nature of, 66

Secret Committee (*Continued*)
  photograph of, 66, *67f*
  Rank on, 85
  Rank's conciliatory letter to, 82–83
  Rank's role and influence in, 66–67
  splintered and turned against Rank, 67, 76,
    81–82, 85, 109, 115
  view of Freud's character, 101
Segal, Robert, 265
Seidenman, Ethel W., 106–107
Seif, Nancy G., 245–246
self
  being a self with others, 6
  differentiation of non-self from, 205. *See also*
    separation–individuation
  dissolution of, 213–214
  rebirthing a new, 145
self-actualization, 11, 107, 183, 245–246. *See
    also* actualizing tendency
self-concepts, unlearning, 61. *See also*
    unlearning
self-consciousness, 153, 163, 165, 218
self-determination
  end phase of therapy and, 111, 201–202
  social work and, 276 n.4
self-disclosure of therapist, 115
self-empowerment, 4, 24
self-in-relationship, 18
self-leadership, xv, 23
  Black liberation and, 62
  capacity for, xx, 4, 10, 51, 128, 137, 162. *See
    also* creative will
  creative will and, 13, 16, 24–26, 51, 106
  difference and, 23, 137
  life force and, 10, 13, 162
  nature of, 10, 13, 51
  Rollo May and, 10
  self-determination and, 276 n.4
  social work and, xx, 22–23, 24–26, 137
  therapy and, 4, 106, 128, 176, 190, 204, 276
    n.5
  women and, xv, 22–23, 24–26, 51, 128
self-realization, 18, 245–246, 251–252. *See also*
    life fear
self-transcendence, 183, 221, 230. *See also*
    agape; transcendence
separateness. *See also* difference;
    Oneness/wholeness
  anxiety related to, 163, 165–166, 210. *See also*
    Angst; birth trauma; separation anxiety
  and empathy, 193
  love and dissolution of, 210
  relationships and, 191, 193–194

  Rogers on, 6, 191, 193–194
  in therapy, 145, 191, 193
separating vs. uniting affects, 161–162
separation anxiety, 113
  birth trauma and, 70–71. *See also under*
    birth trauma
  The Trauma of Birth and, 75, 110, 113
separation–individuation, 113–114, 214. *See
    also* birth trauma; differentiation;
    Oneness/wholeness
  empathy and, 213
  joy in, 70
  from mother, 86
    detachment from ancient primal mother,
      71
    Freud and, 99. *See also under* Freud,
      Amalia
  from therapist, 130, 134, 140, 203–205, 212.
    See also end phase of therapy
    "destroying" the therapist, 204–205
  vs. union, 6, 9, 183, 200. *See also* life fear: vs.
    death fear; microcosm (of individual
    psyche) and macrocosm (of universe)
  will to separate and to unite, 99, 107, 162,
    166, 172, 174, 176, 183, 200
  union and, 70, 145, 210, 254–255, 273–274
  wholeness/Oneness and, 9, 157, 165, 174,
    176, 207
separation phase of relationship therapy, 212.
    See also end phase of therapy;
    time-limited therapy
Severn, Elizabeth, 131–132
sex drive, 151. *See also* id; libido
sexuality, 152. *See also specific topics*
  reducing all feelings to, 116
Sheets-Johnstone, Maxine, 263–264
Shuman, Michael L., 262
Sievers, Burkard, 253–254
Sloterdijk, Peter, 111, 256–257
Smith, Edward W.L., 265–267
Smith, Huston, 252–253
Smith, J.C., 251
Smith, Kenwyn, 250
social oppression and social problems, 16
social work, xiii, xx
  psychology of difference and, xix–xx, 57, 62,
    136–137
  Rank on, 24, 85
  self-leadership and, xx, 22–23, 24–26, 137
  strengths-based approach to, xx, 15–17
social workers
  as connective leaders, 15–16
  contrasted with analysts, 26

female, 16, 22, 25, 122, 123
"immortality," 25
soul, 33, 34f, 154
immortality and belief in, 32–33
Rank on, 32–33, 153–154, 183, 226. *See also*
Psychology and the Soul
willing and, 32
Spencer, Sharon, 247, 267–268
spirituality, 7, 205. *See also* mysticism; soul
Rogers on, 7, 148, 205–208, 214–215
Spiro, Jack D., 245
Spitz, Ellen Handler, 251–252
Sprengnether, Madelon, 251
Stein, Eric, 264–265
Stephenson, Laura, 274–275
Stevens, Richard, 247–248
Stoehr, Taylor, 253–254
Stolorow, Robert D., 245
Stone, Alison, 113, 271
strengths-based approach to social work, xx,
15–17
structural theory (id, ego, super-ego), 19, 104.
See also Ego and the Id
sublimation, 151
suffering, 18, 154, 251–252
difference and, 9, 174
Suler, John, 189, 253
Sullivan, Daniel, 268–269, 270–271, 274–275
super-ego/"above-I" (*Über-Ich*)
father vs. mother as source of, 75, 80–81
female psychology, women, and, 80–81, 124,
154
Freud and, 19, 72–75, 78–79, 86, 124
first use of the term, 72
Oedipus complex and, 19, 25–26, 72–73, 79,
86, 154
origins, 19, 25–26, 72, 75, 88, 154
pre-Oedipal, 88
surgeon, therapist operating like a, 31–32, 116,
120, 189. *See also* indifference
surrender, 208, 213–215
Sward, Keith, 245–246
Symbols of Government (Rank's course), 36–37
systems thinking, 30–31

Taft, Jessie, xx, 26, 121, *137f*
characterizations of, 25
children, self-leadership, and, 24
on emotions, 161
Freud, psychoanalysis, and, 123, 161
on immortality and immortalization, 25
influences on, xx
professional achievements, 136–137

on Rank, 87, 134–136, 145, 187, 234, 241,
280 n.1
Rank's influence on, 25
Rank's relationship with, 37, 57, 134–136,
173, 206, 210, 280 n.1
strengths-based approach to social work
and, xx, 16–17
on therapy, 16–17, 24–25, 37, 135–137, 145,
162, 173
Virginia Robinson and, 135–136
will and, 24–25
women's movement, feminism, and, 136–137
writings, 24, 136–137
Tallis, Frank, 2, 190, 228, 271–272
termination. *See* end phase of therapy;
separation–individuation: from
therapist; time-limited therapy
terror management theory (TMT), 35,
242–243, 273–274
therapeutic relationship, 207. *See also*
mutuality; "real relationship"; *specific*
topics
goal of deepening, 203
healing effect, xvi, 1
therapy. *See also specific topics*
as an art form, xix
forms of, 2
goals of, 200
as microcosm, 174
psychotherapy research, 33–35. *See also*
science
Rogers on curative force in, 4
role of therapist, 145
as creative artist, 31
Thorne, Brian, 190, 205
time-limited therapy, 106, 140, 249, 264–265.
See also brief therapy; relationship
therapy
Todesangst. See also death fear
origin of the term, 38
Todestrieb (death drive), 38, 50, 113, 199
Becker on, 40–41
as cause of resistance, 38, 80, 122, 150, 199
and the daimonic, 199, 202
vs. death fear (*Todesangst*) as cause of
aggression, 12, 38, 40–41, 43, 50, 162
Freud on, 38–39, 73–74, 80, 149–150, 221
overview and nature of, 38
Rank and, 38, 201
Rogers and, 202
why Freud invented, 201
Tookey, Helen, 140, 260

transcendence, 215, 226, 233. *See also* Beyond; mysticism; self-transcendence
  Rogers and, 148, 205–208. *See also* Rogers, Carl: on spirituality
transference, 120, 179, 204
  analyst as God, 211–212
  Becker on, 211
  in client-centered therapy, 192, 211. *See also* Rogers, Carl: on transference
  conceptions of, 103, 179, 192, 211
  creative will suppressed by, 26, 179, 212
  critiques of Freud's concept of and approach to, 26, 30, 102–105, 130, 144, 161, 179, 192, 212
  dangers of, 104
  Ferenczi on, 102–105, 210–211, 279 n.1
  Freud and, 63, 101–104, 178–180, 211
  and healing, 102, 104, 192
  and interminable analysis, 102–103, 179, 192, 212
  interpretation of, 38, 103–105, 149, 180
  meanings, uses, and scope of the term, 104–105, 210–211
  nature of, 102, 130, 211
  as power over (not power with) patients, 26, 120
  racism and, 62–63
  Rank and, 109, 144, 179–180, 242
  Rank on, 103–105, 210–212, 268–269
  vs. real relationship, 26, 30, 104–105, 109, 120–121, 144, 149, 180, 192, 210–212, 242
  Rogers on, 192, 211
  Rollo May on, 192
  and suggestibility, 104
  unresolvable, 103. *See also* interminable analysis
transference love. *See also* love: in relationship therapy; transference
  and dependence (on analyst) vs. independence, 203, 212. *See also* interminable analysis; transference: creative will suppressed by
  Freud on, 102
  lured by analyst, 103, 178–179, 211
  Rank on, 204, 210–212
transforming leadership
  defined, 14–15
  James MacGregor Burns on, 13–15
  social work, Rank, and, 14–15
Trauma of Birth, The (Rank), 59, 71, 250, 255–256. *See also* birth trauma

anxiety and, 70, 75, 81, 86, 110, 113, 242–243. *See also under* separation anxiety
  characterizations of, 59, 68, 74, 82, 83, 248–249, 258–259, 263–264
  culture and, 111, 258–259
  The Development of Psychoanalysis and, 108–109
  existence, being, and, 223
  existential unconscious and, 164
  Ferenczi and, xviii, 71, 76
  Freud and, xviii–xix, 8, 22, 64, 70, 71, 74–76, 82–84, 89, 109, 154, 258–259
  as groundbreaking, 80–81, 82–83, 96, 110, 123
  impact/ramifications, 68, 71, 74, 76, 80
  Inhibitions, Symptoms and Anxiety (Freud) and, xviii, 246–247
  inspiration for, 89
  mothers and, 64, 70, 75–76, 80–81, 91–92, 94
  mystics and, 212
  Oedipus complex and, xviii, 71, 76, 80–81
  Rank's reflections on, 9, 59
  Rank's unwillingness to recant, 82–83
  Richard Neutra and, 261
  Samuel Beckett and, 261
  therapy and, 108–111
  will and, 80–81, 154
  women and, 20–21, 22–23, 80–81
Twain, Mark, 57–58

Über-Ich ("above-I"). *See* super-ego
Ukraine, Russian invasion of, 45–46
unconditional positive regard, 191–192, 194–195, 281 n.3
unconscious. *See also* existential unconscious
  fear of the, 220
  Freud and the, 98
unio mystica. See mystical union
union. *See* mystical union
United States, Freud and, 141
unity. *See* Oneness/wholeness
University of Pennsylvania School of Social Work (Penn School), xx, 24, 149, 234, 263–264
Unknown and the Unknowable, the, 148, 214–215
unlearning, 60–61, 144–145, 265–267
unthought known, 214–215, 218, 222
Urangst (universal primal fear), 12. *See also Angst*; primal fear/primal anxiety
  Freud and, 220
  Lebensangst, Todesangst, and, 12, 162, 211

overcoming/alleviating, 165, 167, 220
relationships and, 167, 212
therapy and, 165, 212
Urmutter (ancient primal mother), 71. *See also*
    Freud, Amalia
separating from, 71, 75, 86

Vanhooren, Siebrecht, 272–274
void, 38, 48, 214–215. *See also* Nothingness
Volosinov, Valentin N., 250

Wadlington, Will, 103, 188, 247–248, 258–259,
    261–262, 265, 275
Wall, John N., 244
Walton, Andre, 268–269
war, 45–46, 50
    heroes, heroism, and, 28, 41, 44
    immortality and, 41, 44, 46
Watt, Stephen, 249
Webber, Andrew, 255–256
Westerink, Herman, 264
Whitaker, Carl, 31
Whites, Whiteness, and psychoanalysis, 55–56,
    62. *See also* racism
wholeness. *See* Oneness/wholeness
will, 33, 152–153. *See also* creative will; love
        and will; women: will of; *specific topics*
    as "free." *See under* destiny/fate; determinism
    to healing and health, 73–75, 200
    "I am" and, 77, 153, 163, 168, 176
    interpreted by Freud as resistance, 140, 174
    to live, 44
    meanings and uses of the term, 77, 150–151
    nature of, 150–151, 156–157, 159–160
    Nietzsche and, 154, 167
    and not-willing, 162
    positive vs. negative, 142
    Rollo May and, 77
    Schopenhauer on suffering and, 154
    vs. sexuality, 152
    softening vs. hardening of, 162
    terminology and related terms, 77, 253
will conflict between therapist and patient, 143,
        199–201, 203–204. *See also* counter-will
will denial, 169–170
will psychology, xix, 16. *See also* will
will therapy, 16. *See also* relationship therapy
    leadership development and, 16
    relationship therapy and, 145, 150, 187
*Will Therapy: An Analysis of the Therapeutic
        Process in Terms of Relationship* (Rank),
        xix, 1, 22, 38, 77, 150

inspiration for, 22
originally titled *Dynamic Therapy*, 145
Winnicott, Donald W., 277 n.8
    on birth experience, 223, 228
    Rank's influence on, 248–249
    on sexual conception, 223
Wirth, Hans-Jürgen, 262, 275–276
Wittgenstein, Ludwig, 230
Wolitzky, David L., 252–253
womb. *See* prenatal psychology and womb
        experience
women. *See also* feminism; Freud, Sigmund;
        patriarchy; social workers: female
    demonization of, 35–36
    ethics and, 19–20, 80–81, 124
    fear of, 35
    Freud on, 22, 80, 123, 245–246. *See also
        under* femininity; Oedipus complex;
        patriarchy
        "stemming the power of the female sex,"
        19–20, 99
    woman as "failed man," 20, 22
    Lebensangst (fear of life) and, 22, 77, 128
    oppression of, 16. *See also* masculine
        ideology
    "war on women" in psychoanalysis, 124
    power, 19, 20–22, 80–81, 126
    powerlessness and, 20, 22–23, 51, 197
    psychoanalysis and, 20
    Rank and female psychology, 250
    self-leadership and, xv, 24–26, 51, 128
    The Trauma of Birth (Rank) and, 20–21,
        22–23, 80–81
    will of, xxi, 26, 122. *See also under* father's
        will
        creative will, xxi, 22, 25–26, 234
        Freud and, 19, 22, 25, 77, 80, 153–154, 234
        Rank and, 25
        Rank on, 19, 77, 80, 154
working through, 116, 144

Yalom, Irvin D., xvii, 200
    death, death anxiety, and, 12, 35, 263–264
    on Rank, xvii, 12, 35, 245–246, 263–264
    Rollo May and, 12, 77
    will and, 77, 200, 245–246, 253
Young, Isaac F., 270–271

Zaretsky, Eli, 268
Zottl, Anton, 245–247

204